CLINICIAN'S GUIDE TO
AHCC®

Evidence-Based Nutritional Immunotherapy

Edited by

Anil D. Kulkarni, Philip Calder and Toshinori Ito

Published by International Congress on Nutrition and Integrative Medicine

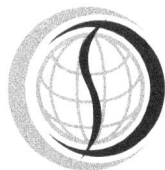

ICNIM

Contents

Introduction

PART 1   Profile Summary of AHCC

PART 2   Basic & Clinical Studies on AHCC

PART 3   Case Reports and Unpublished Studies

Chapter 10. Cancer

Appendix

A Word from the Editors

This book is written for the benefit and education of physicians as well as for patients and their families, with information on AHCC as an evidence-based beneficial supplement in the treatment of various diseases. The book is presented with a general introduction of nutritional immunological state-of-the-art knowledge. It is further subdivided into three sections, providing the following: 1) a general introduction to the manufacture and testing of AHCC with relevant regulatory compliance, 2) an overview of the experimental evidence coming from basic scientific investigations, and 3) clinical case results and efficacious outcome observations in humans. AHCC is used as a supplement in many different clinical situations.

—Anil Kulkarni

This book brings together information on the composition and manufacture of AHCC and on the scientific evidence supporting the use of AHCC in many common clinical conditions. The evidence presented comes from both basic science investigations that detail the effects of AHCC and the underlying mechanisms, and clinical research. There is a focus on modulation of the immune and inflammatory systems, suggesting a role for AHCC in supporting immune function, preventing and treating infections, and combating inflammatory disorders and cancer. The summaries of research on AHCC are placed in a more general context with introductory sections, providing a broader perspective on the influence of nutrition on molecular, cellular, and tissue function and on responses to challenge. Overall, this book provides a comprehensive summary of the current state of knowledge regarding AHCC. As such, it presents a remarkable reference work of value to physicians, patients, and researchers alike.

—Philip Calder

This guidebook is based on evidence obtained through basic and clinical research regarding AHCC conducted over a long period and all over the world. Functional foods, especially mushroom products, can be regarded and positioned as one of the modalities in the field of integrative medicine. AHCC has a wide spectrum of activities, such as immune modulation and some regulatory actions against cancer, infection, and inflammation. I hope this book will serve as an information base and reference on the use of AHCC for patients as well as physicians.

—Toshinori Ito

About the Editors

Anil D. Kulkarni, Ph.D., received his doctorate degree (faculty of medicine) from the Queen's University of Belfast, Belfast, N. Ireland, United Kingdom. He is currently Professor of Surgery in the Department of Surgery at the University of Texas Medical School in the world's largest medical center in Houston, Texas. His research specialization is in nutritional immunology, and has experience in basic and translational research. He also teaches medical students and mentors students from high school to graduate and medical students. He has traveled internationally extensively with numerous research collaborations in several countries in Asia, Europe, and Latin America. He is known internationally for his work in immunonutrition and functional foods and is frequently invited to be a keynote speaker. He mentors medical students for their global health concentration as a part of their curriculum. He has been on the editorial boards of international journals and serves as peer reviewer. He also develops international exchange programs for faculty, staff, and students. He has trained several international and domestic graduate and medical students. One of his current active interests is in Global Health activities and education. Recently, he received two international awards as recognition for his contributions of global work: "Hind Rattan Award" followed by "Fulbright-Nehru Scholarship 2014."

Philip C. Calder, Ph.D., is Professor of Nutritional Immunology within the Human Development and Health Academic Unit of the Faculty of Medicine at the University of Southampton in the United Kingdom. He has broad interests in nutritional modulation of immunity, inflammation, and cardiometabolic disease risk. Much of his work has been devoted to exploring the metabolism and functionality of fatty acids with an emphasis on the roles of omega-3 fatty acids. Dr. Calder has received several awards for his work, including the Sir David Cuthbertson Medal (1995), the Nutricia International Award (2007), the ESPEN Cuthbertson Lecture (2008), the Louisiana State University Chancellor's Award in Neuroscience and Medicine (2011), the German Society for Fat Science's Normann Medal (2012), the American Oil Chemists' Society Ralph Holman Lifetime Achievement Award (2015), the BAPEN Pennington Lecture (2015), the British Nutrition Foundation Prize (2015), and the Danone International Prize in Nutrition (2016). He has served on many committees of professional societies and was President of the International Society for the Study of Fatty Acids and Lipids (2009–2012). Dr. Calder is currently Chair of the Scientific Committee of the European Society for Clinical Nutrition and Metabolism (ESPEN) and President-Elect of the Nutrition Society. He has over 500 scientific publications, his work has been cited over 22,000 times, and he is listed as an ISI Highly Cited Researcher. Dr. Calder was Editor-in-Chief of the *British Journal of Nutrition* from 2006 to 2013, and he is currently an Associate Editor of *Clinical Science, Journal of Nutrition, Clinical Nutrition, Lipids,* and *Nutrition Research.* He is a member of the several other editorial boards of journals in the nutrition, clinical science, and lipidology fields. He receives many invitations to speak and is a consultant to the industry.

Toshinori Ito, M.D., Ph.D., is a Professor in the Department of Integrative Medicine at Osaka University Graduate School of Medicine and in the School of Nursing at Senri Kinran University in Japan. His research areas are in pancreas and islet transplantation, gastroenterological surgery (pancreatic surgery), transplantation immunology, mucosal immunology, tumor immunology, and integrative medicine. He has been in charge of lecture of integrative medicine, which was established in January 2005. In addition, he has worked as a digestive surgeon and a transplant surgeon to develop clinical research using evidence-based medicine (EBM) in the areas of cancer, inflammatory bowel disease, and pancreas and islet transplantation. He has been exploring treatment approaches to improve the effects of current treatment and patients' Quality of Life (QOL) and is interested in the role of complementary and alternative medicine (CAM) in medical treatment. Dr. Ito is a member and a councilor of a number of societies. He also serves as a chief director of a general incorporated association called *evidence*-Based Integrative Medicine (*e*BIM), which provides opportunities to researchers to present their research results. Since June of 2016, he has been appointed as President of International Congress on Nutrition and Integrative Medicine (ICNIM), the publisher of this book.

Contributors List

Masuo Hosokawa, M.D., Ph.D.
President Emeritus, International
Congress on Nutrition and Integrative
Medicine
Professor Emeritus, Hokkaido
University

Satoshi Ohno, M.D., Ph.D.
Associate Professor, Department of
Integrative Medicine, Graduate School
of Medicine, Osaka University

Toshinori Ito, M.D., Ph.D.
President, International Congress on
Nutrition and Integrative Medicine,
Professor, Department of Integrative
Medicine, Graduate School of Medicine,
Osaka University

Noriaki Fujii
Senior Director, Manufacturing
Division, Amino Up Co., Ltd.

Shotaro Kudo
Research & Development Scientist,
Global Strategy Group, Amino Up
Co., Ltd.

Kenji Sato, Ph.D.
Professor, Marine Biological Function,
Division of Applied Biosciences,
Graduate School of Agriculture,
Kyoto University

Maki Kashimoto, MSc.
Marine Biological Function, Division
of Applied Biosciences, Graduate
School of Agriculture, Kyoto
University

Thomas Walshe, M.D.
Assistant Professor of Neurology,
Harvard Medical School
Chief, General Neurology Division,
Department of Neurology, Brigham
and Women's Hospital

Hiroshi Nishioka, Ph.D.
Senior Director, Research &
Development Division, Amino Up
Co., Ltd.

Juan Torrado, Ph.D.
Professor, School of Pharmacy,
Complutense University of Madrid

Philip C. Calder, Ph.D.
Professor, Human Development &
Health Academic Unit, Faculty of
Medicine, University of Southampton

Chantal Matar, Ph.D. RD.
Professor, Faculty of Health Sciences,
University of Ottawa

Emilie Graham, MSc.
Faculty of Health Sciences, University
of Ottawa

Gerald Sonnenfeld, Ph.D.
Vice President for Research and
Economic Development, Professor,
The University of Rhode Island

Sho Hangai, M.D., Ph.D.
Department of Molecular Immunology,
Institute of Industrial Science,
The University of Tokyo

Satoru Iwase, M.D., Ph.D.
Section Chief, Department of Palliative
Medicine, The Institute of Medical
Science, The University of Tokyo

Hiroaki Yanagimoto, M.D., Ph.D.
Assistant Professor, Department of
Surgery, Kansai Medical University

Anil D. Kulkarni, Ph.D.
(Faculty of Medicine) Professor of
Surgery, McGovern Medical School,
The University of Texas at Houston

Shigeru Abe, Ph.D.
Director & Professor, Institute of
Medical Mycology, Teikyo University

Shigeru Tansho-Nagakawa, Ph.D.
Deputy associate professor, Department
of Microbiology & Immunology, Teikyo
University School of Medicine

Kazumi Hayama
Assistant Professor, Institute of Medical
Mycology, Teikyo University

Mikio Nishizawa, M.D., Ph.D.
Professor, Department of Biomedical
Sciences, College of Life Sciences,
Ritsumeikan University

Tominori Kimura, M.D., D.M.Sc.
Professor and Vice Dean, Department
of Pharmacy, College of Pharmaceutical
Sciences, Ritsumeikan University

Judith A. Smith, B.S., Pharm.D., RPh.
Associate Professor, Department
of Obstetrics, Gynecology, and
Reproductive Sciences, The University
of Texas Health Science Center
Medical School

Masaki Fujita, M.D., Ph.D.
Associate Professor, Department
of Respiratory Medicine, Fukuoka
University Hospital

Kentaro Wakamatsu, M.D., Ph.D.
Chief, Department of Respiratory
Medicine, National Hospital
Organization, Omuta Hospital

Koji Wakame, Ph.D.
Associate Professor, Department
of Pharmacology, Hokkaido
Pharmaceutical University School
of Pharmacy

Taisei Nomura, M.D., Ph.D.
Professor Emeritus, National Institutes
of Biomedical Innovation, Health and
Nutrition
Graduate School of Medicine, Osaka
University

Tatsuya Hisajima, Ph.D.
Professor, Faculty of Health Care,
Teikyo Heisei University

Fermín Sánchez de Medina, Ph.D.
Professor, Department of Pharmacology,
CIBERehd, School of Pharmacy,
University of Granada

Olga Martínez-Augustin, Ph.D.
Professor, Department of Biochemistry
and Molecular Biology II, CIBEREHD,
School of Pharmacy, University of
Granada

Tetsuya Okuyama, Ph.D.
Assistant Professor, Department of
Biomedical Sciences, College of Life
Sciences, Ritsumeikan University

Yusai Kawaguchi, M.D.
Director, Kitakawachifujii Hospital

Norbert Szalus, M.D. Ph.D.
Director, ImmunoMedica Clinic

Edwin A. Bien, M.D.
Director, LeBIEN Wellness Specialists

Massimo Bonucci, M.D.
Director, Department Clinical
Pathology and Surgical Pathology,
Integrative Oncology Outpatient,
San Feliciano Hospital
Professor, Scienza della Vita, Marconi
University of Rome

Anuchit Chutaputti, M.D.
Section of Digestive and Liver Diseases,
Phramongkutklao Hospital

Francisco J. Karkow, M.D., Ph.D.
Professor, Fatima's Faculty

Natalia Mikhailichenko, M.D., Ph.D.
General Director, International Medical
Center Nevron

Viacheslav Kulagin, M.D.
Head of the Neurofunctional
Diagnostics Laboratory, International
Medical Center Nevron

Takayuki Yoshizawa, M.D.
Director, Iryouhoujinshadan Aigokai
Kanamecho Hospital (Medical
Corporation Aigokai Kanamecho
Hospital)

Akitaka Yoshizawa, M.D.
Assistant Director, Iryouhoujinshadan
Aigokai Kanamecho Hospital (Medical
Corporation Aigokai Kanamecho
Hospital)

Preface

Masuo Hosokawa

Today, public awareness of health has grown enough for people to maintain their health by themselves rather than leaving it to healthcare institutions. One way to maintain health is to take "functional food" supplements.

In cancer treatment, early detection and early resection are the cornerstones, and radiotherapy may become the first choice in some cases. However, as surgery and irradiation can be applied only to the treatment of localized cancer, chemotherapy will be administered in addition to these treatments for cases where the cancer has already metastasized to other organs and tissues. The side effects of chemotherapy cause severe dysfunction in patients; therefore, immunotherapy is gaining attention now as the fourth therapeutic choice.

Immunotherapies can be classified into four categories: 1) specific active immunotherapy usually with a cancer antigen vaccine, 2) adoptive immunotherapy with lymphocytes sensitized to cancer antigens, 3) passive immunotherapy with cancer-specific antibodies, and 4) non-specific active immunotherapy with immuno-stimulants. AHCC and other supplements are included as therapeutic tools for non-specific active immunotherapy in the fourth category. Increasing attention to supplements shows the fact that quite a few people suffer from diseases that cannot be treated even with advanced modern medicine despite the sharp rise of public awareness to health. Although the scientific evidences of these health foods have been elucidated and accumulated gradually, they are still far from sufficient. In other words, we can find numerous books that introduce the benefits of many health foods; however, they provide few research reports, which deserve researchers' citation. Furthermore, scientific evidences that retain continuous reproducibility of research results are required to evaluate the effects of medicine used in medical treatment, and this requirement also applies to functional foods.

This book introduces the function and effects of the functional food AHCC, a standardized extract of cultured *Lentinula edodes* mycelia. The International Congress on Nutrition and Integrative Medicine (ICNIM) marked its 24th symposium this year where I had served as co-chair of four chairpersons until 2015. I also served as the president of ICNIM and AHCC Research Association over a decade until May, 2016. Having served in these positions, I have a strong interest in the medical applications of AHCC. Fifteen years have passed since *The Basic and Clinical Researches on AHCC*—which I co-edited with fellow ICNIM chairpersons, Dr. Masatoshi Yamazaki and Dr. Yasuo Kamiyama—was published by Life Science, Inc. In that period, research on AHCC has spread throughout the world, and a great deal of new knowledge has been accumulated.

The Clinician's Guide to AHCC has been compiled to present this accumulated knowledge with contributions from the researchers who engaged in the studies. As AHCC is not a medicine, one has to decide its use not by direction from medical doctors but by his or her own judgment. This book introduces the features and benefits of AHCC, which are backed by scientific evidence, to help make the judgment. The effects of AHCC on cancer prevention and cancer treatment have been mainly researched up until now; however, AHCC exerts more functions than just an anti-carcinogenic effect, such as anti-infective benefits against fungi, viruses, and parasites with its immunomodulating effects, anti-stress effect, chemotherapy-enhancing effect, and mitigating effect for immunosuppression. Although the detailed mechanism has not yet been clarified, cell interaction modification effect and suppressive effect on the invasive and metastatic capability of cancer cells have been observed as well.

Additionally, the quality and safety of AHCC as a health food are assured by the sole manufacturer of AHCC and are certified according to Good Manufacturing Practice (GMP) standards for dietary supplements and ISO 9001:2008 and ISO 22000:2005 criteria.

I hope that this book will be helpful to deeply understand AHCC not only for clinicians and healthcare professionals, but also for consumers who will use AHCC in various clinical situations.

INTRODUCTION

Regulations on Functional Foods and Utilization in Clinical Practices

Satoshi Ohno

The Eastern world traditionally advocates the philosophy of "a balanced diet leads to a healthy body" or "source of medicine and food is the same" in which food forms the basis for healing. Similarly, in the Western world, the father of medicine, Hippocrates, left the words, "Let food be thy medicine and medicine be thy food." This means that prevention and treatment of diseases are essentially the same as health maintenance by food. In this chapter, the regulations on functional food in each country are outlined, and applications of functional food and vision for the future medical field are explained.

What Is "Functional Food"?

In the 1980s, the research team of the Ministry of Education, Science and Culture, Government of Japan proposed the food function theory for the first time in the world, and pharmacological effects of food gained attention. In their theory, the tertiary function of food was defined as biological defenses and controls for health maintenance, in addition to the primary function, providing nutrients and calories necessitated for the life, and the secondary function, providing taste and flavor of food. Namely, the research team advocated that food has functions for health maintenance such as biorhythm adjustment, biological defense, disease prevention, disease recovery, and anti-aging, and food having these tertiary functions is defined as "Functional Food." This project has given opportunities for advancement of research on the functions of food.

Health Claim System for Food in Japan

In recent years, people's awareness on health is growing in developed countries due to aging of the societies; the interest in diet is also increasing. Moreover, it has become apparent from the epidemiological studies that excessive nutrition intake and unbalanced diet are factors of lifestyle-related diseases. Therefore, "informed choice," a system that enables consumers to choose food based on appropriate information provided, is required in the current societies.

"Food with Health Claims (FHC)" is a system in Japan enabling the claim of the tertiary function of a food if it meets certain conditions. The FHC is classified into Food for Specified Health Uses (FOSHU), Food with Nutrient Function Claims (FNFC), and Food with Function Claims (FFC), depending on the intended use of food and the differences in requirements by the government.

Food for Specified Health Uses (Established in 1991)

The FOSHU refers to foods containing functional ingredients that impact physiological functions of the body, with health claims contributing to specific health applications, such as maintaining normal levels of blood pressure and cholesterol, and maintaining gastrointestinal condition. To market a product as FOSHU, the efficacy and safety of each product has to be reviewed and its health claim has to be authorized by the government. The number of items approved as of 2015 is approximately 1,150.

Food with Nutrient Function Claims (Established in 2001)

The FNFC indicates foods used to supplement daily intake of essential nutrients such as vitamins and minerals, and functions of the essential nutrients are claimed. The functions can be claimed using the expressions prepared by the government without notifying them if a product contains a certain standard dose of an essential nutrient with scientific evidence. To market a product as FNFC, recommended daily intake of an essential nutrient has to be within the upper and lower limits, and the alerts must be displayed in addition to the nutrient function claims.

Food with Function Claims (Established in 2015)

The FFC requires scientific evidence that has been collected and summarized by business operators, and the evidence on the safety and efficacy has been reported to the Director General of the Consumer Affairs Agency, Japan, prior to marketing of a product. However, unlike in the case of FOSHU, FCC products do not receive individual authorizations from the Director General of the Consumer Affairs Agency.

International Comparison of Health Claim Systems

Health claim systems are in a phase of development throughout the world. In this section, an overview of the health claim systems in the United States, European Union, Australia and New Zealand, China, and South Korea, as well as the guidelines prepared by Codex Alimentarius Comission (CAC), are introduced as typical examples.

The United States

In accordance with the Nutrition Labeling and Education Act (NLEA) of 1990, health claims that show relationship of nutritional substances to diseases or health-related conditions can be made if a product contains a certain amount of a scientifically proven substance and is approved by the Food and Drug Administration (FDA).

Moreover, it became possible to make structure/function claims that show the actions or the roles of nutritional substances by maintaining or affecting normal structure or function of the body, in accordance with the Dietary Supplement Health and Education Act (DSHEA) of 1994. The feature is that post-marketing notification to the FDA is only required for the business operators, and structure/function claims can be made at the manufacture's own responsibility without any review process. However, problems on the safety and claims have been pointed out, and there are demands for revision of the framework of structure/function claims.

In addition, there is a food category called "Medical Food" which is defined as a food product formulated to be consumed or administered under the supervision of a physician for the specific dietary management of a disease with distinct nutritional requirements. Medical foods are exempted from the health claims under the NLEA, and pre-market review or approval by the FDA is not required.

European Union (EU)

In EU, due to presence of their own individual laws of each member state, the Directorate-General for Health and Food Safety of European Commission, which is responsible for the implementation of EU laws on food safety, is taking the central role in the development of a common system. Also, in the basis of "informed choice," which enables consumers to choose a food from given information, the framework for nutrition and health claims was established by Regulation (EC) No 1924/2006, in which the health claims were classified into claims on general function, disease risk reduction, and children's development or health. For the health claims in EU, the European Food Safety Authority evaluates each individual product. Additionally, recommended daily intake and acceptable daily intake of vitamin and minerals in food supplements such as tablet and capsule products was implemented by Directive 2002/46/EC.

Australia and New Zealand

To develop harmonized food standards between the counties, the Food Standards Australia New Zealand (FSANZ) was established by the Food Standards Australia New Zealand Act 1991 as an independent statutory agency. The guidelines for health claims on food products were published in 2003, and a new food standard on nutrition content and health claims was issued in 2013. The claims are classified into the general level (showing an effect on health function) and the high level (showing an effect on a disease or disease biomarker).

China

The regulation on health food labeling was issued in 1996, and functional foods with health claims have to be reviewed individually by the government. Currently, there are twenty-seven types of permitted health claims, such as enhancement of immunity, assistance in blood lipids, reduction of blood sugar, antioxidation, and assistance in memory.

South Korea

The Health Function Food (HFF) Act was issued in 2002 to ensure the safety of HFF. The health claims of the HFF are classified into three categories: nutrient function claims, other function claims, and disease risk claims. Nutrient function claims for some nutrients such as vitamins, minerals, and essential fatty acids, and some traditional ingredients such as ginseng and DHA can be made in accordance with the approved list on the HFF code. The health claims by other functional ingredients has to be reviewed and approved by the government and classified into three grades based on the level of scientific evidence.

Codex Alimentarius Commission (CAC)

The CAC is responsible for establishing the international food standards, guidelines, and codes of practice contributing the safety, quality, and fair trade of food. The CAC has been discussing the health claims on food since the 1990s. Finally, the guidelines for use of nutrition and health claims (CAC/GL 23-1997) were established with the following prerequisites: 1) Consistency and support in health and nutrition policies of the countries, 2) Proof of appropriate and adequate scientific evidences, 3) Provision of accurate information to the consumers, and 4) Support for scientific education to the customers. In accordance with the guidelines, nutrition and health claims are classified into three types: nutrient function claim, other function claims, and reduction of disease risk claims. The summary of the health claim frameworks in each country is shown in Table 1 below. As a global trend, harmonization with the international guidelines prepared by the CAC is promoted now.

TABLE 1 INTERNATIONAL COMPARISON OF HEALTH CLAIM SYSTEMS

NUTRITION	FUNCTION	STRUCTURE/ DISEASE RISK	REDUCTION
Japan	FNFC	FOSHU/FFC	FOSHU
United States	DSHEA		NLEA
EU	Regulation (EC) No 1924/2006		
Australia / New Zealand	FSANZ		
China	Health Food		—
Korea	HFF		
Codex Alimentarius	CAC/GL 23–1997		

Orientation and Agendas in the Medical Field

As shown in Table 1, the health claims of disease risk reduction are allowed as the global standard. However, the claims on the food indicating cure or treatment of diseases are not allowed. In some countries, such as Canada, where the food supplements are classified as medicinal products, the food supplements are classified under different structure of regulatory frameworks.

In addition, the difference in the insurance system in each country should be considered. For example, in Japan, enteral nutrition is considered medicinal, while concentrated nutrient products are considered food products; this difference in the classification leads to differences in insurance reimbursements. On the other hand, in the United States, insurance reimbursement depends on the policies of the health insurance provider. In the European Union, insurance reimbursement policies are different in each member state.

In the future, harmonization of healthcare and insurance systems should be considered to promote utilization of functional food in the medical field.

Outlook for Functional Foods

Recently, the concept of integrative medicine (which combines complementary and alternative medicine, of which safety and efficacy have been proven, with modern Western medicine) is gaining prominence. In the United States, the National Center for Complementary and Integrative Health (NCCIH) is conducting integrative medicine research, including the role of functional food in the reduction of side effects associated with medical treatments and for the management of symptoms associated with disease progression. Their research outcomes are being applied to clinical practices now.

In addition, the proportion of the national health expenditure to the national budget is continually increasing due to the aging of society, and measures against this fact are being required in countries worldwide. As mentioned at the beginning of this section, food is the foundation of health. Therefore, there is no doubt that functional food will lead to the prevention of diseases. Additionally, with regard to medical cost reduction, the application of functional food in preventive healthcare is important. However, mainstream medical treatments are still focused on treating symptoms. Thus, a paradigm shift to preventative healthcare is required within the current medical frameworks.

Integrative Medicine and Functional Food

Toshinori Ito

In recent years, upon the remarkable advancement in medical science, the improvement in disease diagnosis techniques and medical treatments have been highly recognized. In Japan, this improvement has resulted in shift of disease types from acute to chronic disease. In addition, Japanese society is becoming a "super-aged" society. Besides cancer, modern chronic diseases include hypertension, diabetes, dyslipidemia, and obesity, among others. This change in the lifestyle has been gradually increasing the cost of health and medical care, which is threatening to collapse the Japanese medical insurance system.

On the other hand, there have been changes in the awareness of patients. The massive spread of information by technological advance has contributed to the realization that preventive care is important for health. Also, it is clear that patients are increasingly voicing their own opinions regarding their therapy options. In other words, patients' awareness has transferred from being passive to active, and they are requesting medical treatment that deals with quality of life (QOL) as their standard. Based on these changes in medicine and patients' awareness, the field of complementary and alternative medicine (CAM) came under focus.

Shift from Complementary and Alternative Medicine to Integrative Medicine

CAM was defined as the types of therapy that do not fall within the categories of conventional medicine because their efficacies are not clearly proven scientifically. These types may include: 1) manipulative and body-based practice such as massage, chiropractic, reflexology, and acupuncture, 2) mind-body medicine such as yoga, meditation, psychotherapy, art therapy, and music therapy, 3) whole medical system such as Ayurveda, traditional Chinese medicine, and homeopathy, 4) Energy medicine such as qigong, Reiki, and magnetic therapy, and 5) biologically based practices such as herbs, dietary supplements, and special foods, which are the most common category with CAM. CAM spread in the beginning as an alternative medicine used by patients in their end stages of cancer, or other difficult diseases, who would stop receiving common medical treatment and use these types of alternative medicine. However, recently, the trend has changed toward using this type medicine along with conventional medicine in the shape of "integrative medicine" to improve QOL or in the shape of "preventive medicine" to avoid disease before it occurs. Clinically, the list of diseases, preceded by cancer, also includes gynopathy, neuropathy, cardiovascular diseases, and orthopedics.

At first, the interest in CAM originated when a Harvard University study determined that 60 million adults in the United States, which is close to 33.8% of the adult population, use CAM in some form.[1] A later study was conducted that showed the number of users had increased to 83 million, which is equal to 42.1% of the U.S. adult population.[2] Also, it was found that more women (and people in general) who have relatively higher level of education are CAM users and that they use different types of CAM, including Western herbs, chiropractic, and massage.

We can summarize the factors that contribute to the spread of CAM as follows:

1. The mentality that the best type of medicine is to prevent disease and that disease prevention is the ultimate goal of using CAM.

2. The idea that all sorts of conventional medicine is basically the same, and we need to use the healing power available in nature.

3. Conventional medicine is too specialized, and we need comprehensive medicine that looks at the body as a whole.

4. CAM has fewer side effects or risks of medical mistakes, and it is the safest type of treatment.

5. CAM is the type of medicine that allows the patient to have a positive interaction with the therapy methods.

Based on this Harvard University study, the U.S. government decided to establish the Office of Alternative Medicine (OAM) within the National Institutes of Health

(NIH) in 1992, with a start-up annual budget of 2 million U.S. dollars, aiming to conduct further studies. Later, following the increasing demand for CAM, it was decided to upgrade the OAM to the National Center for CAM (NCCAM) and to increase the annual budget to 20 million U.S. dollars. By 2005, the annual budget increased steadily to over 121 million U.S. dollars; an equal budget is established every year thereafter. Three-quarters or more of this cost are for clinical studies. This appropriated enormous budget is regarded as an investment in future medical expenditure reduction.

Likewise in Japan, a cancer research grant by the Ministry of Health, Labour and Welfare was used to create a new research group (The Research Group of Cancer Alternative Therapy in Japan), and Hyodo et al. conducted a field survey related to CAM in which 3,461 cancer cases were investigated (in sixteen cancer centers and forty hospices). The results of this investigation showed that 44.6% of the patients use CAM.[3]

The groups who were taking any source of CAM included women under age 60, university graduates, patients who experienced chemical therapy, patients under palliative care, and people who have just discovered they have cancer. It was found that 89% of the subjects in these groups were using functional food (also known as health food)—67.1% of the cases used CAM with the objective of suppressing the spread of cancer, 44.5% as part of their total therapy, 27.1% to reduce the symptoms, and 20.7% as an alternative to conventional medicine. Interestingly, only 23.3% said that they decided to take CAM based on their awareness of its importance, as the majority stated that they started taking CAM because family members and friends influenced them to do so. Also, 84.5% said that they did not check with their doctors to determine if there would be any problems associated with starting CAM, and 60.7% said that they made the decision on their own without consulting their doctors.

Based on these circumstances, the research group published the *Guidebook for Cancer Complementary and Alternative Medicine,* First Edition, in April 2006. The guidebook was verified basically on medical research papers related to CAM in Japan. It has been revealed that most CAM approaches had poor scientific validation, but actually few clinical trials examining CAM efficacy had been conducted. In February 2012, the same research group, which was taken over by Yamashita Group, published the third revised edition of the guidebook.[4]

In recent years, the concept of integrative medicine (also called integrated medicine)—in which CAM is bound with modern Western medicine—is being advocated as the ideal medical system for looking at the human body as a whole. Based on this, in 2014, NCCAM was renamed, whereby *Alternative* was replaced by *Integrative* and *Medicine* was replaced by *Health,* so that the name of the center became the National Center for Complementary and Integrative Health (NCCIH).

Food and the Immune System

The importance of food to maintain good health has been well known since ancient times by various civilizations such as the Greek Hippocrates and the Japanese Genpaku Sugita. This concept is expressed in Japanese as *Ishoku-dougen* (the idea that to cure illnesses and to have a diet are essentially equal in supporting life and maintaining health).

According to the statistics of 2014, Japan has the highest life expectancy in the world, where women's average life span is 86.61 years (first in the world) and men's average is 79.19 years (fourth in the world). Among the factors that led to these statistics, the Japanese cuisine, which is based on plant proteins from rice and tofu, can be focused on. In December 2013, the Japanese cuisine (Washoku) was designated as an element on the UNESCO Intangible Cultural Heritage list.

Food is originally characterized by three functions: the first function of providing nutrients to maintain and extend life; the second function of stimulating and influencing the three senses of sight, smell, and taste, which are related to appetite; and the third function of physiological control and biological defense. It is thought that these functions take part in adjusting the body rhythm, protecting from disease, anti-aging, and stimulating the immune system. In fact, the fruits and vegetables that we normally eat include different physiologically active components, which are thought to contribute to the third function of food.

Our bodies perform adjustments of their biological functions by continuously linking the endocrine, nervous (autonomic nervous), and immune systems. In particular, the body has its own biological defense system that, via its immune system, reacts against foreign substances trying to enter the body. The prevention of the invasion of foreign substances takes place at the surface of the skin, which has direct contact with the outside world, or the mucous membrane of the respiratory or digestive systems. Among these systems, the digestive system contains the largest part of the immune system, which is able to push away the massive amount of antigens that enter with food via antibodies, such as IgA, that are parts of the mucous membrane.

On the other hand, the immune system has a mechanism that may allow the intake of beneficial foreign substances rather than getting rid of them. This is called oral tolerance, and it is thought to be a special immunity function in the digestive system. When this function performs normally, our bodies can maintain healthy conditions. However, abnormalities in this function may cause allergies or other autoimmune disorders

In 1983, a "functional food" pioneer research group was established by the Japanese Ministry of Education to suggest the theory of food functions. This theory gave special importance to the third function of food, which drew the world's attention. In other words, the expression *functional food* was first used in Japan and later spread globally to indicate which types of food have beneficial effects on physiological control and biological defense.

Consequently, this research group started developing functional food (food with specific functions). In 1991, the expression "food for specific health uses" (FOSHU), abbreviated in Japanese as TOKUHO was established. Based on this, it became possible to make "health claims," such as "food to improve abdominal conditions," "food for people with high blood pressure," or "food for people with concern about blood sugar." To be able to make such claims, approval must be obtained from the Ministry of Health, Labour and Welfare, which evaluates applications that contain clinical data submitted and reviewed by a committee created by the ministry and the National Institute of Health and Nutrition. By the end of January 2015, there were 1,141 items registered as FOSHU.

There is another category called "food with nutrient function claims," which is defined as food that contain specific nutrients and are able to claim the functionality of these specific claims following the standards determined by the Ministry of Health, Labour and Welfare. These nutrients include five minerals (calcium, iron, zinc, copper, and magneium) as well as the twelve different types of vitamins. Accordingly, food with health functionality can be categorized as either "Food for Specific Health Uses" or "Food with Nutrient Function Claims." All other sorts are categorized as general food, including healthy food. However, as of April 2015, a new system that allows making health claims on some items within the food was executed. More details about this new system can be found in the previous section by Satoshi Ohno.

Mucosal Immune System of the Digestive Tract

The number of bacteria living inside a human body exceeds 100 billion of around 500 species. The net weight of these bacteria is 1.0 to 1.5 kg, and they are closely related to the immune function of the digestive system. The enteric bacteria consist of useful bacteria for maintaining a healthy body as well as harmful bacteria. Usually, these two categories of bacteria exist in a proper balance, forming what is called the intestinal flora. However, this balance might be disturbed by different factors, such as aging, medicine (antibiotics), disease, junk food, stress, etc., leading to different types of disease due to the imbalance of the intestinal flora toward the harmful bacteria. Useful bacteria include lactic acid bacteria such as *Lactobacillus*, *Lactococcus*, and *Bifidobacterium*, whereas harmful bacteria include *Clostridium perfringens*, *E. coli*, *Staphylococcus*, and *Pseudomonas aeruginosa*.

Therefore, when there is an imbalance in the intestinal flora toward the harmful bacteria, the idea is to adjust the balance back toward the useful bacteria. This can be achieved with probiotics, prebiotics, or both (synbiotics). Probiotics can be as simple as taking useful bacteria orally. These useful bacteria, which can be represented by the lactic acid bacteria, can be found in dairy products such as yogurt and cheese, as well as in vegetarian products such as miso, natto, and some pickled food.

Probiotics should meet the following conditions:

1. It should be commensal bacteria on the human body.

2. It should be able to survive digestive enzymes, such as gastric acid and bile acid.

3. It should be able to multiply within the digestive system.

4. It should have efficacies to improve constipation and be able to inhibit the production of harmful substances by inhibiting bacterial growth.

5. It should be safe as a food item or medical product.

On the other hand, the use of prebiotics is the method of taking fiber as "food" for the useful bacteria, orally, so as to improve the intestinal environment by allowing the useful bacteria to multiply and accelerate their activities. When both methods are active at the same time, the terminology *synbiotics* is used. Accordingly, the following efficacy should be expected from taking food that target intestinal bacteria:

1. Increasing intestinal peristalsis and improving constipation.

2. Improving the immune function and inhibiting colon cancer.

3. Reducing the blood cholesterol level.

4. Reducing the number of *Helicobacter pylori*, which is a bacteria viewed as responsible for causing stomach cancer or peptic ulcer.

5. Preventing tooth decay and periodontal disease.

6. Reducing blood pressure.

7. Acting as an anti-allergen.

In addition, immunonutrition is one of the medical measures taken to reduce post-surgical complications. After surgery, different types of complications might occur. Therefore, total parenteral nutrition (TPN) used to be given after surgery together with anastomosis in the digestive tract. However, as the fasting period gets longer, the upper layer of the intestinal mucous membrane becomes atrophied, which affects the disease-preventive structure of the membrane. It was, consequently, revealed that the imbalance of intestinal bacteria can lead to serious complications, including bacterial translocation (BT) as well as sepsis. As a result, it was recommended to start enteral nutrition postoperatively as early as possible.

Consequently, the idea of reducing post-surgery complications by increasing the activity of the intestinal mucous membrane during the perioperative period was examined. For example, in the case of an operation due to colon cancer, the immune function of the patient can be reduced due to different factors, including the condition of the cancer, the surgery itself, and the stress resulting from foreign influencers such as anesthesia. For this case, we consider giving immunonutrition that is fortified by different elements such as omega-3 fatty acids, fiber, oligosaccharide, arginine, glutamine, trace minerals (zinc, copper, manganese, and selenium), and nucleic acid.

It was found that omega-3 fatty acid is able to stimulate the cellular immunity and anti-inflammation; fibers and oligosaccharides, being prebiotics, can improve the intestinal flora by inhibiting the growth of harmful bacteria, as well as averting BT by preventing membrane atrophy due to stress caused by surgery; arginine and glutamine, being nucleic acid precursors, are able to synthesize protein and activate cell-mediated immunity; and finally minerals such as zinc, copper, manganese, and selenium play a vital role in maintaining the body membrane, acting as oxygen scavengers.

As a result, there have been different reports on the efficacy of clinical immunonutrition. This is leading to a series of advantages; by reducing post-operative complications, the period in which the patient needs to stay hospitalized can be reduced, which results in reduction of the overall medical expenses.

Cautions of Health Food (Supplements)

Within functional food, the category of what is so-called health food (supplements) occupies the majority of market and is becoming of interest to many people. Because of its availability as well as the current trend of health awareness, the market of supplements has been growing year by year in Japan (1 billion Japanese yens in contrast with 6 billion Japanese yens for pharmaceuticals). Popular supplements include antioxidants such as vitamins C and E, and polyphenols; mushroom components (α- and β-glucans) to support immune system; natural herbs, and animal extracts. The external appearance of most of these supplements is similar to usual medicine (capsules, tablets, powder, etc.), and they usually contain a number of active components. Therefore, it is necessary to have careful management on the production lots to assure the quality of the supplement. Also, safety measures should be strictly taken to avoid the existence of impurities.

However, problems with health hazards related to supplements have been frequently reported. For example, there was one serious case in which an herbal supplement for weight reduction, imported from China, was contaminated with N-nitrosofenfluramine, which caused encephalopathy due to liver dysfunction to two of the users; one of them had to undergo liver transplantation while the other passed away. This was just one case among others that were reported to the Ministry of Health, Labour and Welfare, who in February 2005 prepared guidelines of Good Manufacturing Practice (GMP) based on the one made originally for pharmaceutical products, to assure quality and establish the difference between the various manufacturing players. Additionally, they implemented a certification system to qualify specialists called "Functional Food Consultant."

Also, attention should be drawn to the possible interaction between supplements and medicine. Many types of medicine are metabolized in the liver cytochrome P450 (CYP) and hydroxylase family, and excreted. On the other hand, it is known that some supplements are also metabolized by CYP. If this is the case, it will mean that taking medicine with this certain supplement would interfere with the metabolism of the medicine, which will lead to high concentration of the medicine in the blood. Moreover, some supplements are known to block the function of CYP, which may lead to the same results of a high concentration of medicine in the blood.

Similarly, taking antioxidant supplements (vitamins C and E or polyphenols) along with anticancer treatment may weaken the efficacy of the treatment.[5] For medicine that shows anticancer efficacy by generating active oxygen, such as anthracyclines, alkylating agents, platinum compounds, or topoisomerase inhibitors, it is recommended to refrain from taking antioxidants. This applies to radiotherapy as well. On the other hand, if the anticancer drug is not based on active oxygen, such as antimetabolites, or alkaloids, taking antioxidants may not cause complications.

Summary

This chapter focuses on food, especially functional food that is used in integrative medicine. Within CAM, health food occupies the majority of treatments in Japan. Regardless of safety, there is demand on what is thought to be the efficacy of the functional food. Therefore, the Ministry of Health also launched a project to deliver correct information related to integrative medicine to the public (see "Resources" below.) Also, it was demanded that when a new substance is introduced, an evidence-based structure should be implemented from the basic research until clinical studies show efficacy. In this sense, the biomarker is an important factor used for evaluation. It is also necessary to discuss not only current developments, but also future ideas. Nowadays, it is possible to completely grasp the changes in the metabolite and the expression in protein and mRNA using the omics technique, which was initiated from the genome plan. In the future, the effects of functional food and the development of health food shall be further clarified via the introduction of "neutraceuticals" and "nutrigenomics," which are highlighted as new fields of research. Consequently, medicine based on customized CAM shall no longer be a dream.

As for integrative medicine, it is not going to simply support conventional medicine. Rather, it will provide disease prevention and health-maintenance measures toward potential medical conditions, which are not considered therapy, providing comprehensive adhesion with Western medicine. Finally, integrative medicine is expected to provide comprehensive treatment as an ideal medical system for the upcoming generations.

REFERENCES

1. Eisenberg DM, Kessler RC, Foster C, et al. "Unconventional medicine in the United States. Prevalence, cost, and pattern use." *N. Engl. J. Med.* 328: 246–252, 1993.

2. Eisenberg DM, Davis RB, Ettner SL, et al. "Trends in alternative medicine use in the United States, 1990–1997." *JAMA* 280: 1569–1575, 1998.

3. Hyodo I, Amano N, Eguchi K, et al. "Nationwide survey on complementary and alternative medicine in cancer patients in Japan." *J. Clin. Oncol.* 23: 2645–54, 2005.

4. Cancer Research Fund of the Ministry of Health Labour and Social Welfare. "Research related to the scientific verification and clinical response of cancer alternative therapy." *Guidebook of Cancer Alternative Medicine* (3rd Edition), 2012 (In Japanese).

5. Yasueda A, Urushima H, and Ito T. "Efficacy and interaction of antioxidant supplements as adjuvant therapy in cancer treatment: a systematic review." *Integrative Cancer Therapies* 15(1): 17–39, 2016.

Online Resources

Ministry of Health, Labour and Welfare (Food safety information)
https://www.mhlw.go.jp/topics/bukyoku/iyaku/syoku-anzen/index.html

National Institute of Health and Nutrition
https://www.nibiohn.go.jp/eiken/english/index.html

National Center of Complementary and Integrative Medicine (NCCIM)
https://www.nccih.nih.gov/

Office of Cancer Complementary and Alternative Medicine (OCCAM)
https://cam.cancer.gov

Information Site for Evidence-based Japanese Integrative Medicines
https://www.ejim.ncgg.go.jp/public/index.html

PART 1

PROFILE SUMMARY OF AHCC

Chapter 1

MANUFACTURING PROCESS

Noriaki Fujii, Shotaro Kudo

AHCC is a standardized extract of cultured *Lentinula edodes* mycelia and the trademark of Amino Up Co., Ltd., Japan. It was developed by Amino Up Co., Ltd. (Sapporo, Japan), and Dr. Toshihiko Okamoto (School of Pharmaceutical Sciences, the University of Tokyo, Japan) in 1989. Since then, AHCC has also become available in many other countries outside of Japan. For example, in European Union, an AHCC product has been marketed since 1994.

It is known that AHCC has an immunomodulatory effect, and one of its active components is partially acylated α-glucans, which stimulate the gut immunity, although an immunomodulatory effect of general α-glucans (such as maltodextrin) is not known. Because of this effect, AHCC has been widely used as a supplement among immunocompromised people, including cancer patients, since its launch. It should be noted that modulation of the immunity to the appropriate condition is one of the key factors for health.

Manufacturing Process

Most mushroom products are made from the fruiting bodies of mushrooms by extracting components with a solvent such as water. However, AHCC is made from the mycelia of Shiitake mushroom, which are cultured in a liquid medium. When mushrooms are cultured in a liquid medium, they proliferate and form globular fungal bodies (see Figure 1 on the following page), but not fruiting bodies. The effects of AHCC are achieved through this unique manufacturing process (see Figure 2 on the following page).

In the manufacturing procedure, the mycelium source is obtained from a frozen working culture, and the use of this frozen working culture leads to consistency in AHCC. The mycelium source is cultured in the media by increasing the scales over a period of approximately thirty-seven days, after which the mycelium culture is extracted. The insoluble cell materials are removed from the solution using centrifugal separation techniques to produce a supernatant that contains various nutrients, and the solution is sterilized and freeze-dried to obtain a powder called AHCC-FD. However, due to its hygroscopic property, the powder is formulated and granulated with other ingredients for commercial use to lower its hygroscopic property. This fine granular powder is generally called AHCC.

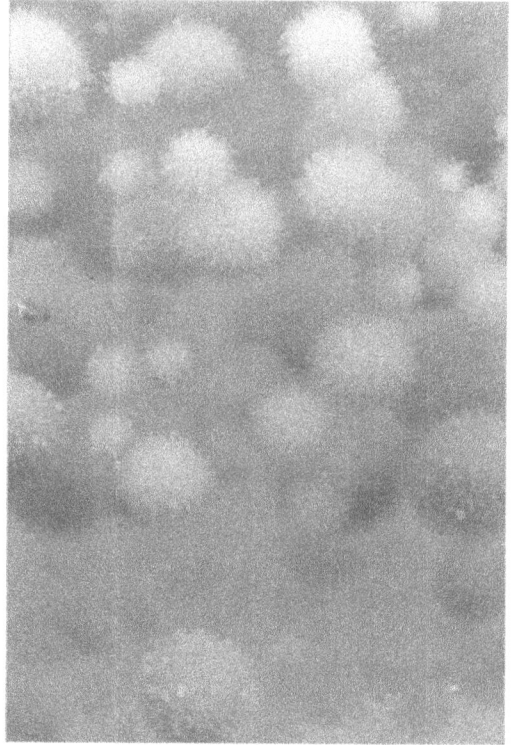

Figure 1. Globular Fungal Bodies

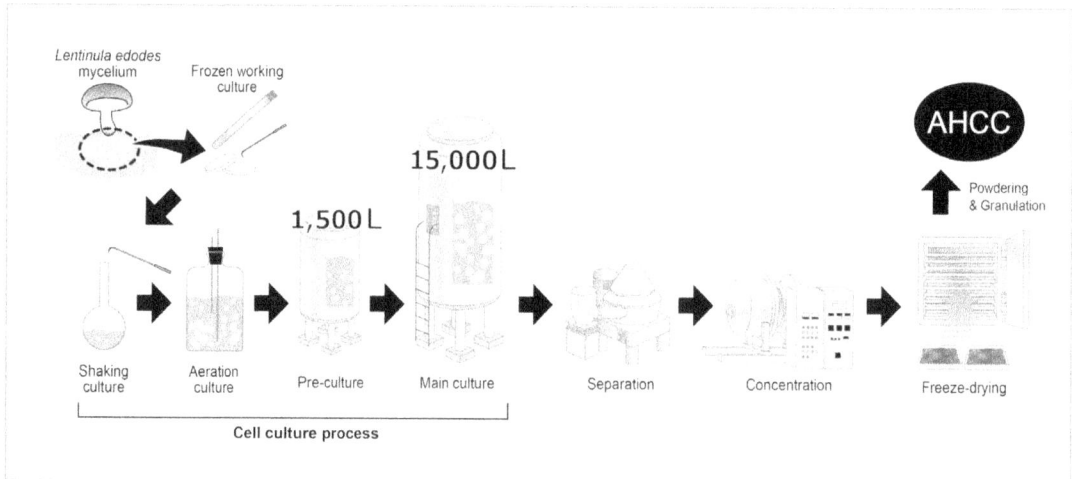

Figure 2. Manufacturing Procedure

Quality Control

AHCC is manufactured in accordance with Good Manufacturing Practice (GMP) for dietary supplements, a standard prepared by the Ministry of Health, Labour and Welfare in Japan and is certified by the Japan Health and Nutrition Food Association. AHCC is also manufactured in accordance with International Organization for Standardization (ISO) 9001:2008 for quality management and also ISO 22000:2005 for safety management, which combine interactive communication, system management, prerequisite programs, and the Hazard Analysis Critical Control Point (HACCP) principles developed by the Codex Alimentarius Commission.

Because the fungi are extremely sensitive to environmental conditions, all critical parameters are controlled through implementation of process controls, which include monitoring of temperature, time, pH, Brix, specific gravity, and microbial contamination to maintain a stable culturing environment for long periods.

As most mushroom products are from the fruiting body, cultivation conditions may be affected by environmental factors such as weather and season, and those nutrient profiles may also be varied. On the other hand, the environmental factors during the manufacturing process of AHCC are controlled using modern technologies. Therefore, it can be said that the quality of AHCC is more consistent than other types of mushroom products.

Chapter 2

COMPOSITION

Kenji Sato, Maki Kashimoto

This chapter introduces the main components of AHCC and addresses compounds with potential biological activities and characteristic structure with regard to those contents. The relationship between these compounds and biological responses by intake of AHCC is also discussed.

Approximate Composition

The approximate composition of AHCC-FD, which is the essential part of AHCC, is shown in Table 1 below and is compared with those of dried fruit bodies of mushrooms (*Agaricus blazei* and *Lentinula edodes*).[1] AHCC is characterized by higher car-

TABLE 1. **APPROXIMATE COMPOSITION OF AHCC-FD AND DRIED FRUIT BODIES OF MUSHROOMS (%)**

	AHCC-FD	*AGARICUS BLAZEI*	*LENTINULA EDODES*
Protein	13.1	40–45	19.3
Lipid	2.2	3–4	3.7
Carbohydrate	71.2	38–45	59.2
Dietary fiber	2.1	6–8	10.0
Ash	8.9	5–7	3.9

See Reference 1.

bohydrate content and lower fiber content than the dried mushrooms. AHCC-FD is a crude extract obtained through cultures of *Lentinula edodes* mycelia. For cultivation of the mycelia, some nutritional ingredients, such as rice bran extract, are used. The unique manufacturing process achieves the high carbohydrate content of AHCC-FD.

Carbohydrate

Monosaccharides in AHCC-FD were derivatized with 1-phenyl-3-methyl-5-pyra-zolone (PMP), and the derivatives were detected by liquid chromatography-tan-dem mass spectrometry (LC-MS/MS). The precursor ions, which yield fragment ion derived from PMP (m/z = 175), were detected by a precursor scan. This scan allows specific detection of reducing sugars. By scanning mass-to-charge ratio (m/z) cor-responding to monosaccharides, some aldoses were detected. By comparison of retention time of standard sugars, monosaccharides in AHCC-FD were identified as shown in Figure 1 below.

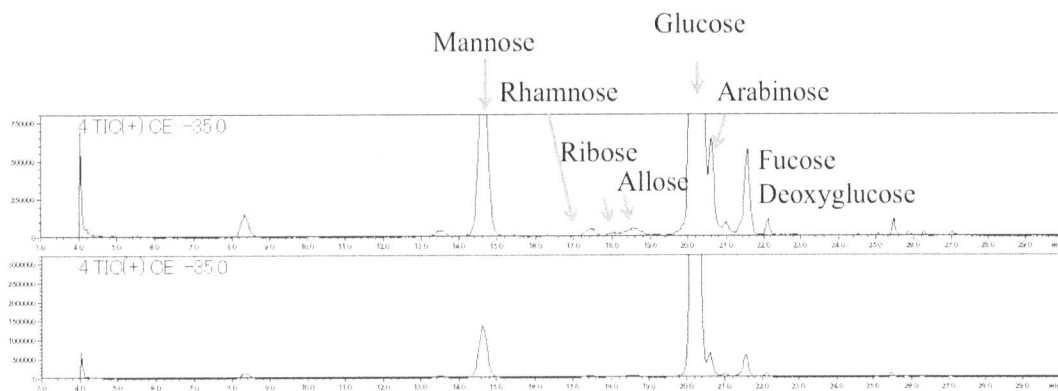

Figure 1. Estimated aldoses in water extract of AHCC-FD. Aldoses were detected by precursor scan yielding fragment ion (m/z = 175) in monosaccharide range. (Unpublished data).

Glucose and mannose are major constituents. In addition, arabinose, fucose, ribose, allose, rhamnose, and some unidentified aldoses are present as minor com-ponents, which may be derived from the nutritional ingredients used in the culture process (see Table 2 on the following page). While the presence of partially acylated α-1,4-glucan has been suggested in AHCC as described below, no acetylated hexose was detected as monosaccharide by this procedure. However, this approach can only detect reducing sugars (aldose). If a hydroxyl group of carbon 1 of pyranose form of

TABLE 2. **MONOSACCHARIDE CONTENT IN AHCC-FD**

Glucose	187.7	Rhamnose	0.4
Mannose	22.7	Fucose	0.4
Arabinose	4.0	Allose	0.6
Ribose	0.3		

(mg/g dry matter)

glucose is acetylated or esterified with other organic acids, the pyranose ring cannot open and thus cannot be detected by PMP-derivatization-LC-MS/MS technique. To solve this problem, monosaccharides in AHCC-FD were fractionated by size exclusion chromatography (SEC) and subjected to the sugar analysis. As shown in Figure 2, only a negligible level of PMP-glucose was detected in a SEC fraction before acid hydrolysis, while glucose peak extensively increased after acid hydrolysis of the same SEC fraction. In addition, organic acids were also liberated by the acid hydrolysis of same SEC fraction. These facts suggest presence of *O*-esterified glucose at carbon 1.

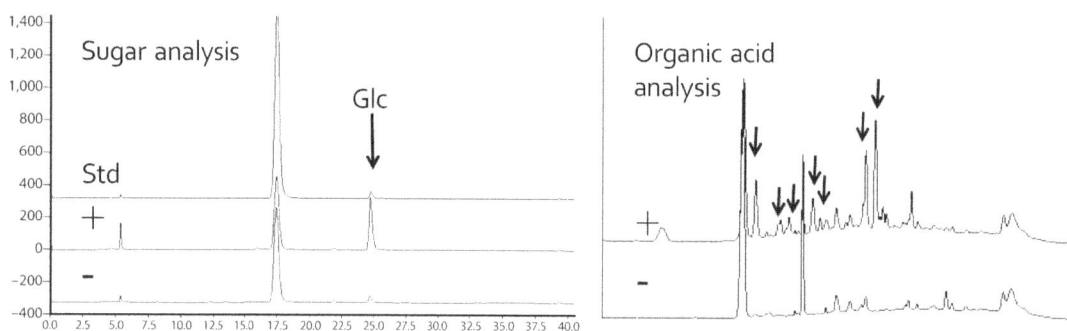

Figure 2. Detection of glucose and organic acids before (−) and after hydrolysis (+) of a size exclusion chromatography fraction of AHCC-FD. Components of AHCC-FD were fractionated by size exclusion chromatography by using superdex Peptide 10/30 equilibrated with 30% acetonitorile-0.1% trifluoroacetic acid at 0.5 mL/min. Fraction eluted from 40–41 min was collected and subjected to sugar and organic acid analyses. After acid hydrolysis, glucose (Glc) and some organic acids (arrows) were liberated. (Unpublished data)

Disaccharides were also detected by PMP-precolumn derivatization and LC-MS/MS. As shown in Figure 3, at least four disaccharides consisting of two hexoses were detected, which indicates the presence of disaccharides in addition to maltose and isomaltose. Interestingly, the disaccharide marked with arrow in Figure 3 is stable against acid hydrolysis. Structures of these disaccharides remain to be solved.

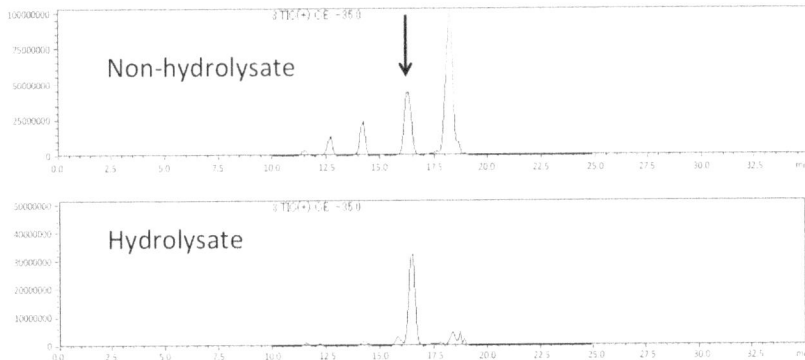

Figure 3. Disaccharides in water extract of AHCC-FD. Disaccharides were detected by precursor scan yielding fragment ion (m/z = 175) in disaccharide range. All disaccharides consist of two hexoses. The peak marked with an arrow resists acid hydrolysis. (unpublished data)

Components of AHCC-FD were fractionated by the method as illustrated in Figure 4.[1] The polysaccharide fraction was further characterized by monosaccharide analysis based on techniques such as alditol acetate derivatization-gas chromatography, SEC, nuclear magnetic resonance (NMR) spectroscopy. These analyses revealed

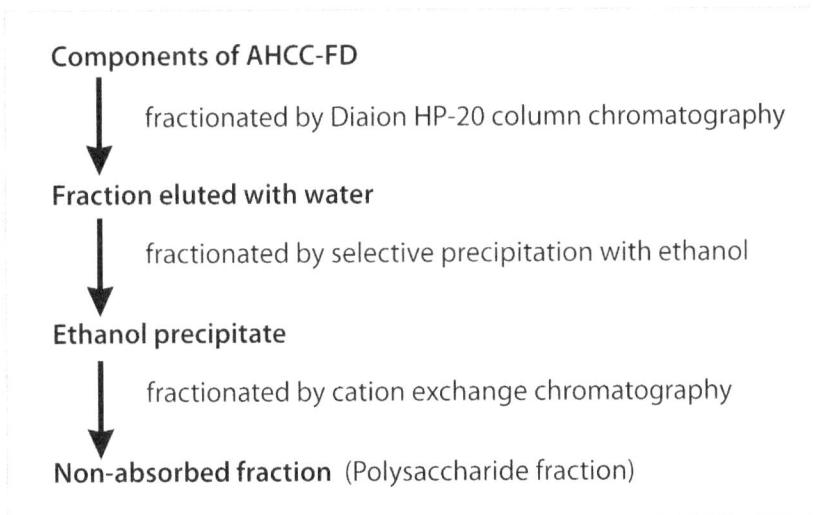

Components of AHCC-FD

↓ fractionated by Diaion HP-20 column chromatography

Fraction eluted with water

↓ fractionated by selective precipitation with ethanol

Ethanol precipitate

↓ fractionated by cation exchange chromatography

Non-absorbed fraction (Polysaccharide fraction)

Figure 4. Preparation of polysaccharide fraction from AHCC-FD. (From Fujii and Nakagawa, 2003)

that main polysaccharide is α-1,4-glucan with average molecular mass of 5,000. Sugar chain analysis after digestion with isoamylase revealed that this glucan has branched chains, which are linked to main chain by α-1,6 bond. In addition, NMR spectrometric analysis has suggested the presence of acylated hydroxyl group in the α-glucan.

Taken together, the main polysaccharide in AHCC has been assumed as illustrated in Figure 5.[1] The "acylated α-glucan" is one characteristic compound in AHCC compared to mushroom fruit body, of which the main soluble polysaccharides are β-glucans.[2,3] The specific "acylated α-glucan" can be derived from starch in the medium and modified during the culture process of *Lentinula edodes* mycelia. The "acylated α-glucan" has been suggested to be responsible for the immunostimulatory activity of AHCC. On the other hand, monosaccharides and disaccharides analyses have indicated the presence of a couple of monosaccharides and disaccharides in addition to glucose, maltose, and isomaltose. Therefore, there is a possibility that some novel sugar chain structure is present in AHCC polysaccharide, and it may play a significant role in exerting biological activity by intake of AHCC.

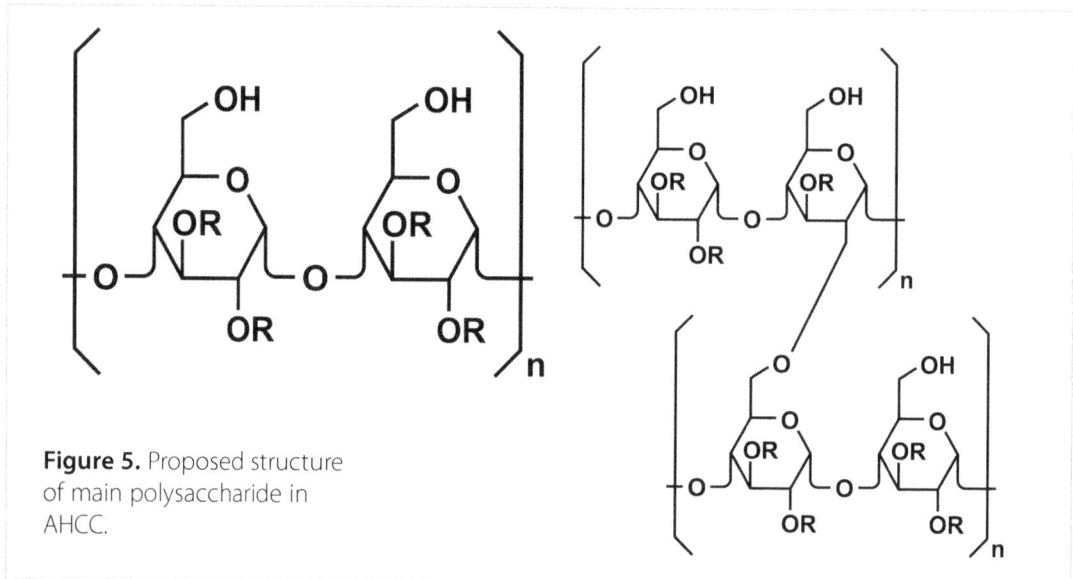

Figure 5. Proposed structure of main polysaccharide in AHCC.

Amino Acids and Peptides

Free amino acid composition in AHCC-FD is shown in Figure 6 compared with those of dried fruit bodies of mushrooms.[1] The amino acid composition of AHCC-FD is different from those of fruit bodies of *Agaricus blazei* but also *Lentinula edodes.* Compared

28

to the dried fruit body of *Lentinula edodes,* AHCC-FD has higher aspartic acid, pro-line, and valine and lower glutamic acid, histidine, and arginine. These differences can arise from nutritional ingredients used in the culture medium and also metabolism during liquid culture.

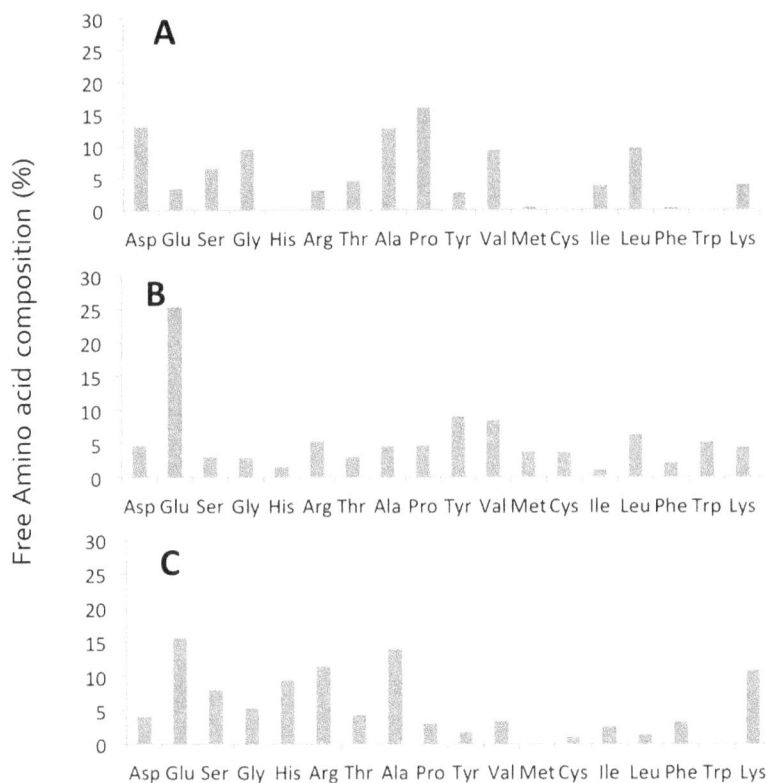

Figure 6. Free amino acid compositions of AHCC-FD (A), dry fruit bodies of mushrooms: Agariscus blazei (B) and Lentinula edodes (C). (From Fujii and Nakagawa, 2003)

There are few data on proteins and peptides in AHCC. These compounds might be responsible for the biological activities of AHCC. Recently, pyroglutamyl-leucine (pEL) was found in AHCC-FD (90 µg/g). Pyroglutamyl residue is generated from amino-terminal glutaminyl residue by cyclization.[4] In vitro experiments using rat macrophage[5] and primarily cultured hepatocyte[6] have demonstrated that pEL has anti-inflammatory activity. In addition, it has been demonstrated that pEL attenuates hepatitis[7] and colitis[8] in animal models and also normalizes microbiota in mice with colitis.[8] These facts suggest that pEL could contribute to the beneficial effects of AHCC. Further studies on identification and biological activities of peptides in AHCC are necessary.

Vitamins

As shown in Table 3 below,[1] AHCC-FD has detectable but an extensively lower level of ergosterol and lower vitamin B_2 than the dried fruit body of *Lentinula edodes*. Negligible amounts of vitamins K_1, K_2, and D_2 may be present in AHCC-FD. Hypervitaminosis is caused by excess consumption of fat-soluble vitamins, especially vitamin A, but also water-soluble ones such as niacin. In addition, patients taking warfarin, an anticoagulant normally used in the prevention of thrombosis, are advised to avoid excess consumption of vitamin K to prevent excess clotting. AHCC is sometimes consumed for a long period. However, even consumption of high dose AHCC (6 g/day) does not cause niacin-induced hypervitaminosis[9] (300 mg/day) and is safe for patients taking warfarin.

TABLE 3. **VITAMIN CONTENT IN AHCC-FD AND FRUIT BODIES OF MUSHROOMS**

	AHCC-FD	*AGARICUS BLAZEI*	*LENTINULA EDODES*
Vitamin B_1	3	6	5
Vitamin B_2	3	51	14
Vitamin K_1 and K_2	N.D.	—	N.D.
Niacin	550	430	170
Ergosterol	21	—	2570
Vitamin D_2	N.D.	—	0.85

(µg/g of dry matter)   *N.D.: Not detectable.*   *See Reference 1.*

Purine Bases

The content of purine bases in AHCC-FD is shown in Table 4 on the facing page; adenine, guanine, and xanthine are present in AHCC.[1] However, their contents are lower than those of dried fruit body *Lentinula edodes*. In humans, these purine bases are metabolized into uric acid, which is excreted into urine. When uric acid is generated beyond excretion capability from the kidneys (300 mg/day), the blood uric acid level increases higher than 7 mg/dl, which is referred to hyperuricemia. In such case, uric acid can form crystals and induce severe inflammation, namely gout. Purine base intake by consumption of high dose AHCC is less than 10 mg/day.

It has been demonstrated that AHCC suppresses interleukin 1β-induced nitric oxide (NO) production.[10] An activity-guided fractionation study revealed that adenosine, a nucleoside consisting of adenine, primarily contributes to the in vitro anti-inflammatory activity, while adenine and other nucleosides exert less anti-inflammatory activity.[11] There is a possibility that adenosine in AHCC-FD (250 μg/g) could contribute, at least partially, to the beneficial effect of AHCC intake.

TABLE 4. CONTENT OF PURINE BASES IN AHCC-FD AND DRIED FRUIT BODY OF *LENTINUS EDODES*

	AHCC-FD	*LENTINUS EDODES*
Adenine	0.6	2.0
Guanine	0.4	1.7
Xanthine	0.2	0.1
Hypoxanthine	N.D.	N.D.

(mg/g of dry matter)   *N.D.: Not detectable.*   *See Reference 1.*

Minerals

Mineral content in AHCC-FD and dried fruit bodies of *Agaricus blazei* and *Lentinula edodes* is shown in Table 5 on the following page.[1] In comparison to the dried fruit bodies of mushrooms, AHCC-FD contains higher sodium and phosphorus, which can be derived from rice bran and other ingredients. However, intakes of sodium and phosphorus by consumption of high dose AHCC (6 g/day) are less than 50 mg and 100 mg, respectively, which are considerably less than the Tolerable Upper Intake Level (2.3 g for sodium and 4 g for phosphorus).[12]

Discussion

AHCC is a standardized extract of cultured *Lentinula edodes* mycelia. As shown in the above discussions, the composition of AHCC-FD is considerably different from dried fruit bodies of *Lentinula edodes* and other mushrooms. For mycelia culture, nutrient ingredients are added, and compounds in these ingredients are used by the mycelia and changed to other compounds. Therefore, AHCC is not just dried

TABLE 5. MINERAL CONTENT IN AHCC-FD AND DRIED FRUIT BODIES OF MUSHROOMS

	AHCC-FD	*AGARICUS BLAZEI*	*LENTINUS EDODES*
Potassium	20.0	46.0	21
Sodium	8.4	0.44	0.13
Phosphorus	15.0	13.0	3.1
Calcium	0.069	1.35	0.10
Iodine	N.D.	—	—

(mg/g of dry matter)   *N.D.: Not detectable.*   *See Reference 1.*

mushroom powder, but a mixture of compounds generated by the liquid culture of the mycelia.

Ingestion of AHCC exerts many beneficial activities as shown in other chapters in this book. As AHCC exerts beneficial effects against chronic diseases such as cancer, relatively high doses of AHCC (3 – 6 g/day) are commonly consumed for a long period. Therefore, it is important that the nutritional status of patients is not disturbed by the consumption of AHCC. As explained in this chapter, excess intake of specific nutrient over daily upper limit does not generally occur even when high doses of AHCC are consumed.

In vitro studies of AHCC have indicated that AHCC stimulates cells involved in immune responses, such as monocyte,[13] and simultaneously suppresses excess inflammation response by cells in non-immune system such as hepatocyte,[10] which is big advantage of AHCC in comparison to other drugs and functional foods with single immunostimulatory or anti-inflammatory activity. It has been suspected that polysaccharide fraction of AHCC, "acylated α-1,4-glucan," is responsible for its immunostimulatory activity. However, sugar motif, which directly acts on the cells in immune system, has not been identified. Further studies on identification of the structure of the active sugar motif are necessary. For anti-inflammatory activity to primary cultured hepatocyte, adenosine and pyroglutamyl-leucine have been identified in AHCC. The potential hepatoprotective activity of these compounds should be confirmed by animal and human studies. In addition, little is known regarding the structure and biological activities of peptides in AHCC, which should be explored.

REFERENCES

1. Fujii H and Nakagawa T. "Composition of AHCC." Basic and clinical studies on AHCC, 2003.

2. Usui T, Iwasaki Y, and Mizuno T. "Isolation and characterization of antitumor active β-D-glucans from the fruit bodies of *Ganoderma applanatum.*" *Carbohydr. Res.* 115, 273–280, 1983.

3. Kiho T, Yoshida I, Nagai K, Ukai S, and Hara C. "(1—>3)-α–D-glucan from an alkaline extract of *Agrocybe cylindracea,* and antitumor activity of its O-(carboxymethyl)ated derivatives." *Carbohydr. Res.* 189, 273–279, 1989.

4. Sato K, Nishimura R, Suzuki Y, Motoi H, Nakamura Y, Ohtsuki K, and Kawabata M. "Occurrence of indigestible pyroglutamyl peptides in an enzymatic hydrolysate of wheat gluten prepared on an industrial scale." *J. Agric. Food Chem.* 46, 3403–3405, 1998.

5. Hirai S, Horii S, Matsuzaki Y, Ono S, Shimmura Y, Sato K, and Egashira Y. "Anti-inflammatory effect of pyroglutamyl-leucine on lipopolysaccharide-stimulated RAW 264.7 macrophages." *Life Sci.* 117, 1–6, 2014.

6. Oishi M, Kiyono T, Sato K, Tokuhara K, Tanaka Y, Miki H, Nakatake R, Kaibori M, Nishizawa M, Okumura T, and Kon M. "PyroGlu-Leu inhibits the induction of inducible nitric oxide synthase in interleukin-1β-stimulated primary cultured rat hepatocytes." *Nitric Oxide* 44, 81–87, 2015.

7. Sato K, Egashira Y, Ono S, Mochizuki S, Shimmura Y, Suzuki Y, Nagata M, Hashimoto K, Kiyono T, Park EY, Nakamura Y, Itabashi M, Sakata Y, Furuta S, and Sanada H. "Identification of a hepatoprotective peptide in wheat gluten hydrolysate against D-galactosamine-induced acute hepatitis in rats." *J. Agric. Food Chem.* 61, 6304–6310, 2013.

8. Wada S, Sato K, Ohta R, Wada E, Bou Y, Fujiwara M, Kiyono T, Park EY, Aoi W, Takagi T, Naito Y, and Yoshikawa T. "Ingestion of low dose pyroglutamyl leucine improves dextran sulfate sodium-induced colitis and intestinal microbiota in mice." *J. Agric. Food Chem.* 61, 8807–8813, 2013.

9. Dietary Reference Intakes for Japanese, 2015.

10. Matsui K, Ozaki T, Oishi M, Tanaka Y, Kaibori M, Nishizawa M, Okumura T, and Kwon AH. "Active hexose correlated compound inhibits the expression of proinflammatory biomarker iNOS in hepatocytes." *Eur. Surg. Res.* 47, 274–283, 2011.

11. Tanaka Y, Ohashi S, Ohtsuki A, Kiyono, T, Park EY, Nakamura Y, Sato K, Oishi M, Miki H, Tokuhara K, Matsui K, Kaibori M, Nishizawa M, Okumura T, and Kwon AH. "Adenosine, a hepatoprotective component in active hexose correlated compound: Its identification and iNOS suppression mechanism." *Nitric Oxide* 40, 75–86, 2014.

12. Dietary Reference Intakes (DRIs): Tolerable Upper Intake Levels, Vitamins. Food and Nutrition Board, Institute of Medicine, National Academies, 1997.

13. Lee WW, Lee N, Fujii H, and Kang I. "Active hexose correlated compound promotes T helper (Th) 17 and 1 cell responses via inducing IL-1β production from monocytes in humans." *Cell Immunology* 275, 19–23, 2012.

Chapter 3

SAFETY ASSESSMENT

Thomas Walshe, Hiroshi Nishioka

Basidiomycetes used for AHCC are the mycelia of widely eaten shiitake mushrooms. From the experience of consumption, AHCC is considered to be safe as a food. Nevertheless, various safety evaluations were conducted to scientifically demonstrate that AHCC is a safe and reliable food, as discussed in this chapter.

Pre-Clinical Studies

Rat Single Dose Oral Toxicity Test (GLP Complied)[1]

Crj:CD Sprague-Dawley (SD) rats were used for the toxicity test, and a single oral dose of 12,500 mg/kg AHCC freeze-dried powder (AHCC-FD) was administered to the AHCC group at day 0. The rats were observed up to fourteen days post administration. The control group received a single oral dose of purified water as a vehicle at day 0. The number of animals in both groups was ten male rats (five weeks old) and ten female rats (six weeks old).

There were no deaths observed in either the control group or the AHCC group. The general observation findings indicated that all male rats of the AHCC group experienced an onset of reduction in the spontaneous motor activity from around 30 minutes after administration; and they started drinking more water and accompanied diarrhea. However, the male rats recovered from these symptoms at the end of the observation period on the day of administration. Then, it was observed that the female rats started drinking more water and suffering from diarrhea around 30 minutes after the administration of AHCC-FD. The female rats also recovered from these symptoms at the end of observation on the day of administration. No abnormalities were observed in the male and female rats of the control group through the test period including the administration day. In the autopsy findings, none of the male rats in either group showed abnormalities. Although dilatation of the renal pelvis was observed in one of the females undergoing AHCC-FD, no other abnormalities were detected.

As described above, all ten cases of both sexes in the 12,500 mg/kg AHCC-FD administration group survived with no severe symptoms. Thus, it was determined that the LD_{50} (lethal dose, 50%) value for a single oral dose of AHCC-FD was higher than 12,500 mg/kg.

Repeated-dose 90-day Oral Toxicity Test in Rats (GLP and OECD408 Complied)[1]

AHCC-FD was repeatedly administered to Slc:SD rats (five weeks old) at doses of 0 mg/kg (control group), 1,000 mg/kg (low-dose group), 3,000 mg/kg (middle-dose group), and 6,000 mg/kg (high-dose group) once daily for ninety days. Each group consisted of ten male and ten female rats. Toxicological evaluations were as follows: clinical observation, body weight, food consumption, ophthalmological examination, urinalysis, hematology, blood chemistry, necropsy, organ weight, and histopathological examination.

In urinalysis, the changes related to the administration of AHCC-FD were significant decrease in pH value and increase in protein excretion in the high-dose group of male rats and the middle- and high-dose groups of female rats, and then elevation of the specific gravity of urine was observed in the high-dose group of male rats. In necropsy, black patch in the mucosa of glandular stomach and white mass in the limiting ridge of stomach were observed in the male and female rats of the high-dose group. Also, in histopathology squamous cell hyperplasia and hyperkeratosis in the limiting ridge of stomach were slightly observed in the male and female rats of the high-dose group, and fatty changes of the centrilobular hepatocytes were observed in the male rats of the high-dose group.

Particularly, since an increase in the excretion of urinary proteins was observed in the AHCC-FD administration groups, a more detailed histopathological examination of the kidney was conducted. The result indicated vascular dilatation of the glomerulus, which was considered to be the impact of the test substance administration, in only two cases of male rats from the high-dose group; however, the finding was not observed in the male and female rats of the dose groups below 3,000 mg/kg.

It was concluded from the above results that the no-observed-adverse-effect level (NOAEL) of AHCC-FD was 3,000 mg/kg/day in both male and female rats under the conditions of this test.

Bacterial Reverse Mutation Test (GLP Complied)[1]

For evaluating the potential of AHCC-FD to induce genetic mutation in bacteria, the reverse mutation test (Ames test) was carried out using *Salmonella typhimurium* TA102, TA1535, and TA1537 strains. The test was estimated in the absence or presence of metabolic activation (S9 mix). The highest concentration of the test substance was 5,000 μg/plate, and a total of six concentrations were set with a two-fold dilution step (156, 313, 625, 1,250, 2,500, and 5,000 μg/plate).

The average number of revertant colonies of each tester strain in the test substance-treated groups was less than twice that of the negative control group and no concentration-dependent increase was observed in the assay without or with metabolic activation, demonstrating that the result was negative.

Based on the above results, it was determined that AHCC-FD was not mutagenic to the tester strains under the current test conditions.

Mouse Micronucleus Assay (GLP Complied)[1]

The micronucleus assay was performed to evaluate the potential of AHCC-FD to induce chromosomal aberration in vivo. The test substance was orally administered to seven-week-old Crlj:CD-1 (ICR) male mice at 500, 1,000, and 2,000 mg/kg/day twice at a 24-hour interval. In the negative and positive control groups, purified water as a vehicle was orally administered and a single dose of 1 mg/kg mitomycin C was intraperitoneally administered, respectively. Each group had six animals, and the evaluation was carried out 24 hours after the final administration.

There were no significant differences observed between all the AHCC-FD administered groups and the negative control group in the percent of micronucleated erythrocytes to total polychromatic erythrocytes. On the other hand, the percent of micronucleated erythrocytes in the positive control group was significantly higher when compared to the negative control group. No significant differences were observed between the negative control, the positive control, and the test substance groups in the ratio of polychromatic erythrocytes to total erythrocytes.

From the above results, it was concluded that AHCC-FD did not induce micronuclei under the conditions in this assay and showed no potential to induce chromosomal aberration in vivo.

Clinical Studies

Phase I Safety Study[2]

The phase I study was conducted using healthy individuals based on the U.S. Food and Drug Administration (FDA) guidelines to assess the safety of AHCC in humans. Twenty-six (eleven male and fifteen female) healthy volunteers (age 18–61, average age 34) were given a 50-mL AHCC drink containing 3 g of AHCC-FD three times a day (9 g of AHCC-FD per day) for fourteen days. Medical interviews, questionnaires, electrocardiogram, and hematology and blood biochemistry tests were used to evaluate the safety.

In the study, the average compliance for the twenty-six subjects was 99%. During the test period, four subjects reported the adverse events such as headache, toe cramps, diarrhea, abdominal bloating, and fatigue; however, they were mild and transient. Also, abnormalities were not observed in the electrocardiogram and hematology and blood biochemistry tests.

Taken together, serious adverse events were not observed in the phase I study using three- to nine-fold dosage compared to the recommended dose, concluding that AHCC is safe as a food used in clinical practice.

Prospective Cohort Study[3]

The cohort study was performed over a period of nine years and eleven months in 222 postoperative patients with hepatocellular cancer, who were divided into the AHCC group (113 subjects) and the control group (109 subjects). The AHCC group received 3 g/day of AHCC fine granule (AHCC-FG). The purpose of this study was to investigate whether AHCC intake improved the prognosis in hepatocellular cancer patients after surgery, as well as to identify the side effects of AHCC.

Only three subjects in the AHCC group reported slight nausea, while no other side effects were observed. Although not directly related to safety evaluation, the recurrence rate of cancer and the patient survival in the AHCC group were significantly improved compared to the control group. Furthermore, AHCC treatment significantly improved the activities of serum aspartate transaminase (AST), γ-glutamyltransferase (GGT), and cholinesterase.

From the above, it can be considered that AHCC-FG is a functional food with high safety and no serious side effects, even when ingested over a long period.

Conclusion

To assess the safety of AHCC, pre-clinical studies and clinical trials were carried out using AHCC-FD or AHCC-FG. The data from each test have not indicated any concern about the safety of AHCC. Therefore, it is evident that AHCC is a safe and reliable functional food capable of a long-term supplementation.

REFERENCES

1. Fujii H, et al. "Genotoxicity and subchronic toxicity evaluation of Active Hexose Correlated Compound (AHCC)." *Regul. Toxicol. Pharmacl.* 59, 237–250, 2011.

2. Spierings EL, et al. "A phase I study of the safety of the nutritional supplement, active hexose correlated compound, AHCC, in healthy volunteers." *J. Nutr. Sci. Vitamino.* 53, 536–539, 2007.

3. Matsui Y, et al. "Improved prognosis of postoperative hepatocellular carcinoma patients when treated with functional foods: a prospective cohort study." *J. Hepatol.* 37, 78–86, 2002.

Conventional and Water-Soluble AHCC Formulations

Juan Torrado

Amino Up Co., Ltd., is the manufacturer of the immunomodulator complex known as AHCC, extracted from Shiitake fungus (*Lentinula edodes*) through a growth-controlled process at its industrial facilities in Sapporo, Japan. The well-controlled industrial process allows the company to standardize AHCC production and to minimize inter-batch variability. Amino Up Co., Ltd. has patented the product and its industrial production process.

AHCC is a complex mixture mainly composed of α-glucans. The presence of low molecular weight glucans and partially acylated-α-glucans is characteristic of AHCC. AHCC is sold in different countries as a functional food to improve the immune system, especially for cancer patients. Furthermore, AHCC is also indicated as coadjuvant for the treatment of different infections, inflammatory processes, and other diseases. Interestingly, AHCC is useful not only to treat, but also to prevent, cancer and infections. Obviously, dosage requirements are very different depending on the health conditions of the consumers and may vary from milligrams to grams per day.

Although many scientific studies have been performed by different independent research laboratories around the world, the active components of AHCC have not been clearly elucidated. Identification of the active components of AHCC is a topic of ongoing research. It is accepted that its biological activity depends not only on a unique individual component but also on many of them. The biological activity of AHCC is related to both direct and indirect actions on the immune system. For instance, the prebiotic activity of AHCC has been proved as an indirect way to interact on the immune system. During the last years, special interest has been observed on the combinations of AHCC with other natural products to obtain synergic effects, particularly combinations with probiotic, nucleotides, and extracts of other natural products such as garlic.

The standard AHCC products developed by Amino Up Co., Ltd., are prepared for consumers from many different countries. Great efforts have been taken to guarantee the stability of AHCC at different extreme environmental conditions such as very high-humidity circumstances. Usually, water uptakes of these powder products are closely related to instability that can compromise its activity. For stability reasons, the conventional standard AHCC products are prepared to avoid water uptake. These formulations can be defined as hydrophobic AHCC formulations. Conventional AHCC marketed formulations are hydrophobic formulations of sachets and capsules. Sachets for direct oral consumption without water are the standard method of AHCC intake in Japan. However, in Western countries, sachets are usually related to extemporaneous oral suspensions/solutions. When the Japanese sachets were intended to suspend in water, most of the product was floating and with poor wet ability characteristics. Moreover, for the treatment of cancer, high doses of AHCC are usually required, and deglutition capacities (or swallowing ability) of these patients can be compromised. For these consumers, water-soluble AHCC formulations have been recently developed and are available from Amino Up Co., Ltd. These water-soluble formulations are easier to swallow than conventional hydrophobic formulations.

Water-soluble formulations are prepared with exactly the same active AHCC raw materials contained in the conventional formulations. To improve water uptake, some of the hydrophobic components of the conventional AHCC formulations have been replaced by natural hydrophilic products. Moreover, the final production process of these water-soluble AHCC formulations has been adapted to increase water affinity. Stability characteristics of these new formulations have been carefully studied during the formulation development process. Water-soluble AHCC preparations are not only easy to dissolve but easier to swallow even at very high doses (3 g) as well.

Apart from this, AHCC has a pleasant taste. Pure AHCC is a mushroom extract that is appreciated and used by sophisticated gourmets and chefs. Water-soluble AHCC formulations have been developed not only to maintain its activity but also to offer the consumer the genuine natural taste of AHCC.

PART 2

BASIC & CLINICAL STUDIES ON AHCC

Chapter 4

IMMUNE MODULATION

Nutrition and the Immune Response

Philip C. Calder

Humans exist in an environment that is threatening to health. One major threat is the presence of invasive organisms that can damage host tissues, causing illness and, in some cases, death. These organisms include bacteria, viruses, parasites, and fungi. Humans have evolved elaborate protective mechanisms to enable survival in the face of the threat of pathogenic invasive organisms; collectively, these protective mechanisms are termed *the immune system.* The mechanisms of protection include physical and chemical barriers that restrict entry of the organisms into the body; a sophisticated cellular and chemical response that aims to identify and eliminate threatening organisms that manage to penetrate the protective barriers; maintenance of "memory" of immunological encounters in order to make any subsequent response more effective; and activities to repair any damage done to host tissues during the course of the immune response.

Mounting an immune response requires energy sources, building blocks, biochemical substrates, enzymatic cofactors, and regulatory factors. These must come from the diet or from body stores. Hence, nutrition is important in assuring adequate delivery of the substances needed to support the immune system to achieve its protective role. Consequently, poorly nourished individuals or individuals with specific nutrient deficiencies have impaired immune responses and increased susceptibility to infection.[1-3] These can both be reversed by tackling the nutritional defect.[1-3] The immune response is highly regulated, and "balances" are maintained by cross-regulation of the different types of cellular responses. A breakdown in these regulatory patterns can result in disease, the exact nature of which is determined by the nature of the immune imbalance. Clinical outcomes include inability to cope with being infected (leading to sepsis), poor wound healing, inappropriate immune responses to foods (leading to allergic disease, celiac disease, and so on), inappropriate responses to commensal microorganisms (leading to skin diseases and inflammatory bowel diseases, for example), and inappropriate responses to "self" (leading to autoimmune diseases). Hence, while there is much interest in finding strategies to support an appropriate immune response to a threatening organism, or other legitimate target such as a cancer cell, there is also much interest in finding ways to control inappropriate immune responses. Nutrition and specific food components can play a role in both supporting a protective immune response and in controlling adverse immunological activities. The aim of this chapter is to provide an overview of the immune system and how it functions normally and to describe, in outline, the influence of nutrition on the immune response. This is a large topic and interested readers are directed to several multi-author books devoted to it.[4-6] This chapter is based in part upon a previously published article.[7]

Overview of the Immune System

The role of the immune system is to protect the host from infectious agents that exist in the environment, such as bacteria, viruses, fungi, and parasites; from other noxious environmental insults; and from cancer (tumor) cells. The immune system is complex and involves many different cell types that are distributed across many locations throughout the body and travel between those locations in the lymph and the bloodstream. In some locations in the body, immune cells are organized into discrete lymphoid organs, classified as primary lymphoid organs where immune cells arise and mature (bone marrow and thymus) and secondary lymphoid organs (e.g., lymph nodes, spleen, gut-associated lymphoid tissue) where mature immune cells interact and respond to antigens. The immune system has two broad functional divisions called the innate (or natural) immune system and the acquired (or specific or adaptive) immune system.

Innate Immunity

Components of the innate immune system include physical barriers, soluble factors in the bloodstream and in secretions like saliva and tears, and phagocytic cells, which include granulocytes (neutrophils, basophils, and eosinophils), monocytes, and macrophages. Innate immunity has no memory and so is not affected by prior exposure to an organism or other immune trigger. The soluble factors of innate immunity include complement proteins. Phagocytic cells recognize certain common structures on bacteria and other microorganisms via surface receptors called pattern recognition receptors; the structures they recognize are called microbe-associated molecular patterns. Binding of the organism to one of these receptors triggers phagocytosis (engulfing) and subsequent destruction of the pathogenic microorganism by toxic chemicals, such as superoxide radicals and hydrogen peroxide. Natural killer cells also possess surface receptors and destroy their target cells by the release of cytotoxic proteins. In this way, innate immunity provides a first line of defense against invading pathogens. However, an immune response often requires the coordinated actions of both innate and acquired immunity.

Acquired Immunity

In contrast to innate immunity, which is not very specific, acquired immunity involves the specific recognition of molecules (termed *antigens*) derived from an invading pathogen and that distinguish it as being foreign to the host. Acquired immunity is also involved in assuring tolerance to sources of non-threatening antigens such as non-pathogenic bacteria, food, and the host's own tissues. The main cells involved in acquired immunity are the lymphocytes, which are classified into T and B lymphocytes (also called T cells and B cells). B lymphocytes undergo development and maturation in the bone marrow before being released into the circulation, while T lymphocytes mature in the thymus. From the bloodstream, lymphocytes can enter secondary lymphoid organs, like the spleen and lymph nodes. Immune responses occur largely in these lymphoid organs, which are highly organized to favor the interactions between cells and antigens that are required for an effective immune response.

The acquired immune response is highly specific and becomes effective over several days after its initial activation. It also persists for some time after the removal of the initiating antigen. This persistence gives rise to immunological memory, which is also a characteristic feature of acquired immunity. Memory is the basis for a stronger, more effective immune response upon re-exposure to an antigen (i.e., reinfection with the same pathogen) and is the rationale for vaccination. Eventually, the immune system will reestablish homeostasis using self-regulatory mechanisms.

B lymphocytes produce antibodies (soluble antigen-specific immunoglobulins).

This form of immune protection is called *humoral immunity*. Antibodies bind to the surface of microorganisms bearing the antigen the antibody was raised against, and this promotes the recognition and phagocytosis of the organism by phagocytic cells. The organisms being dealt with by humoral immunity are extracellular until they are phagocytosed. However, some pathogens, particularly viruses, but also certain bacteria, infect individuals by entering cells. These pathogens will escape humoral immunity and are instead dealt with by cell-mediated immunity, which is conferred by T lymphocytes. T lymphocytes express antigen-specific T-cell receptors on their surface. They are only able to recognize antigens that are presented to them on another cell surface (the cell presenting the antigen to the T lymphocyte is termed an *antigen presenting cell,* or APC). Activation of the T-cell receptor results in proliferation of the T cell and secretion of the cytokine interleukin (IL)-2, which promotes proliferation and differentiation. This process greatly increases the number of antigen-specific T lymphocytes.

There are three principal types of T lymphocytes; cytotoxic T cells, helper T cells, and regulatory T cells. Cytotoxic T lymphocytes carry the surface protein marker CD8 and kill infected cells and tumor cells by secretion of cytotoxic enzymes, which cause lysis of the target cell. Helper T lymphocytes carry the surface protein marker CD4 and eliminate pathogens by stimulating the phagocytic activity of macrophages and the proliferation of, and antibody secretion by, B lymphocytes. Helper T lymphocytes have traditionally been subdivided into two broad categories according to the pattern of cytokines they produce. Th1 cells produce IL-2 and interferon (IFN)-γ, which activate macrophages, natural killer cells, and cytotoxic T lymphocytes. Antigens derived from bacteria, viruses, and fungi tend to induce a Th1-dominant response. Th2 cells produce IL-4, which stimulates immunoglobulin (Ig)E production, and IL-5, an eosinophil-activating factor. Th2 cells are responsible for defense against helminthic parasites, which is due to IgE-mediated activation of mast cells and basophils. Other categories of helper T cells, including Th17 cells, have been described. Regulatory T cells produce IL-10 and transforming growth factor-β and suppress the activities of B cells and other T cells, preventing inappropriate activation.

The Gut-Associated Immune System

Mucosal surfaces have a strong immune component, as they are sites of interaction with the environment. The immune system of the gut (sometimes termed *the gut-associated immune system* or *gut-associated lymphoid tissue*) is extensive and is believed to contain up to 70% of the immune cells in the human body. This makes sense because it is the site of continuous exposure to pathogenic and non-pathogenic microorganisms from within the gut lumen and to food-borne antigens. The gut-associated immune system includes the physical barrier of the intestine, as well as components of the innate and acquired immune systems. The physical barrier includes acid in the stomach, mucus, and tightly connected epithelial cells, which collectively prevent the entry of pathogens. The cells of the gut-associated immune system are organized into specialized structures, termed *Peyer's patches,* which are located directly beneath the epithelium in the lamina propria. This also contains so-called M cells, which sample small particles from the gut lumen; these particles can be derived from food or from microorganisms. The gut-associated immune system has a vital role in assuring host defense against pathogens within the gastrointestinal lumen, but also in generating tolerogenic responses to harmless microorganisms and to food components.[8]

The Immune System Over the Life Course

Babies are born with an immature immune system. After birth, immunologic competence is gained partly as a result of the many maturation factors present in breast milk and partly as a result of exposure to antigens (from the mother's skin, from food, and from environmental microorganisms, the latter starting during the birth process itself).[9,10] Some of the early encounters with antigens play an important role in assuring tolerance, and a breakdown in this system of "immune education" can lead to disease.[9,10] At the other end of the life course, older people experience a progressive dysregulation of the immune system, leading to decreased acquired immunity and a greater susceptibility to infection.[11–14] This age-related decline in acquired immunity is termed *immunosenescence.* Innate immunity appears to be less affected by aging than acquired immunity, although there can be an increase in low-grade inflammation.

An Activated Immune System
Has Increased Nutritional Demands

The immune system is functioning at all times. However, specific immunity becomes activated by the presence of pathogenic organisms, which are direct immune stimulants. This results in a significant increase in the demand of the immune system for substrates and nutrients to provide a ready source of energy, which can be supplied from exogenous sources (i.e., from the diet) and/or from endogenous pools (see Figure 1 below). The cells of the immune system are metabolically active and are able to utilize glucose, amino acids, and fatty acids as fuels.[15] Many of the enzymes involved in energy generation have metal ions at their active site or as cofactors, while electron carriers and coenzymes are usually derivatives of vitamins. Activation of the immune response induces the production of proteins (including immunoglobulins, cytokines, cytokine receptors, adhesion molecules, and acute-phase proteins) and lipid-derived mediators (including prostaglandins and leukotrienes).

To respond optimally to an immune challenge, there must be the appropriate

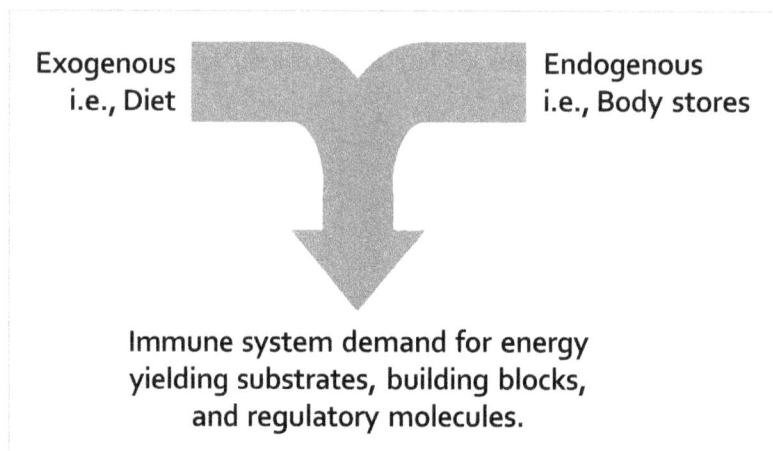

Exogenous
i.e., Diet

Endogenous
i.e., Body stores

Immune system demand for energy yielding substrates, building blocks, and regulatory molecules.

Figure 1. An activated immune response increases demand for energy, for building blocks, and for regulatory molecules.

enzymic machinery in place for RNA and protein synthesis and their regulation and ample substrate available (including nucleotides for RNA synthesis, the correct mix of amino acids for protein synthesis, and polyunsaturated fatty acids for eicosanoid synthesis). An important component of the immune response is oxidative burst, during which superoxide anion radicals are produced from oxygen in a reaction linked to the oxidation of glucose. The reactive oxygen species produced can be damaging to host tissues and thus antioxidant protective mechanisms are necessary. Among these are the classic antioxidant vitamins (vitamins E and C), glutathione, the antioxidant enzymes superoxide dismutase and catalase, and the glutathione recycling enzyme glutathione peroxidase. The antioxidant enzymes all have metal ions at their active site (manganese, copper, zinc, iron, and selenium).

Cellular proliferation is a key component of the immune response, providing amplification and memory: before division, there must be replication of DNA and then of all cellular components (proteins, membranes, intracellular organelles, etc.). In addition to energy, this clearly needs a supply of nucleotides (for DNA and RNA synthesis), amino acids (for protein synthesis), fatty acids, bases and phosphate (for phospholipid synthesis), and other lipids (e.g., cholesterol) and cellular components. Some of the cellular building blocks cannot be synthesized in mammalian cells and must come from the diet (e.g., essential fatty acids, essential amino acids, and minerals). Amino acids (e.g., arginine) are precursors for the synthesis of polyamines, which have roles in the regulation of DNA replication and cell division. Various micronutrients (e.g., iron, folic, zinc, and magnesium) are also involved in nucleotide and nucleic acid synthesis. Some nutrients, such as vitamins A and D, and their metabolites are direct regulators of gene expression in immune cells and play a key role in the maturation, differentiation, and responsiveness of immune cells.

The Importance of Nutrition in Supporting the Immune Response

The roles for nutrients in immune function are many and varied, and it is easy to appreciate that an adequate and balanced supply of these is essential if an appropriate immune response is to be mounted (see Figure 2 below). In essence, good nutrition creates an environment in which the immune response is able to respond appropriately to challenge, regardless of the nature of the challenge. The response may be an active destructive one, or a more passive tolerogenic one. Such good nutrition would provide adequate amounts of energy yielding fuels, essential amino acids, essential

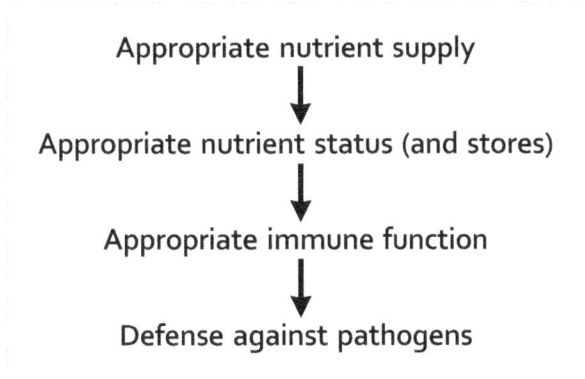

Appropriate nutrient supply

↓

Appropriate nutrient status (and stores)

↓

Appropriate immune function

↓

Defense against pathogens

Figure 2. Relationship between good nutrition, an appropriate immune response, and resistance to infection.

fatty acids, and the full range of vitamins and minerals. These should be provided through a balanced and varied diet, but there may be situations where this is not feasible—for example, in situations of food shortage or where an individual is unable to eat. Here, well-balanced formulas providing a mix of nutrients—perhaps in an energy-dense format—are useful.

There may be situations where an individual has a deficiency in one or more essential nutrients; in such situations, provision of the nutrient(s) in modest amounts through a supplement is appropriate. However, care must be taken to avoid creating nutritional imbalances, which can impact adversely upon host metabolism and the host immune response. A number of other, non-nutritive, food components are now recognized to also be important in supporting the immune system and in controlling the adverse immune responses that occur as a result of imbalances in the immune system. These include a number of the immune factors found in breast milk and numerous phytochemicals, including polyphenolic compounds.

The Role of Gut Microbiota

Humans have a wide diversity of live organisms in their gut lumen; these are collectively referred to as the *gut microbiota.* The number of organisms varies along the length of the gastrointestinal tract, the greatest number being in the colon (10^{11} to 10^{12} per gram of colonic contents), and varies between individuals, or at least sub-groups of individuals.[16] Variation in number and type of organisms within the gut microbiota has been associated with many diseases including metabolic and immunologic diseases.[17] It is known that the gut microbiota is modified according to diet.[17] This has opened the way to strategies aimed at specifically modifying the gut microbiota in a health-promoting way. The gut microbiota interacts with the host's immune system through several mechanisms, including the production of metabolites such as short chain fatty acids, the production of proteins that influence the immune system, and direct contact between cells of the gut-associated lymphoid tissue and specific gut organisms.[18] Hence, modifying gut microbiota is believed to influence the host's immune response.

It is likely that many foods and many dietary components influence the gut microbiota (number and type of organisms present). However, two strategies have been especially explored. The first is simply to provide modest numbers of specific live organisms orally and trust that they will take hold in, or colonize, the gastrointestinal tract, particularly the colon. This is the probiotic approach,[17] and favored organisms are typically members of the lactobacillus or bifidobacteria genus. A number of studies have examined the influence of various probiotic organisms, either alone or in combination, on immune function, infection, and inflammatory conditions in humans.[19] Probiotics appear to enhance innate immunity (particularly phagocytosis and natural killer cell activity), but have weaker effects on acquired immunity. The second approach is to provide substrate that will enable preferential growth of an already existing favored organism; this is the prebiotic approach and the substrates are usually, though not always, carbohydrates, which are not digestible by mammalian enzymes but which are selectively fermented by gut microbiota. Although there is growing evidence for potential immunomodulatory effects of prebiotics,[20] it is not clear whether they are direct effects, or manifested through alteration of the gut microbiota.

Summary

A well-functioning immune system is key to providing good defense against pathogenic organisms and to providing tolerance to non-threatening organisms, food components, and self. The immune system works by providing an exclusion barrier, by identifying and eliminating pathogens and by identifying and tolerating non-threatening sources of antigens, and by maintaining a memory of immunological encounters. The immune system is complex, involving many different cell types distributed throughout the body and many different chemical mediators, some of which are involved directly in defense while others have a regulatory role. Babies are born with an immature immune system that fully develops in the first years of life. This immune maturation requires the presence of specific immune factors and exposure to antigens from food and from microorganisms. Immune competence can decline with age. This process is termed *immunosenescence*. The suboptimal immune competence that occurs early and late in life increases susceptibility to infection. Undernutrition impairs immune defenses, making an individual more susceptible to infection. The gut-associated lymphoid tissue is especially important in health and well-being because of its close proximity to a large and diverse population of organisms in the gastrointestinal tract and its exposure to food constituents. Probiotic bacteria and prebiotics, which modify the gut microbiota, may enhance immune function in humans.

REFERENCES

1. Chandra RK. 1990 McCollum Award lecture. "Nutrition and immunity: lessons from the past and new insights into the future." *Am. J. Clin. Nutr.* 53, 1087–1101, 1991.

2. Scrimshaw NS and SanGiovanni JP. "Synergism of nutrition, infection, and immunity: an overview." *Am. J. Clin. Nutr.* 66, 464S-477S, 1997.

3. Calder PC and Jackson AA. "Undernutrition, infection and immune function." *Nutr Res Rev* 13, 3–29, 2000.

4. Suskind RM and Tontisirin K. *Nutrition, Immunity, and Infection in Infants and Children,* Vevey/Philadelphia: Nestec/Lippincott Williams and Wilkins, 2001.

5. Calder PC, Field CJ, and Gill HA. *Nutrition and Immune Function,* Wallingford: CAB International, 2002.

6. Calder PC and Yaqoob P. *Diet, Immunity and Inflammation,* Cambridge: Woodhead Publishing, 2013.

7. Calder PC. "Feeding the immune system." *Proc. Nutr. Soc.* 72, 299–309, 2013.

8. Mowat AM. "Anatomical basis of tolerance and immunity to intestinal antigens." *Nature Rev. Immunol.* 3, 331–341, 2003.

9. Bernt KM and Walker WA. "Human milk as a carrier of biochemical messages." *Acta. Paed. Suppl.* 88, 27–41, 1999.

10. Calder PC, Krauss-Etschmann S, de Jong EC, Dupont C, Frick J-S, Frokiaer H, Garn H, Koletzko S, Lack G, Mattelio G, Renz H, Sangild PT, Schrezenmeir J, Stulnig TM, Thymann T, Wold AE, and Koletzko B. "Early nutrition and immunity—progress and perspectives." *Brit. J. Nutr.* 96, 774–790. 2006.

11. Castle SC. "Clinical relevance of age-related immune dysfunction." *Clin. Infect. Dis.* 31: 578–585, 2000.

12. Burns EA. "Effect of aging on immune function." *J. Nutr. Health Aging* 8, 9–18, 2004.

13. Agarwal S and Busse PJ. "Innate and adaptive immunosenescence." *Ann Allergy Asthma Immunol* 104, 183–190, 2010.

14. Pawelec G, Larbi A, and Derhovanessian E. "Senescence of the human immune system." *J. Comp. Pathol.* 142 (Suppl 1), S39-S44, 2010.

15. Calder PC. "Fuel utilization by cells of the immune system." *Proc. Nutr. Soc.* 54, 65–82, 1995.

16. Wu GD, Chen J, Hoffmann C, Bittinger K, Chen YY, Keilbaugh SA, Bewtra M, Knights D, Walters WA, Knight R, Sinha R, Gilroy E, Gupta K, Baldassano R, Nessel L, Li H, Bushman FD, and Lewis JD. "Linking long-term dietary patterns with gut microbial enterotypes." *Science* 334, 105–108, 2011.

17. Hill C, Guarner F, Reid G, Gibson GR, Merenstein DJ, Pot B, Morelli L, Canani RB, Flint HJ,

Salminen S, Calder PC, and Sanders ME. "Expert consensus document: The International Scientific Association for Probiotics and Prebiotics consensus statement on the scope and appropriate use of the term probiotic." *Nat. Rev. Gastroenterol. Hepatol.* 11, 506–514, 2014.

18. Hemarajata P and Versalovic J. "Effects of probiotics on gut microbiota: mechanisms of intestinal immunomodulation and neuromodulation." *Therap. Adv. Gastroenterol.* 6, 39–51, 2013.

19. Lomax AR and Calder PC. "Probiotics, immune function, infection and inflammation: a review of the evidence from studies conducted in humans." *Curr. Pharmaceut. Design* 15, 1428–1518, 2009.

20. Lomax AR and Calder PC. "Prebiotics, immune function, infection and inflammation: a review of the evidence." *Brit. J. Nutr.* 101, 633–658, 2009.

Immune Modulatory Function

Chantal Matar, Emilie Graham

AHCC is a standardized extract of cultured *Lentinula edodes* mycelia used as a complementary and alternative medicine (CAM) for immune support worldwide. Previous reports in animal models and in clinical settings have indicated that AHCC is associated with an enhanced response to infection and increased survival.[1,2] Studies have indicated that AHCC supplementation clearly affects immune outcomes and immune cell populations, suggesting that it has potent anti-inflammatory effects. Moreover, available data have demonstrated that AHCC reduces symptoms, improves survival, and shortens recovery time in animal models infected with viruses, bacteria, and even fungal infections.[3-6] AHCC was proven to be a good adjunct therapy for vaccines, as it was reported for a randomized controlled trial and improved immune response to the influenza B vaccine.[7] AHCC was also shown to exert immunosurveillance control against many types of neoplasia. Furthermore, many studies have pointed out common mechanisms by which AHCC maintains immune homeostasis in the body.

AHCC in Immunoprotection against Infection

AHCC may serve as an immunoprotectant against infection. It decreased mortality and improved bacterial clearance of mice infected with *Pseudomonas aeruginosa*.[8] Furthermore, supplementation with AHCC was found to increase the number of IgA⁺ cells in the intestinal epithelium as well as secretory IgA (sIgA) production.[9] Nutritional interventions appear to impact sIgA production as well as enhance mucosal defenses and reduce infection risk.[10,11] Additionally, supplementation with AHCC yielded minor, but significant, alterations in inflammatory cytokine production at the epithelium and inside the lungs.[9]

AHCC can also exert immunoprotection in healthy individuals against the common cold. In a randomized trial, healthy individuals were given 1 g/day of either a placebo or AHCC over the course of four weeks, extending from the beginning to the middle of winter.[12] Immune function is correlated with air temperature, which could be due to cooled nasal airways, limiting local defenses. Additionally, natural killer (NK) cells have been shown to decrease in numbers in the winter months.[13] The study showed that AHCC maintained immune function throughout the winter compared to the placebo group, which demonstrated a decline.

AHCC in Compromised Immune Response

The cumulative evidence points toward a strong ability for immunomodulation by AHCC, which could be beneficial for high-risk populations, such as those with impaired immune function: human immunodeficiency virus (HIV), post-traumatic stress disorder (PTSD), stress after space flight conditions, and immunosenescence.[14–16]

One at-risk population includes those infected with HIV and suffering from acquired immune deficiency syndrome (AIDS). Since AHCC has been shown to be particularly effective in those with an impaired immune system,[14] HIV/AIDS patients could benefit from taking AHCC as they are susceptible to infection and illness.[15] AHCC has been shown to improve CD4+ T cell numbers,[17] which are the most affected immune cells in HIV/AIDS.[18] Lee et al. discovered that AHCC enhanced interleukin-1 beta (IL-1β) production in human monocytes and also IL-17 and interferon-gamma (IFN-γ) production in autologous CD4+ T cells.[17] When monocytes from the innate immune system produce more IL-1β, this can influence the creation of type 1 helper T (Th1) cells and Th17 cells, which are known to mostly produce IFN-γ and IL-17, respectively. IL-17 allows for neutrophil-mediated responses against extracellular pathogens by activating cytokines like IL-8.[17] IL-8 modulates neutrophil activation and migration from tissue to blood.[19]

Other at-risk groups that are proposed to benefit from AHCC supplementation include patients with PTSD, depression, and anxiety. All of these illnesses are stress-inducing and hence can result in a compromised immune system. In particular, PTSD has been associated with a decrease in NK cell activity.[20–22] NK cell activity can be hindered by stress caused by accidents, surgery, medical treatments, nutritional deficiencies, emotional trauma, grief, and hormone imbalances.[15] Specifically,

NK cell activity may be influenced by stress through neuropeptide Y (NPY) and/or norepinephrine. NPY is a neuropeptide involved in activating the sympathetic nervous system and has been shown to suppress NK cell activity.[23] Norepinephrine is a neurotransmitter and has also been shown to inhibit NK cell activity.[24]

NK cells are part of the first line of defense in the innate immune system. They are filled with granules and target antigens, which also may include abnormal cells and tumor cells.[15] However, unlike cytotoxic T cells, they do not target specific antigens before destroying a defective cell. They work by attaching to the defective cell and insert chemicals that break down the membranes of the abnormal cells, causing them to burst.[15]

AHCC may counter reduced NK cell frequency by increasing its activity.[12,25–29] An in-office, nonrandomized, open-label trial determined that AHCC was the only supplement that could statistically and consistently increase the activity of NK cells, with an average increase of 249%.[25] Other studies have also confirmed the benefits of AHCC on NK cell activity.[15,26] AHCC may increase NK cell activity by enhancing NK cells to secrete more IFN-γ and IL-2 cytokines, which have previously been shown to be overexpressed by AHCC.[30,31] As mentioned previously, AHCC increases IFN-γ production in CD4+ cells. Therefore, taking AHCC as a supplement could be beneficial for those experiencing high levels of stress, such as PTSD patients.

Additionally, individuals who are subjected to space flight conditions may experience a compromised immune system.[14] Hence, in 2004, Aviles et al. examined the effects of AHCC on a hindlimb-unloading model in mice for space flight conditions. Mice were orally given AHCC one week prior to and throughout infection conditions. Spleen and peritoneal cells were primed with concanavalin A (Con A) or lipopolysaccharide (LPS). The study found that AHCC improved spleen cell proliferation as well as increased cytokine production in the spleen and nitric oxide (NO) production in peritoneal cells. Specifically, AHCC increased production of cytokines, including IFN-γ, IL-2, IL-4, IL-6, IL-10, and tumor necrosis factor-alpha (TNF-α) in spleen cells and TNF-α and IL-1β in peritoneal cells, particularly after LPS stimulation. Further, AHCC enhanced peritoneal macrophage function, which can help clear bacterial load. This study suggests that AHCC acts as an immune enhancer for immune systems deteriorated by hindlimb-unloading model for space flight conditions.

As another example, individuals undergoing surgery could benefit from taking AHCC because of the prolonged inflammation experienced as a result of hypovolemia, hemorrhage, or infection.[32] A study on female Swiss-Webster mice pretreated with AHCC or water by gavage ten days prior to cecal ligation and puncture (CLP) found that AHCC decreased cortisol levels and lowered plasma norepinephrine (NE) concentration after twenty-four hours.[32] By reducing stress hormones, AHCC again acted as an immune enhancer.

In fact, there are several mechanisms of action that we can derive from these studies. As mentioned previously, stress-related hormones like NE can cause a decrease in NK cell activity. Because AHCC stimulates NK cells to produce cytokines such as IFN-γ and IL-2, this enhances the innate and adaptive immune responses, given that IFN-γ and IL-2 can act as messengers to adaptive pathways.[30]

Immunosenescence refers to the gradual deterioration of the immune system from natural aging. This makes older adults more susceptible to infection and disease. It occurs because of many years of exposure to antigens such as viruses, pathogenic bacteria, allergens, pollution, and foods.[16] With age, the thymus atrophies, leading to higher cortisol levels and decreased levels of dehydroepiandrosterone (DHEA) and some other hormones.[16] Immunosenescence may also be caused by malnutrition and a sedentary lifestyle, which often accompanies old age. These conditions can lead to a decrease in function of NK cells, T cells, and macrophages, suppression of IL-2, and an overproduction of IL-6.[16] In particular, NK cells play a major role in preventing immunosenescence.[16]

As evidenced by many reports, AHCC could be beneficial to this risk group because of its ability to increase NK cell, T cell, and cytokine function. One study examined the effects of AHCC on subjects age 50 and above and found that AHCC taken orally daily over a thirty-day period increased the frequency of CD4+ and CD8+ T cells producing IFN-γ and TNF-α compared to baseline values.[33] The effect remained for thirty days following the discontinued treatment. Enhancing the adaptive immune system through increased T cell activity could help protect older adults from infection, as well as against inflammaging, or continuous low-grade inflammation seen in older adults. Inflammaging can lead to cancer, perhaps explaining why 77% of cancer is diagnosed in individuals over the age of 55.[34]

AHCC and Immunosurveillance

Immune system failure can lead to tumoral cells escaping immunosurveillance. Many studies have examined the benefits of AHCC on cancer prevention and treatment, particularly as a complementary medicine to chemotherapy treatments. It has been shown to improve quality of life, enhance anti-tumor activities of chemotherapy agents, and protect the immune system from adverse effects, such as chemotherapy-induced neutropenia.[27,35,36] In one study on twelve Korean cancer patients with different types of cancer, patients took 3–6 g of AHCC per day orally while continuing their chemotherapy regimens. AHCC was shown to increase the ratio of NK cells to total lymphocytes, which could prevent bone marrow depression caused by chemotherapy.[29] In another study, albino rats were pretreated with AHCC by gavage for two weeks before and during a thirty-four-week submandibular salivary gland neoplasm induction period.[30] Findings from Badawi et al. suggested that AHCC induces the overexpression of IFN-γ and IL-2 cytokines in the submandibular gland and lymph nodes. Furthermore, AHCC did not cause any negative side effects and slowed tumor progression. It was proposed that since AHCC stimulates NK cells to produce IFN-γ and IL-2 cytokines, it might activate an innate immune response through toll-like receptors (TLRs) and the downstream nuclear factor-κB (NF-κB) pathway, which are additionally involved in adaptive immune response regulation.

A clinical trial was conducted using thirty-eight cancer patients who were in stage IV of their cancer with unsuccessful chemotherapy treatments and one hundred seventeen healthy controls.[28] Uno et al. administered 6 g of AHCC daily to patients, taking a dose after each meal over a six-month period. Measurements revealed an increased NK cell percentage, increased IFN-γ concentration, and increased IL-12 secretion. Only 4 patients reported feverish symptoms, which could be attributed to immune stimulation. IFN-γ and IL-12 are cytokines relating to Th1. IL-12 is a pro-inflammatory cytokine mainly produced by macrophages, monocytes, and dendritic cells that responds to LPS from bacteria and pathogens, and from connecting to active T cells (such as Th1); hence, it creates a bridge between the innate and adaptive immune systems.[37] IL-12 can induce NK cells and Th1 cells to produce IFN-γ, which can activate CD8+ T cells to develop a memory response.[28] CD8+ T cells also produce both IFN-γ and TNF-α and direct cytotoxicity. Therefore, these cells can infiltrate a tumor and remove the abnormal cells.

Moreover, AHCC was shown to enhance the NO production and cytotoxicity of peritoneal macrophages, as well as NK cell activity in mammary cancer in rats when added to the chemotherapy agent tegafur-uracil (UFT).[27] Additionally, AHCC restored mRNA expression of IL-1α and TNF-α, which was lowered by the chemotherapy treatment. Furthermore, when AHCC was orally administered to C57BL/6 mice prior to and following injection with B16F0 melanoma or EL4 lymphoma tumor cells,[26] delayed tumor growth and antigen-specific activation and proliferation of CD4+ and CD8+ T cells, as well as increased the number of tumor antigen-specific

IFN-γ-producing CD8[+] T cells, were noticed. These results suggested that AHCC modulated the adaptive immune system. Further, AHCC increased NK cell and γδ T cell counts. γδ T cells, like NK cells, are part of the innate immune system and do not require presentation of antigens by MHC cells.[38] γδ T cells have an important role in activating dendritic cells.[38] It has been proposed that these innate T cells may play an important role in tumor immune surveillance.[39] By enhancing immune responses, both IFN-γ and lymphocytes have been shown to be necessary components of tumor immune surveillance.

AHCC and Inflammation

Many of the above-mentioned studies have demonstrated that AHCC modulates cytokine expression in various tissues. These include IL-1α, IL-1β, IL-2, IL-6, IL-8, IL-10, IL-17, TNF-α, and IFN-γ.[14,17,27,28,30,40,41] Cytokines are important immune and inflammatory pathway messengers that play a role in illnesses such as colitis and inflammatory bowel disease (IBD). In the canonical NF-κB signaling pathway, pro-inflammatory cytokines (such as some of those mentioned above) activate the IκB kinase (IKK) complex (combination of kinases), which phosphorylate IκB proteins, causing their ubiquitination and degradation and freeing NF-κB/Rel complexes. These complexes are also activated by post-translational modifications (phosphorylation, acetylation) and move to the nucleus where they may interact with other transcription factors (e.g., STAT), causing target gene expression.[42,56] In particular, it regulates genes involved in inflammation, including those for cytokines.[40] The NF-κB pathway is important in gut immune health because it is involved in maintaining intestinal barrier integrity by stimulating defensin production.[43]

One study conducted on AHCC in mice with induced colitis found that AHCC decreased the secretion of pro-inflammatory cytokines for TNF-α and IL-1β, while normalizing the production of IL-6, IL-10, and IL-17.[41] It also decreased STAT4 and IκB-α phosphorylation in splenic CD4[+] cells. Interestingly, this study demonstrates that although AHCC sometimes increases the production of TNF-α and IL-1β, it can decrease these cytokines in conditions of induced inflammation. In fact, this is in agreement with previous observations in infectious models in which AHCC was shown to exhibit an effector response, such as increased NK cell activity, only when the animals were challenged with an infection.[5] Therefore, AHCC may play a role in maintaining immune balance and enhancing mucosal barrier function that can prevent IBD.

Potential Mechanisms of Action

AHCC is a standardized extract of cultured *Lentinula edodes* mycelia that contains polysaccharides, amino acids, lipids, and minerals and is rich in α-glucan and acylated α-glucan. One hypothesis that underlies the beneficial and pleiotropic effects of AHCC involves combinations of cell-signaling pathways on global cell regulators and is related to bioactive substance appearance. The main active component of AHCC has been proposed to be the acylated α-1,4-glucan.[44] The quantity of α-glucan to β-glucan in AHCC is almost 30:1, and the low molecular weight of α-glucans may aid in their absorption, but whether this is necessary for activity is not yet established.[45]

The culturing process of AHCC favors the release of small bioactive molecules that act as nontoxic agonists for TLRs, specifically TLR-4, initiating a systemic anti-inflammatory response. For instance, β-glucans are known as ligands to TLR-2 and TLR-4 activation. TLRs are a key family of microbial sensors in the innate and adaptive immunity involved in inflammatory signaling. Dysregulation of TLR signaling causes pathological inflammation underlying not just infection, but also cancer, suggesting that TLR-mediated mechanisms are pivotal in cancer too. Therefore, TLRs are thought to be the cellular gate to control inflammation. They are very important in stimulating the host's innate immune system to defend against many pathogens.[46] In particular, TLR-2 binds an array of ligands, including lipoteichoic acid, peptidoglycan, and bacterial lipoproteins that are located in the cell wall of both gram-positive and -negative bacteria.[47] A well-studied TLR ligand, LPS, is found on the surface of bacteria and is recognized by TLR-4, which induces a potent, pro-inflammatory immune response through the NF-κB pathway.[48] In the context of neoplasia-associated inflammation, TLR-4-mediated signaling has been implicated in metastasis in a variety of cancers.[49] High TLR-4 expression correlated with deeper tumor invasion in oral squamous cancer.[50]

As such, TLR activation makes important contributions to immediate innate self and non-self-discrimination and the subsequent immune response. Administration of AHCC to Balb/c mice by gavage found that it increased IgA+ cells in the intestine, as well as elevated sIgA, IL-10, and IFN-γ concentrations in intestinal fluid of the mice.[51] Intestinal epithelial cells (IECs) collected from the mice for ex vivo studies demonstrated an increase in IL-6 production, but not to the pro-inflammatory level of the positive controls (LPS and *E. coli*). Furthermore, blocking of TLR-2 and TLR-4 reduced AHCC-activated IL-6 production, implying that these TLRs may be involved in IEC immune response to AHCC. TLR-2 and TLR-4 are expressed on the apical surface of IECs.[52] These two TLRs may be involved in immune priming and homeostasis, while remaining capable of pathogen-recognition and effector response induction when necessary.[53,54] AHCC may prime TLR-2 and TLR-4 because of a response to AHCC's food-associated molecular patterns (FAMPs), also found in other mushrooms (see Figure 1 below).

Therefore, it is clear that the immunomodulatory activities of AHCC are mediated at least in part through contact with pattern-recognition receptors present on the intestinal epithelium. A large family of complex food products, including not only yeast glucans, mushrooms, and dairy peptides, but also probiotics, polyphenols and their metabolites, and certain fatty acids, may also participate in innate immune recognition as a special category of FAMPs. These common food patterns serve as non-pathogenic, non-danger signals that, instead of eliciting a strong and potentially damaging response, are involved in keeping the immune response primed, balanced, and tolerant.

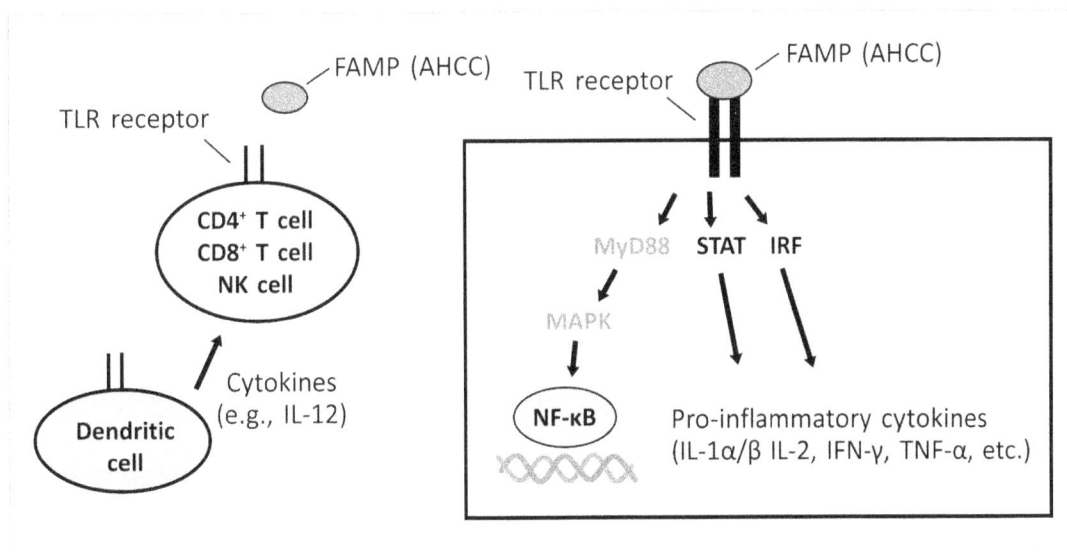

Figure 1. AHCC binds toll-like receptors (TLRs) and acts as an immune enhancer. Immune cells such as CD4+ and CD8+ T cells and natural killer (NK) cells will produce cytokines by either cytokine stimulation by dendritic cells or ligand binding to TLRs. When ligands such as food-associated molecular patterns (FAMPs) (e.g., AHCC oligosaccharides) bind to TLRs, it initiates pathways, such as the TLR/MyD88 and NF-κB/MAPK pathways. NF-κB is a transcription factor, which allows for the expression of pro-inflammatory cytokines necessary for innate and adaptive immune system responses.[40,55]

Summary

AHCC is a promising natural compound for immunomodulation and immune enhancement with well-documented studies on a variety of diseases. AHCC may play a role in orchestrating the host immune response, maintaining immune homeostasis, and providing systemic immunoprotection related to infections, in compromised immune response or in immunosurveillance. Such a response is likely due to the recognition of FAMPs, such as those associated with other mushroom or yeast-derived compounds at the gate of TLRs. By controlling the systemic inflammatory response, AHCC is able to exhibit a large array of immunoprotective activities, consolidating its use for immune support.

REFERENCES

1. Nogusa S, Gerbino J, and Ritz BW. "Low-dose supplementation with active hexose correlated compound improves the immune response to acute influenza infection in C57BL/6 mice." *Nutr. Res.* 29, 139–143, 2009. doi:10.1016/j.nutres.2009.01.005

2. Ritz BW. "Supplementation with active hexose correlated compound increases survival following infectious challenge in mice." *Nutr. Rev.* 66, 526–531, 2008. doi:10.1111/j.1753–4887.2008.00085.x

3. Aviles H, O'Donnell P, Sun B, and Sonnenfeld G. "Active hexose correlated compound (AHCC) enhances resistance to infection in a mouse model of surgical wound infection." *Surg. Infect.* 7, 527–535, 2006. doi:10.1089/sur.2006.7.527

4. Ishibashi H, Ikeda T, Tansho S, Ono Y, Yamazaki M, Sato A, Yamaoka K, Yamaguchi H, and Abe S. "Prophylactic efficacy of a basidiomycetes preparation AHCC against lethal opportunistic infections in mice." *Yakugaku Zasshi* 120, 715–719, 2000.

5. Ritz BW, Nogusa S, Ackerman EA, and Gardner EM. "Supplementation with Active Hexose Correlated Compound increases the innate immune response of young mice to primary influenza infection." *J. Nutr.* 136, 2868–2873, 2006.

6. Wang S, Welte T, Fang H, Chang GJJ, Born WK, O'Brien RL, Sun B, Fujii H, Kosuna K, and Wang T. "Oral administration of active hexose correlated compound enhances host resistance to West Nile encephalitis in mice." *J. Nutr.* 139, 598–602, 2009. doi:10.3945/jn.108.100297

7. Roman BE, Beli E, Duriancik DM, and Gardner EM. "Short-term supplementation with active hexose correlated compound improves the antibody response to influenza B vaccine." *Nutr. Res.* 33, 12–17, 2013. doi:10.1016/j.nutres.2012.11.001

8. Aviles H, Belay T, Fountain K, Vance M, Sun B, and Sonnenfeld G. "Active hexose correlated compound enhances resistance to *Klebsiella pneumoniae* infection in mice in the hindlimb-unloading model of spaceflight conditions." *J. Appl. Physiol.* (Bethesda, Md : 1985) 95, 491–496, 2003. doi:10.1152/japplphysiol.00259.2003

9. Mallet JF, Graham E, Ritz B, Homma K, and Matar C. "Role of intestinal epithelial cells and involvement of TLRs in immune effects of AHCC (638.4)." *FASEB J* 28, 638.4, 2014.

10. Brandtzaeg P. "Induction of secretory immunity and memory at mucosal surfaces." *Vaccine* 25, 5467–5484, 2007. doi:10.1016/j.vaccine.2006.12.001

11. Mantis NJ, Rol N, and Corthésy B. "Secretory IgA's complex roles in immunity and mucosal homeostasis in the gut." *Mucosal Immunol.* 4, 603–611, 2011. doi:10.1038/mi.2011.41

12. Takanari J, Hirayama Y, Homma K, Miura T, Nishioka H, and Maeda T. "Effects of active hexose correlated compound on the seasonal variations of immune competence in healthy subjects." *J. Evid.-Based Complement Altern Med* 20, 28–34, 2015. doi:10.1177/2156587214555573

13. Lévi FA, Canon C, Touitou Y, Reinberg A, and Mathé G. "Seasonal modulation of the circadian time structure of circulating T and natural killer lymphocyte subsets from healthy subjects." *J. Clin. Invest.* 81, 407–413, 1988. doi:10.1172/JCI113333

14. Aviles H, Belay T, Vance M, Sun B, and Sonnenfeld G. "Active hexose correlated compound enhances the immune function of mice in the hindlimb-unloading model of spaceflight conditions." *J. Appl. Physiol.* (Bethesda, Md. : 1985) 97, 1437–1444, 2004. doi:10.1152/japplphysiol.00259.2004

15. Kenner D. "Treatment for immune dysfunction from post-traumatic stress disorder and chronic disease with AHCC." *Townsend Lett. Dr. Patients* 68–72, 2001.

16. Pescatore F. "Reversing immunosenescence: The key to anti-aging?" *Int. J. Anti-Aging Med.* 47–49, 2000.

17. Lee WW, Lee N, Fujii H, and Kang I. "Active Hexose Correlated Compound promotes T helper (Th) 17 and 1 cell responses via inducing IL-1β production from monocytes in humans." *Cell. Immunol.* 275, 19–23, 2012. doi:10.1016/j.cellimm.2012.04.001

18. Kasang C, Kalluvya S, Majinge C, Kongola G, Mlewa M, Massawe I, Kabyemera R, Magambo K, Ulmer A, Klinker H, Gschmack E, Horn A, Koutsilieri E, Preiser W, Hofmann D, Hain J, Müller A, Dölken L, Weissbrich B, Rethwilm A, Stich A, and Scheller C. "Effects of prednisolone on disease progression in antiretroviral-untreated HIV infection: A 2-year randomized, double-blind placebo-controlled clinical trial." *PloS One* 11, e0146678, 2016. doi:10.1371/ journal.pone.0146678

19. Müzes G, Molnár B, Tulassay Z, and Sipos F. "Changes of the cytokine profile in inflammatory bowel diseases." *World J. Gastroenterol.* 18, 5848–5861, 2012. doi:10.3748/wjg.v18.i41 .5848

20. Inoue-Sakurai C, Maruyama S, and Morimoto K. "Posttraumatic stress and lifestyles are associated with natural killer cell activity in victims of the Hanshin-Awaji earthquake in Japan." *Prev. Med.* 31, 467–473, 2000. doi:10.1006/pmed.2000.0744

21. Ironson G, Wynings C, Schneiderman N, Baum A, Rodriguez M, Greenwood D, Benight C, Antoni M, LaPerriere A, Huang HS, Klimas N, and Fletcher MA. "Posttraumatic stress symptoms, intrusive thoughts, loss, and immune function after Hurricane Andrew." *Psychosom. Med.* 59, 128–141, 1997.

22. Kawamura N, Kim Y, and Asukai N. "Suppression of cellular immunity in men with a past history of posttraumatic stress disorder." *Am. J. Psychiatry* 158, 484–486, 2001. doi:10.1176/appi.ajp.158.3.484

23. Nair MP, Schwartz SA, Wu K, and Kronfol Z. "Effect of neuropeptide Y on natural killer activity of normal human lymphocytes." *Brain Behav. Immun.* 7, 70–78, 1993.

24. Vredevoe DL, Moser DK, Gan XH, and Bonavida B. "Natural killer cell anergy to cytokine stimulants in a subgroup of patients with heart failure: relationship to norepinephrine." *Neuroimmunomodulation* 2, 16–24. 1995.

25. Belanger J. "An in-office evaluation of four dietary supplements on natural killer cell activity." *Townsend Lett. Dr. Patients* 84–85, 2005.

26. Gao Y, Zhang D, Sun B, Fujii H, Kosuna KI, and Yin Z. "Active hexose correlated compound enhances tumor surveillance through regulating both innate and adaptive immune responses." *Cancer Immunol. Immunother.* 55, 1258–1266, 2006. doi:10.1007/s00262–005–0111–9

27. Matsushita K, Kuramitsu Y, Ohiro Y, Obara M, Kobayashi M, Li YQ, and Hosokawa M. "Combination therapy of active hexose correlated compound plus UFT significantly reduces the metastasis of rat mammary adenocarcinoma." *Anticancer Drugs* 9, 343–350, 1998.

28. Uno K, Kosuna K, Fujii H, Wakame K, Chikumaru S, Hosokawa G, and Ueda Y. "Active Hexose Correlated Compound (AHCC) improves immunological parameters and performance status of patients with solid tumors." *Biotherapy* 14, 303–309, 2000.

29. Won JS. "The hematoimmunologic effect of AHCC for Korean patients with various cancers." *Biotherapy* 16, 560–564, 2002.

30. Badawi TA, Khalil NA, Abdelrahman AH, and Aly ZH. "Immunoprophylactic effect of Active Hexose Correlated Compound on normal and induced submandibular salivary gland neoplasm in albino rats." *Cairo Dent. J.* 28, 485–490, 2012.

31. Rudnicka K, Matusiak A, and Chmiela M. "CD25 (IL-2R) expression correlates with the target cell induced cytotoxic activity and cytokine secretion in human natural killer cells." *Acta Biochim. Pol.* 62, 885–894, 2015. doi:10.18388/abp.2015_1152

32. Love KM, Barnett RE, Holbrook I, Sonnenfeld G, Fujii H, Sun B, Peyton JC, and Cheadle WG. "A natural immune modulator attenuates stress hormone and catecholamine concentrations in polymicrobial peritonitis." *J. Trauma Acute Care Surg.* 74, 1411–1418, 2013. doi:10.1097/TA.0b013e31829215b1

33. Yin Z, Fujii H, and Walshe T. "Effects of active hexose correlated compound on frequency of CD4+ and CD8+ T cells producing interferon-γ and/or tumor necrosis factor–α in healthy adults." *Hum. Immunol.* 71, 1187–1190, 2010. doi:10.1016/j.humimm.2010.08.006

34. Cancer Facts & Figures 2014—acspc-042151.pdf [WWW Document], 2014. URL http://www.cancer.org/acs/groups/content/@research/documents/webcontent/acspc-042151.pdf (accessed 2/6/16).

35. Cowawintaweewat S, Manoromana S, Sriplung H, Khuhaprema T, Tongtawe P, Tapchaisri P, and Chaicumpa W. "Prognostic Improvement of patients with advanced liver cancer after Active Hexose Correlated Compound (AHCC) treatment." *Asian Pac. J. Allergy Immunol.* 24, 33–45, 2010.

36. Hangai S, Iwase S, Kawaguchi T, Kogure Y, Miyaji T, Matsunaga T, Nagumo Y, and Yamaguchi T. "Effect of active hexose-correlated compound in women receiving adjuvant chemotherapy for breast cancer: a retrospective study." *J. Altern. Complement. Med. N.Y. N* 19, 905–910, 2013. doi:10.1089/acm.2012.0914

37. Trinchieri G. "Interleukin-12: a proinflammatory cytokine with immunoregulatory functions that bridge innate resistance and antigen-specific adaptive immunity." *Annu. Rev. Immunol.* 13, 251–276, 1995. doi:10.1146/annurev.iy.13.040195.001343

38. Gao Y and Williams AP. "Role of innate T cells in anti-bacterial immunity." *Front. Immunol.* 6, 302, 2015. doi:10.3389/fimmu.2015.00302

39. Legut M, Cole DK, and Sewell AK. "The promise of γδ T cells and the γδ T cell receptor for cancer immunotherapy." *Cell. Mol. Immunol.* 12, 656–668, 2015. doi:10.1038/ cmi.2015.28

40. Daddaoua A, Martínez-Plata E, Ortega-González M, Ocón B, Aranda CJ, Zarzuelo A, Suárez MD, de Medina FS, and Martínez-Augustin O. "The nutritional supplement Active Hexose Correlated Compound (AHCC) has direct immunomodulatory actions on intestinal epithelial cells and macrophages involving TLR/MyD88 and NF-κB/MAPK activation." *Food Chem.* 136, 1288–1295, 2013. doi:10.1016/j.foodchem.2012.09.039

41. Mascaraque C, Suárez MD, Zarzuelo A, Sánchez de Medina F, and Martínez-Augustin O. "Active hexose correlated compound exerts therapeutic effects in lymphocyte driven colitis." *Mol. Nutr. Food Res.* 58, 2379–2382, 2014. doi:10.1002/mnfr.201400364

42. Hayden MS and Ghosh S. "Shared principles in NF-kappaB signaling." *Cell* 132, 344–362, 2008. doi:10.1016/j.cell.2008.01.020.

43. Voss E, Wehkamp J, Wehkamp K, Stange EF, Schröder JM, and Harder J. "NOD2/CARD15 mediates induction of the antimicrobial peptide human beta-defensin-2." *J. Biol. Chem.* 281, 2005–2011, 2006. doi:10.1074/jbc.M511044200

44. Spierings ELH, Fujii H, Sun B, and Walshe T. "A Phase I study of the safety of the nutritional supplement, active hexose correlated compound, AHCC, in healthy volunteers." *J. Nutr. Sci. Vitaminol.* (Tokyo) 53, 536–539, 2007.

45. Shah SK, Walker PA, Moore-Olufemi SD, Sundaresan A, Kulkarni AD, and Andrassy RJ. "An evidence-based review of a *Lentinula edodes* mushroom extract as complementary therapy in the surgical oncology patient." *J Parenter. Enter. Nutr.* 35, 449–458, 2011. doi:10.1177/0148607110380684

46. Kay E, Scotland RS, and Whiteford JR. "Toll-like receptors: Role in inflammation and therapeutic potential." *BioFactors* May–Jun;40(3):284-94, 2014. http://www.ncbi.nlm.nih.gov/pubmed/24375529.

47. Akira S, Uematsu S, and Takeuchi O. "Pathogen Recognition and Innate Immunity." *Cell* 124, 783–801, 2006. doi:10.1016/j.cell.2006.02.015

48. Tapping RI, Akashi S, Miyake K, Godowski PJ, and Tobias PS. "Toll-like receptor 4, but not Toll-like receptor 2, is a signaling receptor for Escherichia and Salmonella lipopolysaccharides." *J. Immunol.* 165, 5780–5787, 2000.

49. Kidd LCR, Rogers EN, Yeyeodu ST, Jones DZ, and Kimbro KS. "Contribution of toll-like receptor signaling pathways to breast tumorigenesis and treatment." *Breast Cancer,* Dove Med. Press 5, 43–51, 2013. doi:10.2147/BCTT.S29172

50. Mäkinen LK, Atula T, Häyry V, Jouhi L, Datta N, Lehtonen S, Ahmed A, Mäkitie AA, Haglund C, and Hagström J. "Predictive role of Toll-like receptors 2, 4, and 9 in oral tongue squamous cell carcinoma." *Oral Oncol.* 51, 96–102, 2015. doi:10.1016/j.oraloncology.2014.08.017

51. Mallet JF, Graham É, Ritz BW, Homma K, and Matar C. "Active Hexose Correlated Compound (AHCC) promotes an intestinal immune response in BALB/c mice and in primary intestinal epithelial cell culture involving toll-like receptors TLR-2 and TLR-4." *Eur. J. Nutr.* 1–8, 2015. doi:10.1007/s00394–015–0832–2

52. Abreu MT, Thomas LS, Arnold ET, Lukasek K, Michelsen KS, and Arditi M. "TLR signaling at the intestinal epithelial interface." *J. Endotoxin Res.* 9, 322–330, 2003. doi:10.1179/096805103 225002593

53. Otte JM, Cario E, and Podolsky DK. "Mechanisms of cross hyporesponsiveness to Toll-like receptor bacterial ligands in intestinal epithelial cells." *Gastroenterology* 126, 1054–1070, 2004.

54. Vinderola G, Matar C, and Perdigón G. "Role of intestinal epithelial cells in immune effects mediated by Gram-positive probiotic bacteria: involvement of Toll-like receptors." *Clin. Diagn. Lab. Immunol.* 12, 1075–1084, 2005. doi:10.1128/CDLI.12.9.1075–1084. 2005.

55. Adib-Conquy M, Scott-Algara D, Cavaillon JM, and Souza-Fonseca-Guimaraes F. "TLR-mediated activation of NK cells and their role in bacterial/viral immune responses in mammals." *Immunol. Cell Biol.* 92, 256–262, 2014. doi:10.1038/icb.2013.99.

56. Perkins ND. "Post-translational modifications regulating the activity and function of the nuclear factor kappa B pathway." *Oncogene* 25: 6717–6730, 2006. doi: 10.1038/sj.onc.1209937.

Spaceflight Models and AHCC

Gerald Sonnenfeld

Exposure to spaceflight conditions results in changes in immune response in humans and animals that have been exposed to space flight.[1–3] These changes primarily occur in cell-mediated immune response, such as cytokine production and production of cell colonies of immunologically important cells. Although the biomedical significance and importance of these changes have not been fully established, the alterations in immune status induced by spaceflight conditions could lead to changes in the ability to resist infections.[1–3] That risk could possibly increase as the space flights become longer and there is no easy way to return to earth in an emergency situation, for example in a flight to Mars. These very long duration space flights are being considered at the present time by several space agencies.

Models have been developed that simulate some aspects of spaceflight conditions. For rodents, the model is hindlimb unloading.[1–3]. In this model, there is no load bearing on the hind limbs and a six degree head-tilt. This simulates some of the effects that occur during spaceflight, including the effects of microgravity (very low gravity found during low-earth orbit spaceflight) on supporting hind limbs and pooling of blood in the brain. It has been used to demonstrate effects similar to some of those that occur during spaceflight exposure, including changes in the immune system. Changes in resistance to infection have also been shown using the hindlimb-unloading model.

We were able to show that mice maintained in the hindlimb-unloading model had decreased resistance to infection with *Klebsiella pneumoniae,* a species of bacteria that can cause infections.[4] Pretreatment with AHCC prior to infection combined with continued AHCC treatment during the infection increased resistance to infection compared to control mice that were infected but did not receive AHCC. This was shown to coordinate with enhanced cellular immune function in the mice that received AHCC.[5]

The preliminary data suggests that AHCC can enhance the immune responses in mice that have alterations in immune responses in a ground-based model of some aspects of spaceflight conditions. The data also suggest that AHCC may be helpful in moderating infections in mice that are maintained in the hindlimb-unloading model. There are preliminary data and would have to be confirmed in other studies in the model. Additionally, effects of AHCC would have to be tested during actual spaceflight to determine if there is an effect of AHCC on immune responses and infections during actual spaceflight. Also, these studies were carried out in mice, and human studies would have to be performed to determine if the results observed apply to humans in the spaceflight environment. While interesting preliminary data have been obtained, additional studies will have to be carried out to confirm the validity of the studies and applications beyond the specific hindlimb-unloading model used.

REFERENCES

1. Sonnenfeld G, and Shearer WT. "Immune function during space flight." *Nutrition* 18:899–903, 2002.

2. Rose A, Steffen JM, Musacchia XJ, Mandel AD, and Sonnenfeld G. "Effect of antiorthostatic suspension on interferon production by the mouse." *Proc. Soc. Expt'l. Biol. Med.* 177: 253–256, 1984.

3. Gould CL, and Sonnenfeld G. "Enhancement of viral pathogenesis in mice maintained in an antiorthostatic suspension model—coordination with effects on interferon production." *J. Biological Regulation and Homeostatic Agents* 1: 33–36, 1987.

4. Aviles H, Belay T, Vance M, Sun B, and Sonnenfeld G. "Active Hexose Correlated Compound enhances the immune function of mice in the hindlimb-unloading model of space flight conditions." *J. Appl. Physiol.* 97: 1437–1444, 2004.

5. Aviles H, Belay T, Fountain K, Vance M, Sun B, and Sonnenfeld G. "Active Hexose Correlated Compound enhances resistance to Klebsiella pneumoniae infection in mice in the hindlimb-unloading model of space flight conditions." *J. Appl. Physiol.* 95: 491–496, 2003.

Chapter 5

CANCER

Cancer Treatment and Functional Food

Satoshi Ohno, Toshinori Ito

Randomized controlled trials are the gold standard to verify the efficacy of any pharmaceutical development. Moreover, this type of primary research is subjected to systematic reviews to reassess the compilation of the research. On the other hand, research on functional food has advanced in the recent years around the world, and the number of clinical trials on human subjects has increased enormously (see Figure 1 on the following page). This chapter introduces the current situations of the scientific proofs regarding functional food in cancer treatment and their current issues.

Scientific Verification of Functional Food

In PubMed, which runs and organizes the U.S. National Library of Medicine (https://pubmed.ncbi.nlm.nih.gov/), the categories of diagnosis and treatment are categorized in MeSH (https://www.ncbi.nlm.nih.gov/mesh/), where functional food can be traced back within the category of "Dietary supplements." We searched the Internet for research findings concerning functional food and their relationship with cancer treatment according to the following conditions and arrived at the following:

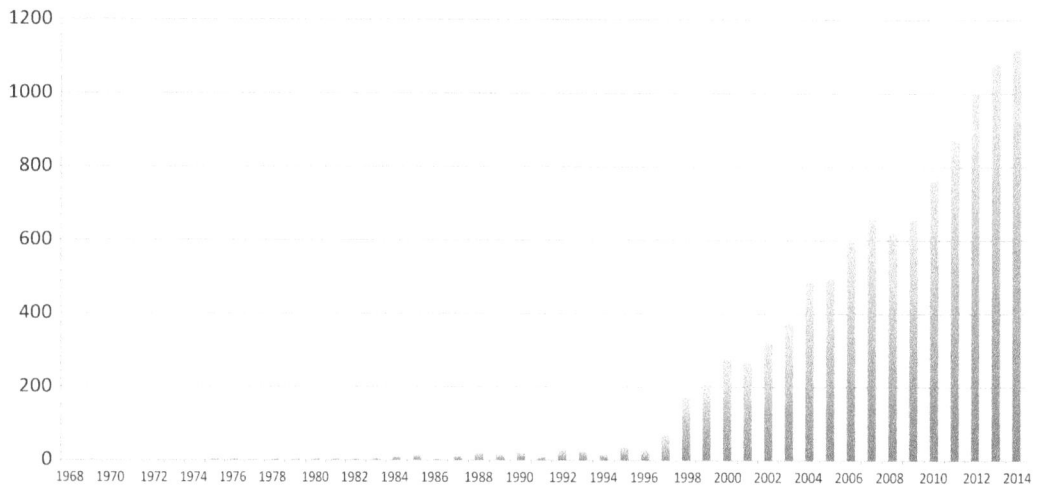

Figure 1. The Number of Randomized Controlled Trials (RCTs) for Dietary Supplements

Randomized Controlled Trials—Searching keywords: Dietary Supplements AND (Randomized Controlled Trial[pt] OR Randomized Controlled Trial[ti] OR Randomized Controlled Trial[ti]) AND Cancer AND 2000/01/01[dp]:2014/12/31[dp]
Searching period: January 1, 2000–December 31, 2014
Searching day: June 1, 2015
Searching results: 548 articles

Systematic Review—Searching keywords: Dietary Supplements AND (cochrane database syst rev[ta] OR meta-analysis[pt] OR meta-analysis[ti] OR systematic review[ti]) AND Cancer AND 2000/01/01[dp]:2014/12/31[dp]
Searching period: January 1, 2000–December 31, 2014
Searching day: June 1, 2015
Searching results: 140 articles

Among the above, screening the abstracts and articles related to systematic reviews revealed that there are twenty-one research articles that verified "functional food in cancer treatment." We arranged these articles according to their clinical question and to the actual clinical situation. Consequently, we arranged the question and topics as follows regarding the usage of functional food.

Do the cancer symptoms get relieved?

We found that there were two articles related to weight reduction, and two articles were related to cachexia. On the other hand, there were no articles related to symptoms such as pain, digestive symptoms, respiratory symptoms, urological symptoms, or sleeping.

Weight Reduction

There were two systematic reviews that addressed this issue.

In Baldwin et al.,[1] in a meta-analysis of twelve randomized control trials (RCTs), which included nutrition advice, the mean difference (MD) was 1.86 kg (95% confidence interval (CI): 0.25 – 3.47). However, as there was high heterogeneity ($I^2 = 76\%$), the analysis in seven RCTs were repeated ($I^2 = 0\%$). This resulted in an MD of 0.31 (95% CI: –0.60 – 1.21), which meant that there was no statistically significant difference.

In Meji et al.,[2] among seven RCTs that used omega-3 fatty acid, the weight was found to be increased in three trials. However, as for the other four, there was no significant difference in comparison with placebo. Accordingly, it is difficult to conclude that there is efficacy of nutrition intervention or omega-3 fatty acid on controlling the weight reduction of cancer patients.

Cachexia

There were two systematic reviews addressing this issue.

Ries et al.[3] studied the literature of three systematic reviews and twenty-seven clinical studies (ten RCTs, eleven non-RCTs, four dose-finding studies, and other.[2] They aimed to understand the effect of omega-3 fatty acid on cachexia and found that the efficacy was demonstrated in small-scale RCTs and in non-RCT cases, whereas large-scale RCTs did not demonstrate any significance. The adverse events investigated included abdominal discomfort, belch, rotten aftertaste, nausea, and diarrhea, where no serious symptoms were particularly found. Also, as this article was part of cachexia guideline by the European Palliative Care Research Collaborative (EPCRC), the authors placed omega-3 fatty acid as "weak negative GRADE recommendation for cachexia" as their conclusion.

Colomer et al.[4] investigated the literature of eighteen clinical studies (nine RCTs and nine non-RCTs), which used omega-3 fatty acid to find out its efficacy on cachexia. They concluded that taking 1.5 g of omega-3 per day can contribute to improvements in the symptoms of cachexia. However, none of the investigations conducted a meta-analysis, which means that it is difficult to draw conclusions regarding the efficacy of omega-3 fatty acid on improving cachexia for cancer patients.

Do the mental conditions associated with cancer get relieved?

There was no systematic review addressing mental conditions such as anxiety and depression in relation to cancer.

Does the quality of life (QOL) improve?

There was only one systematic review addressing this issue.

Baldwin et al.[1] studied the meta-analysis of nine RCTs in which nutrition advices were conducted. They found that the evaluation of QOL has improved as MD was 24.02 (95% CI: 14.3 – 33.72), by applying the scale of the European Organization for Research and Treatment of Cancer Global Quality of Life. However, as heterogeneity was high (I^2 = 98%), the analysis was redone using five RCTs only. Although the MD was as small as 5.53 (95% CI: 0.73 – 10.33), the results were considered statistically significant. Accordingly, it was possible to conclude that introducing nutrition guidance can improve the overall QOL of the cancer patient.

Are any undesired symptoms caused?

Only one systematic review was found addressing this issue.

Alsanad et al.[5] studied five research articles that investigated the mutual actions of drugs and functional food. They found that among 806 cancer patients, there were 433 patients (53.7%) who take functional food along with drugs, and that 60 patients of the 433 (13.9%) said that there might be risk of mutual actions. In total, they raised 167 possible cases of risks. As for the functional food, they mentioned garlic, green tea, mistletoe, Chinese herbs, iron, *Hypericum perforatum* (St. John's wort), ginger, ginseng, and others as food material that should be considered as drug-interfering substances.

Do the adverse events accompanied with therapies get relieved?

Digestive Symptoms

There were six systematic reviews addressing this issue.

Tocuchefeu et al.[6] investigated the literature of seven RCTs of patients under therapy (five trials of radiotherapy, and two trials of anticancer drugs). They looked for the effects of improving the symptom of diarrhea by taking probiotics, and found that in five trials (three of the radiotherapy, and the two of anticancer drugs) the frequency and severity improved.

Henson et al.[7] investigated the meta-analysis of four RCTs of nutritional interference (fat, lactose, and fiber) for patients undergoing radiotherapy. They also looked for the effects of improving the symptoms of diarrhea and found that the risk of diarrhea had reduced 0.66 (95% CI: 0.51 – 0.87, n = 413, I^2 = 14%). However, cases in their last stages were not covered.

Likewise, Ben-Arye et al.[8] investigated the nutritional interference (three cases of glutamine, one case of melatonin, and two cases of probiotics) for patients undergoing both radiotherapy and chemotherapy to investigate the effects on improving diarrhea symptoms, by studying the literature of the published articles. They found that efficacy was demonstrated in one case of glutamine, and two cases of probiotics, while melatonin did not show any efficacy.

Wedlake et al.[9] studied the literature of sixteen RCTs of nutritional intervention for patients under radiotherapy. This included adjusting dietary components (four trials), adjusting fat (four trials), adjusting fiber (two trials), reducing lactate (one trial), and probiotics (five trials); aiming to understand the effects on the digestive symptoms. The results showed efficacy in one, three, one, and four trials of adjusting dietary components, adjusting fat, adjusting fiber, and probiotics respectively. Whereas, reducing lactate did not show efficacy.

Gibson et al.[10] studied the literature of 251 clinical research studies, which they found online. These studies used twenty-nine different types of interventions (including medical drugs) to find the effects of improving any mucous membrane disorders in the digestive system, which may occur due to radiotherapy or chemotherapy. They found that probiotics, such as lactic acid bacteria, has efficacy in preventing diarrhea that may be caused by either radiotherapy or chemotherapy and that high-pressure oxygen therapy has efficacy in preventing rectum inflammation caused by radiotherapy.

Block et al.[11] studied the literature of four RCTs of taking antioxidant supplements (one trial of each; glutathione, melatonin, N-acetylcysteine, and selenium) for cancer patients undergoing radiotherapy. However, they did not find any statistical significance in any of these trials.

Concluding these six research works, there was evidence that probiotics can improve the symptoms of diarrhea in patients undergoing radiotherapy.

Peripheral Nerve Disorder

There were three systematic reviews addressing this issue.

Ben-Arye et al.[8] studied the literature of twelve cases of nutritional intervention for patients under chemotherapy (five cases of vitamin E and glutathione, and one case of glutamine and melatonin). They studied their efficacy in preventing peripheral nerve disorder and found that the efficacy was found in four, three, and one case of vitamin E, glutamine, and melatonin respectively; whereas there was no efficacy confirmed using glutamine.

Schloss et al.[12] studied the literature of twenty-three clinical studies that used nine types of interventions to examine their effects in relieving the peripheral nerve disorder induced by chemotherapy. These types included magnesium, calcium, vitamin E, lipoic acid, N-acetylcysteine, glutathione, glutamine, acetyl-L-carnitine, vitamin B_6, and omega-3 fatty acid. They found that there was not enough proof to support the argument that any of these interventions can improve the symptoms of peripheral nerve disorder caused by anticancer drugs.

Block et al.[11] also studied the literature of eighteen RCTs in which antioxidant supplements were given to patients undergoing chemotherapy. They included nine trials of glutathione, five trials of melatonin, three trials of vitamin E, and one case of each N-acetylcysteine and a blend. Although the following trials showed efficacies, the study did not include meta-analysis (six trials of glutathione, four trials of melatonin, three trials of vitamin E, and one trial of N-acetylcysteine).

The results of these three studies showed that it is difficult to conclude that functional food has efficacy on peripheral nervous disorder in cancer patients undergoing chemotherapy.

Weight Reduction

There were five systematic reviews related to this problem.

Kiss et al.[13] studied the literature of three RCTs in which nutritional intervention was applied on patients undergoing chemotherapy so as to understand the efficacy in controlling weight reduction. This included instructions to adjust the calorie intake as well as the type of nutrients. They found that there was no statistical significance obtained by comparing the subjects with the control group. In another study where they used historical data,[13] they found that there is efficacy in controlling weight reduction by nutritional intervention for patients undergoing radiotherapy as the weight of the subject group dropped –0.56 kg, while the control group dropped –3.9 kg (p-value = 0.027).

Henson et al.[7] conducted a meta-analysis to study the effect of nutritional intervention to control weight reduction in patients undergoing radiotherapy using two RCTs. They found that there was no statistical significance as the difference between the subject and control groups was –0.57 kg (95% CI: –1.22 – 0.09, n = 235, I^2 = 29%).

Similarly, Langius et al.[14] studied the literature of three RCTs to examine the efficacy nutritional intervention on patients with cervical cancer undergoing radiotherapy and chemotherapy. They found that there was efficacy in two out of the three cases.

Garg et al.[15] studied the literature of three RCTs in which nutritional intervention was introduced to patients with cervical cancer undergoing radiotherapy. These included Sustacal®, Ensure®, as well as nutritional guidance aiming to investigate their effects on weight-reduction control. Although Ensure® and nutritional guidance showed efficacy, none of these three studies was subjected to systematic review.

Block et al.[11] studied the literature of three RCTs that used antioxidants to investigate the effects on controlling weight reduction in patients undergoing chemotherapy. They used glutathione in once case and melatonin in the other two cases, and although they found efficacy in all cases, none of them underwent meta-analysis.

These five studies show that it is difficult to conclude that functional food has efficacy in controlling weight reduction in patients undergoing radiotherapy or chemotherapy.

Postoperative Complications

There were two systematic reviews that addressed this issue.

Elia et al.[16] conducted meta-analysis to study the effects of giving nutrition to patients undergoing surgery as cancer therapy both parenterally and enterally. They studied the following cases: the period of admission (eight RCTs), with postoperative complications (twelve RCTs), postoperative infections (twelve RCTs), and with sepsis (two RCTs). The results showed that there were improvements in all the cases as follows: the period of admission was reduced by 1.72 days (95% CI: 0.90 – 2.54), the postoperative complications improved by 0.62 (95% CI: 0.50 – 0.77), the postoperative infections improved by 0.69 (95% CI: 0.57 – 0.85), and sepsis score reduced to 2.21 (95% CI: 1.49 – 2.92).

He et al.[17] conducted meta-analysis to study the effects of giving probiotics or synbiotics to patients waiting to undergo elective surgery related to colorectal cancer.

The effects on diarrhea (two RCTs), intestinal obstruction (two RCTs), period of admission (two RCTs), postoperative infection (four RCTs), postoperative pneumonia (three RCTs), sepsis (two RCTs), and wound contamination (four RCTs) were examined (the control groups underwent different procedures according to the study, including a combination of neomycin and preoperative bowel treatment, enteral nutrition, and maltodextrin).

The results showed that diarrhea (OR: 0.29, 95% CI: 0.14 – 0.62), intestinal obstruction (OR: 0.39, 95% CI: 0.19 – 0.78), postoperative contamination (OR: 0.39, 95% CI: 0.22 – 0.58), and pneumonia (OR: 0.32, 95% CI: 0.11 – 0.93) improved; whereas no indication of positive influence on the period of admission (MD: –1.06, 95% CI: –2.71 – 0.60), sepsis (OR: 0.28, 95% CI: 0.03–2.74), or wound contamination.

The results from these two studies show that there is a possibility for enteral nutritional drugs or probiotics to prevent postoperative complications.

QOL

There are two systematic reviews that address this issue.

Kiss et al.[13] studied the literature of two RCTs in which nutritional intervention was introduced to patients undergoing chemical therapy. By guiding food habits that include the amount of calories and the type of nutrition, they studied the patient's QOL improvement. They found that this intervention did not show any statistical significance in comparison with the control groups in all the trials. On the other hand, the same authors had one case series of nutrition intervention for patients under radiotherapy,[29] in which they found that the QOL improved for some of the patients.

Langius et al.[14] also studied the literature of two RCTs on the effect of nutrition intervention on cervical cancer patients undergoing radiotherapy. They compared one group that was subjected to individual nutrition guidance to another group that had no nutrition guidance to evaluate the QOL based on EORTC QLQ30 (a questionnaire developed to assess the quality of life of cancer patients). Although both cases showed efficacy, functional food was not used in these two trials.

These two studies showed that no conclusion could be drawn on the efficacy of functional food on the QOL of cancer patients.

Disorder of Oral Mucosa

There were two systematic reviews addressing this issue.

Ben-Arye et al.[8] studied the literature of fifteen studies regarding nutrition intervention for patients undergoing chemotherapy (one case of vitamin E and fourteen cases of glutamine). They investigated the efficacy in preventing or improving the oral mucosa disorder. Although they found that there was efficacy in the case of vitamin E and in seven of the cases of glutamine, meta-analysis was not conducted.

Block et al.[11] studied the literature of four RCTs of giving antioxidants to patients undergoing chemotherapy. They were two trials of melatonin, and one trial of each glutathione and vitamin E aiming to investigate the efficacy on controlling disorder of the oral mocosa. Although efficacy was demonstrated in one case of each antioxidant, meta-analysis was not conducted.

These two studies showed that no conclusion could be drawn on the efficacy of functional food on preventing or improving oral mucosa disorder of cancer patients.

Hematopenia

There was only one case of systematic review addressing this issue.

Block et al.[11] studied the literature of four RCTs of giving antioxidant supplements to patients undergoing chemotherapy. Their objective was to investigate the efficacy of controlling the decrease in blood cells using antioxidants such as glutathione (one trial), melatonin (five trials), ellagic acid (one trial), N-acetylcysteine (one trial), selenium (one trial). Although efficacy was found in the case of glutathione, three cases of melatonin, the case of ellagic acid, and in the case of selenium, meta-analysis was not conducted.

These results showed that no conclusion could be drawn on the efficacy of antioxidants on controlling hematopenia in cancer patients.

Does prognosis improve?

Total Mortality

There were four systematic reviews addressing this issue.

Harris et al.[18] conducted a meta-analysis regarding the efficacy of vitamin C supplement on the overall survival rate of breast cancer patients (after diagnosis) in five RCTs. They found that the relative risk of death was 0.81 (95% CI: 0.72 – 0.91, n = 13203).

Baldwin et al.[1] conducted a meta-analysis on fifteen RCTs in which nutrition guidance was given to cancer patients. They did not find statistically significant difference in the death rate, as the risk ratio was 1.06 (95% CI: 0.92 – 1.22, I^2 = 0%).

Buttigliero et al.[19] conducted a meta-analysis regarding the efficacy of giving vitamin D supplement to patients with advanced prostate cancer in three RCTs. They found that the risk ratio of the death rate was 1.07 (95% CI: 0.93 – 1.23, heterogeneity: high).

Davies et al.[20] conducted a meta-analysis regarding the effects on death percentage at three different scenarios. They were; guiding the food habits of cancer patients (seven RCTs), giving antioxidant supplements (seven RCTs), and giving retinol (four RCTs). The results were that the relative risk was equal to 0.90 for the trials of food habits guidance (95% CI: 0.46 – 1.77, I^2 = 18.6%), 1.01 for the trials of antioxidant supplement (95% CI: 0.88 – 1.15, I^2 = 0.0%), and 0.97 for the trials of retinol (95% CI: 0.83 – 1.13, I^2 = 0.0%).

The results of these four studies show that some types of functional food (vitamin C) are showing contribution in improving the efficacy of the anticancer drugs. However, more research is required.

Cause-Specific Mortality

There are two systematic reviews that address this issue.

Harris et al.[18] conducted a meta-analysis regarding the efficacy of giving vitamin C supplement to breast cancer patients in six RCTs on death rate caused by breast cancer. They found that the relative risk factor dropped to 0.85 (95% CI: 0.74 – 0.99, n = 13203).

Davies et al.[20] conducted a meta-analysis regarding the effect on cancer-specific death rate in three scenarios. These were guidance of food habits for cancer patients (three RCTs), giving an antioxidant supplement (two RCTs), and giving retinol (two RCTs). They found that the odds ratio of cancer-specific death was 0.53 in the trials of food habits guidance (95% CI: 0.16 – 1.79, I^2 = 0.0%), 0.81 in the trials of antioxidants (95% CI: 0.39 – 1.71, I^2 = 70.1%), and 0.92 in the trials of retinol (95% CI: 0.65 – 1.31, I^2 = 0.0%).

The results of these two studies show that some types of functional food are showing contribution in improving the efficacy of the anticancer drugs. However, more research is required.

Disease-Free Survival, Progression-Free Survival, Tumor Response Rate

There were two systematic reviews addressing this issue.

Posdazki et al.[21] studied the literature of eight RCTs that had prostate cancer patients as their subjects. They examined the effect of different nutrients including, calcitriol, genistein, daidzein, vitamin B, vitamin C, vitamin E, CoQ10, selenium, tea extract, isoflavone, lycopene, zinc, etc. on the tumor marker (PSA). They found that it was difficult to draw conclusions that support the argument that functional food can lower PSA.

Block et al.[11] studied the literature of seventeen RCTs in which giving antioxidants to patients undergoing chemotherapy aiming to understand the effect on tumor response. The antioxidants examined were glutathione (seven trials), melatonin (five trials), vitamin E (one trial), blended product (two trials), ellagic acid (one trial), and N-acetylcysteine (one trial). They found that efficacy was demonstrated in three trials of both glutathione and melatonin, and in the trial of acetylcysteine. However, meta-analysis was not conducted.

The results of these two studies show that some types of functional food are showing contribution in improving the efficacy of the anticancer drugs on the tumor response rate. However, more research is required.

Future Steps

In order to use functional food clinically for cancer treatment, it will be necessary to unify the standards of the products of functional food. However, the current indications show that the contents of the active components in these products differ according to the manufacturing companies. Also, to demonstrate the efficacy of the functional food in the body, it is essential to start considering the factors that may affect the processes of absorption and metabolism in the body.

Conclusion

Although research in the field of functional food has shown an increasing trend of applying methods such as randomized controlled trials and systematic reviews, there are many issues at the current stage that still need to be addressed. In addition, many patients take functional food for the satisfaction of being in control of their own sickness and symptoms — even when the therapeutic efficacy is not well understood or determined. In this chapter, we based our evaluation on the systematic reviews that are considered as the most reliable interpretation of information. That is because of the high importance of scientific verification in this field.

Nevertheless, the results of these reviews cannot be used to make decisions straightaway. What is so-called evidence-based medicine (EBM) is defined as the consideration of research evidence, patient's preferences and actions, clinical expertise, and clinical state and circumstances to make the best decision regarding the patient's care. To make use of the clinical results collected from RTCs and systematic reviews, it is most important to take into consideration what the patient values and to have adequate communication with the patient.

REFERENCES

1. Baldwin C, Spiro A, Ahern R, and Emery PW. "Oral nutritional interventions in malnourished patients with cancer: a systematic review and meta-analysis." *J. Natl. Cancer Inst.* 104(5): 371–85, 2012.

2. van der Meij BS, van Bokhorst-de van der Schueren MA, Langius JA, Brouwer IA, and van Leeuwen PA. "n-3 PUFAs in cancer, surgery, and critical care: a systematic review on clinical effects, incorporation, and washout of oral or enteral compared with parenteral supplementation." *Am. J. Clin. Nutr.* 94(5): 1248–65, 2011.

3. Ries A, Trottenberg P, Elsner F, Stiel S, Haugen D, Kaasa S, and Radbruch L. "A systematic review on the role of fish oil for the treatment of cachexia in advanced cancer: an EPCRC cachexia guidelines project." *Palliat Med.* 26(4): 294–304, 2012.

4. Colomer R, Moreno-Nogueira JM, García-Luna PP, García-Peris P, García-de-Lorenzo A, Zarazaga A, Quecedo L, del Llano J, Usán L, and Casimiro C. "N-3 fatty acids, cancer and cachexia: a systematic review of the literature." *Br. J. Nutr.* 97(5): 823–31, 2007.

5. Alsanad SM, Williamson EM, and Howard RL. "Cancer patients at risk of herb/food supplement-drug interactions: a systematic review." *Phytother. Res.* 28(12): 1749–55, 2014.

6. Touchefeu Y, Montassier E, Nieman K, Gastinne T, Potel G, Bruley des Varannes S, Le Vacon F, and de La Cochetière MF. "Systematic review: the role of the gut microbiota in chemotherapy- or radiation-induced gastrointestinal mucositis—current evidence and potential clinical applications." *Aliment Pharmacol. Ther.* 40(5): 409–21, 2014.

7. Henson CC, Burden S, Davidson SE, and Lal S. "Nutritional interventions for reducing gastrointestinal toxicity in adults undergoing radical pelvic radiotherapy." *Cochrane Database Syst. Rev.* 2013 Nov 26;11:CD009896.

8. Ben-Arye E, Polliack A, Schiff E, Tadmor T, and Samuels N. "Advising patients on the use of non-herbal nutritional supplements during cancer therapy: a need for doctor-patient communication." *J. Pain Symptom Manage.* 46(6): 887–96, 2013.

9. Wedlake LJ, Shaw C, Whelan K, and Andreyev HJ. "Systematic review: the efficacy of nutritional interventions to counteract acute gastrointestinal toxicity during therapeutic pelvic radiotherapy." *Aliment Pharmacol. Ther.* 37(11): 1046–56, 2013.

10. Gibson RJ, Keefe DM, Lalla RV, Bateman E, Blijlevens N, Fijlstra M, King EE, Stringer AM, van der Velden WJ, Yazbeck R, Elad S, and Bowen JM. "Mucositis Study Group of the Multinational Association of Supportive Care in Cancer/International Society of Oral Oncology (MASCC/ISOO). Systematic review of agents for the management of gastrointestinal mucositis in cancer patients." *Support Care Cancer* 21(1): 313–26, 2013.

11. Block KI, Koch AC, Mead MN, Tothy PK, Newman RA, and Gyllenhaal C. "Impact of antioxidant supplementation on chemotherapeutic toxicity: a systematic review of the evidence from randomized controlled trials." *Int. J. Cancer* 123(6): 1227–39, 2008.

12. Schloss JM, Colosimo M, Airey C, Masci PP, Linnane AW, and Vitetta L. "Nutraceuticals and chemotherapy induced peripheral neuropathy (CIPN): a systematic review." *Clin. Nutr.* 32(6): 888–93, 2013.

13. Kiss NK, Krishnasamy M, and Isenring EA. "The effect of nutrition intervention in lung cancer patients undergoing chemotherapy and/or radiotherapy: a systematic review." *Nutr. Cancer* 66(1): 47–56, 2014.

14. Langius JA, Zandbergen MC, Eerenstein SE, van Tulder MW, Leemans CR, Kramer MH, and Weijs PJ. "Effect of nutritional interventions on nutritional status, quality of life and mortality in patients with head and neck cancer receiving (chemo)radiotherapy: a systematic review." *Clin. Nutr.* 32(5): 671–8, 2013.

15. Garg S, Yoo J, and Winquist E. "Nutritional support for head and neck cancer patients receiving radiotherapy: a systematic review." *Support Care Cancer* 18(6): 667–77, 2010.

16. Elia M, Van Bokhorst-de van der Schueren MA, Garvey J, Goedhart A, Lundholm K, Nitenberg G, and Stratton RJ. "Enteral (oral or tube administration) nutritional support and eicosapentaenoic acid in patients with cancer: a systematic review." *Int. J. Oncol.* 28(1): 5–23, 2006.

17. He D, Wang HY, Feng JY, Zhang MM, Zhou Y, and Wu XT. "Use of pro-/synbiotics as prophylaxis in patients undergoing colorectal resection for cancer: a meta-analysis of randomized controlled trials." *Clin. Res. Hepatol. Gastroenterol.* 37(4): 406–15, 2013.

18. Harris HR, Orsini N, and Wolk A. "Vitamin C and survival among women with breast cancer: a meta-analysis." *Eur. J. Cancer* 50(7): 1223–31, 2014.

19. Buttigliero C, Monagheddu C, Petroni P, Saini A, Dogliotti L, Ciccone G, and Berruti A. "Prognostic role of vitamin D status and efficacy of vitamin D supplementation in cancer patients: a systematic review." *Oncologist* 16(9): 1215–27, 2011. doi:10.1634/theoncologist. 2011–0098. Epub 2011 Aug 11.

20. Davies AA, Davey Smith G, Harbord R, Bekkering GE, Sterne JA, Beynon R, and Thomas S. "Nutritional interventions and outcome in patients with cancer or preinvasive lesions: systematic review." *J. Natl. Cancer Inst.* 98(14): 961–73, 2006.

21. Posadzki P, Lee MS, Onakpoya I, Lee HW, Ko BS, and Ernst E. "Dietary supplements and prostate cancer: a systematic review of double-blind, placebo-controlled randomised clinical trials." *Maturitas* 75(2): 125–30, 2013.

Effect of AHCC in Women Receiving Adjuvant Chemotherapy for Breast Cancer: The Present and Near Future

Sho Hangai, Satoru Iwase

Breast cancer is the most common malignant tumor in women in both the United States and Japan.[1,2] Recent advances in the development of adjuvant therapy combined with surgery and radiotherapy have prolonged survival of patients with breast cancer.[3] Anthracyclines and taxanes are key drugs of chemotherapy for breast cancer.[4] These drugs, however, are often associated with various adverse events, such as bone marrow suppression, hepatotoxicity, nephrotoxicity, peripheral neuropathy, cardiac toxicity, lipid disorders, nausea, and hair loss.

These adverse events not only diminish the intensity of treatments but also impair quality of life (QOL).[5,6] Several treatments are proposed for those adverse events. Pegylated or non-pegylated granulocyte colony stimulating factor (G-CSF) is available for bone marrow suppression, though it is quite expensive.[7,8] Liver supporting therapy such as ursodeoxycholic acid has been applied to hepatotoxicity, which results in limited effectiveness.[9] Several other therapies are recommended; however, efficient treatments are not well defined yet.

AHCC is a standardized extract of cultured *Lentinula edodes* mycelia, a fungus of the basidiomycota family. One of the active components of AHCC is α-glucan. This component is thought to provide a carbohydrate that stimulates immune response.[10,11] In addition, a nucleoside adenosine is thought to be responsible for the liver-protecting effect of AHCC.[12]

Beneficial effects of AHCC have been demonstrated in several studies. Animal experiments have shown that AHCC reduces adverse events by chemotherapeutic agents, such as bone marrow suppression, hepatotoxicity, and nephrotoxicity.[13–15]

The safety and tolerability for humans were shown by studies involving healthy adults.[10,16] Furthermore, Matsui et al. revealed the reduction of the recurrence of hepatocellular carcinoma and adverse events associated with chemotherapy in a human prospective cohort study by administration of AHCC.[17] However, effects of AHCC on patients receiving chemotherapy for breast cancer remain elusive.

We performed a retrospective study exploring the effects of AHCC on adverse events in female patients receiving adjuvant chemotherapy for breast cancer.[18] The eligibility criteria were as follows: (1) aged between 20 and 64; (2) with pathologically proven breast cancer; (3) receiving doxorubicin and cyclophosphamide (AC therapy), followed by taxane-based regimens. Forty-one women were eligible by the above criteria. We then compared the occurrence of adverse events in patients who received AHCC with those who did not. The patients' characteristics in the AHCC group and the control group were well balanced in terms of age, tumor size, clinical stage, and estrogen receptor positivity.

Comparisons of worst-grade adverse events between the two groups, defined as grade 2 or more by the National Cancer Institute Common Toxicity Criteria for Adverse Events (NCI-CTCAE) ver 4.0, revealed that patients in the AHCC group had fewer adverse events associated with triglyceride (TG) than patients in the control group, though statistically not significant (5.5% in the AHCC group and 34.6% in the control group, $p = 0.054$). A similar trend was also found in total cholesterol (T-Chol) (5.5% in the AHCC group and 17.3% in the control group, $p = 0.363$). Of note, patients in the AHCC group had a tendency toward more adverse events in gamma-glutamyl transpeptidase (γ-GTP) (28% in the AHCC group and 13% in the control group, $p = 0.267$).

We then utilized generalized estimating equations (GEEs) to analyze longitudinal changes in the occurrence of adverse events (grades 2–4). We found that the patients in the AHCC group had significantly fewer adverse neutrophil events than the control group (odds ratio, 0.30; 95% confidence interval [CI], $0.1 - 0.80$; $p = 0.016$). The above observation supports the notion that AHCC can alleviate bone marrow suppression via its one of the active components, acylated α-glucan. Indeed, we found that the patients in the AHCC group had significantly lower usage of G-CSF per administration of taxane therapy than the control group (0.14 in the AHCC group and 0.41 in the control group, $p = 0.008$).

As stated above, our study indicated the beneficial effects of AHCC on bone marrow suppression. These results are in agreement with previous studies, which revealed improvement of bone marrow suppression by supplementation of AHCC in mice treated with several anticancer drugs, including adriamycin and cyclophos-phamide.[13] The mechanism by which AHCC alleviates bone marrow suppression remains unclear. A previous study showed that maitake β-glucans (MBG) promoted bone marrow cell viability and protected the bone marrow stem cell colony for-mation unit from adriamycin-induced toxicity.[19] It is speculated that the effects of AHCC on neutrophil count and G-CSF usage may be mediated by a mechanism similar to that of MBG, although the predominant component of AHCC is acy-lated α-glucans. Whatever the mechanism, these results suggest that AHCC has the potential to increase the neutrophil count during chemotherapy. It might be possible to increase the intensity of chemotherapy and achieve better clinical outcome by the administration of AHCC.

We also found that the patients in AHCC group had fewer adverse events in TG and T-Chol, which was not statistically significant. She-Fang Ye et al. reported that AHCC suppressed the increase of serum corticosterone level induced by oxida-tive stress.[20] It might be possible that AHCC improves lipid abnormalities through modulation of the serum corticosterone level, which can also be affected by antican-cer drugs and antiemetic steroids.[21] Lipid abnormalities during chemotherapy are thought to be induced by anticancer drugs and steroids, which are used as antiemetic drugs. Steroids are widely used to treat chemotherapy-induced nausea and vomit-ing.[22] Therefore, AHCC might be effective for patients undergoing chemotherapy for various cancers.

Previous animal studies have revealed that AHCC improves hepatotoxicity by anticancer drugs, defined as elevated liver enzymes such as alanine transaminase (ALT) and aspartate transaminase (AST).[13] Moreover, it has been shown that AHCC improves AST, γ-GTP, and cholinesterase abnormalities in patients with hepatocellular carcinoma after surgery. Our study, however, did not find significant effects of AHCC on hepatotoxicity during chemotherapy. Of note, the patients in the AHCC group in our study had fewer grade 1 or higher ALT abnormalities than the control group (55.5% vs. 73.8%, $p = 0.322$). It is possible that our small sample size failed to detect the beneficial effect of AHCC on hepatotoxicity.

Although the difference was not statistically significant, the patients in the AHCC group had more adverse events in γ-GTP. In contrast, Matsui et al. revealed that AHCC improved the γ-GTP level in postsurgical patients with hepatocellular carci-noma.[17] One possible explanation is that the patients in the AHCC group had more grade 2 or higher γ-GTP events at the beginning of chemotherapy than patients in the control group (10% in AHCC group and 4% in the control group). Further studies are required to fully elucidate the effects of AHCC on γ-GTP levels during adjuvant chemotherapy for breast cancer.

The above study has several limitations, including a small sample size and the retrospective nature of the study. Moreover, no data was available on the compliance of AHCC intake. To further elucidate the effects of AHCC, we are now performing a double blind, randomized controlled study (UMIN CTR: UMIN000015455). Female patients with breast cancer undergoing taxane-based chemotherapy after anthracycline-based chemotherapy are enrolled. A total of 1.0 g of AHCC will be self-administered by each patient orally after each meal for twelve weeks. Fifty patients will be recruited at three medical institutions, with the registration periods of two years. The primary endpoint will be the occurrence of adverse events (grade 2 or higher) associated with white blood cell (WBC) count, neutrophil count, hemoglobin (Hb) concentration, platelet (PLT) count, total bilirubin (T-bil), alkaline phosphatase (ALP), AST, ALT, γ-GTP, TG, HDL cholesterol, LDL cholesterol, and creatinine, according to NCI CTCAE v4.0. The secondary endpoints will be EORTC QLQ-C30 and BR23 score, adherence, the use of G-CSF, and treatment success rate. A data center and independent data monitoring committee will carry out the central monitoring during the trial. This trial will further address the issue regarding AHCC's alleviating effects on chemotherapy-induced adverse events, which might provide patients receiving chemotherapy a better solution.

REFERENCES

1. Siegel RL, Miller KD, and Jemal A. "Cancer statistics, 2016." CA. *Cancer J. Clin.* 66, 7–30, 2016.

2. Center for Cancer Control and information Services, National Cancer Center, Japan, at http://ganjoho.jp/reg_stat/statistics/stat/summary.html.

3. Henderson IC, et al. "Improved outcomes from adding sequential paclitaxel but not from escalating doxorubicin dose in an adjuvant chemotherapy regimen for patients with node-positive primary breast cancer." *J. Clin. Oncol.* 21, 976–983, 2003.

4. Martin M, et al. "Adjuvant docetaxel for node-positive breast cancer." *N. Engl. J. Med.* 352, 2302–2313, 2005.

5. Montazeri A. "Health-related quality of life in breast cancer patients: A bibliographic review of the literature from 1974 to 2007." *J. Exp. Clin. Cancer Res.* 27, 32, 2008.

6. Browall M, et al. "Health-related quality of life during adjuvant treatment for breast cancer among postmenopausal women." *Eur. J. Oncol. Nurs.* 12, 180–9, 2008.

7. Crawford J, et al. "Reduction by granulocyte colony-stimulating factor of fever and neutropenia induced by chemotherapy in patients with small-cell lung cancer." *N. Engl. J. Med.* 325, 164–70, 1991.

8. Vogel CL, et al. "First and subsequent cycle use of pegfilgrastim prevents febrile neutropenia in patients with breast cancer: a multicenter, double-blind, placebo-controlled phase III study." *J. Clin. Oncol.* 23, 1178–84, 2005.

9. Mohammed Saif M, Farid SF, Khaleel SA, Sabry NA, and El-Sayed MH. "Hepatoprotective efficacy of ursodeoxycholic acid in pediatrics acute lymphoblastic leukemia." *Pediatr. Hematol. Oncol.* 29, 627–32, 2012.

10. Spierings ELH, Fujii H, Sun B, and Walshe T. "A Phase I study of the safety of the nutritional supplement, active hexose correlated compound, AHCC, in healthy volunteers." *J. Nutr. Sci. Vitaminol.* (Tokyo) 53, 536–539, 2007.

11. Terakawa N, et al. "Immunological effect of active hexose correlated compound (AHCC) in healthy volunteers: a double-blind, placebo-controlled trial." *Nutr. Cancer* 60, 643–651, 2008.

12. Tanaka Y, et al. "Adenosine, a hepato-protective component in active hexose correlated compound: its identification and iNOS suppression mechanism." *Nitric Oxide—Biol. Chem.* 40, 75–86, 2014.

13. Shigama K, Nakaya A, Wakame K, Nishioka H, and Fujii H. "Alleviating effect of active

hexose correlated compound (AHCC) for anticancer drug-induced side effects in non-tumor-bearing mice." *J. Exp. Ther. Oncol.* 8, 43–51, 2009.

14. Hirose A, et al. "The influence of active hexose correlated compound (AHCC) on cisplatin-evoked chemotherapeutic and side effects in tumor-bearing mice." *Toxicol. Appl. Pharmacol.* 222, 152–158, 2007.

15. Sun B, et al. "The effect of active hexose correlated compound in modulating cytosine arabinoside-induced hair loss, and 6-mercaptopurine- and methotrexate-induced liver injury in rodents." *Cancer Epidemiol.* 33, 293–299, 2009.

16. Yin Z, Fujii H, and Walshe T. "Effects of active hexose correlated compound on frequency of CD4+ and CD8+ T cells producing interferon-g and/or tumor necrosis factor-a in healthy adults." *Hum. Immunol.* 71, 1187–1190, 2010.

17. Matsui Y, et al. "Improved prognosis of postoperative hepatocellular carcinoma patients when treated with functional foods: a prospective cohort study." *J. Hepatol.* 37, 78–86, 2002.

18. Hangai S, et al. "Effect of active hexose-correlated compound in women receiving adjuvant chemotherapy for breast cancer: a retrospective study." *J. Altern. Complement. Med.* 19, 905–910, 2013.

19. Lin H, She YH, Cassileth BR, Sirotnak F, and Rundles SC. "Maitake beta-glucan MD-fraction enhances bone marrow colony formation and reduces doxorubicin toxicity in vitro." *Int. Immunopharmacol.* 4, 91–99, 2004.

20. Ye SF, Wakame K, Ichimura K, and Matsuzaki S. "Amelioration by active hexose correlated compound of endocrine disturbances induced by oxidative stress in the rat." *Endocr. Regul.* 38, 7–13, 2004.

21. Morrow GR, Hickok JT, Andrews PL, and Stern RM. "Reduction in serum cortisol after platinum based chemotherapy for cancer: a role for the HPA axis in treatment-related nausea?" *Psychophysiology* 39, 491–495, 2002.

22. Ioannidis JPA, Hesketh PJ, and Lau J. "Contribution of dexamethasone to control of chemotherapy-induced nausea and vomiting: a meta-analysis of randomized evidence." *J. Clin. Oncol.* 18, 3409–3422, 2000.

Pancreatic Cancer Chemotherapy and AHCC (Significance as Supportive Care)

Hiroaki Yanagimoto

The treatment of cancer consists of surgery, radiation therapy, and chemotherapy that target cancer, and supportive care, which is equivalent to, or more important than, the modality of these treatments. The proper measures and treatment for the side effects associated with the treatment for cancer, local and systemic symptoms due to infiltration of cancer, and paraneoplastic syndrome are not only able to alleviate the symptoms of the patients, but can also improve the recovery rate by completing the cancer treatment as per the schedule, and prolong life in case of advanced and recurrent cancer. On the other hand, cancer in the elderly continues to increase and is often accompanied by geriatric syndrome complications in addition to the reduction in the physiological functions of the mind and body. Therefore, careful planning that appropriately incorporates supportive care is required for the treatment.

It is possible to implement safe and effective cancer treatment by providing high-quality supportive care to cancer patients, and improvement in survival can be observed. Also, cancer therapy is performed for alleviation of symptoms even when healing is difficult, and high-quality supportive care is required specifically for chemotherapy with the objective to prolong life while maintaining a high QOL.

Interest in chemotherapy-related supportive care is growing; the Multinational Association of Supportive Care in Cancer (MASCC) is supporting global education and research to provide high-quality supportive care based on combined modality therapy, regardless of the disease stage. So far, as the central role of supportive care, the measure for nausea and vomiting associated with chemotherapy and febrile neutropenia that occurs frequently with intensive chemotherapy was considered important. These symptoms have been overcome with the progress of support-ive-care drugs, but the supportive care for various pains such as hair loss, numbness, and taste disorder has not been established yet at present.

The role of health food in cancer patients is to help in the prevention and treat-ment of cancer with functions such as:

1. Immunity-enhancing effect to enhance the function of the immune cells for elimi-nating the cancer cells.

2. Antioxidant effect to remove the active oxygen and free radicals that causes aggra-vation of cancer.

3. Antiangiogenic effect to stop the growth of cancer by inhibiting angiogenesis that feeds the cancer.

4. Apoptosis-inducing effect to promote natural killing of the cancer cells.

5. Effects such as improving bowel movement by increasing the good intestinal bac-teria to improve the intestinal environment.

6. Effect of replenishing insufficient nutrients, and activation and adjustment of body functions.

In the field of complementary and alternative medicine (CAM), dietary sup-plements are widely used by cancer patients, and these foods are taken along with chemotherapeutic agents in cancer treatments. In a survey carried out by the Japan Ministry of Health, Labour and Welfare research group, AHCC was listed among the commonly used dietary supplements in Japanese cancer patients. In addition to many other botanical polysaccharides, AHCC has been developed with the expecta-tion of an immune modulation effect.

As the basic and clinical research on AHCC and cancer treatment has pro-ceeded, AHCC came to be used along with conventional therapies. Matsui et al. reported that AHCC contributes to the prevention of cancer recurrence, liver func-tion improvement, and prolongation of postoperative survival rate as an adjunctive therapy following hepatectomy in patients with hepatocellular carcinoma.[1] Since the safety of AHCC and its interactions with chemotherapeutic agents have been confirmed by the various research mentioned in the other chapters of this book, AHCC can be used widely as a dietary supplement in patients not only with hepa-tocellular carcinoma but also with other types of cancer, such as advanced liver cancer,[2] breast cancer,[3,4] gastric cancer and colon cancer,[5] lung cancer and colon cancer,[6] early stage prostate cancer,[7] head and neck cancer,[8] and non-small cell lung cancer.[9]

Ito et al. reported that administration of AHCC significantly decreased the levels of human herpes viruses (HHV-6) in saliva, which are reactivated by physical and psychological stresses as a possible biomarker of fatigue during chemotherapy. It was also reported that AHCC improved not only QOL scores in the EORTC QLQ-C30 questionnaire but also hematotoxicity and hepatotoxicity in patients during chemotherapy with pancreatic, ovarian, lung, and colorectal cancers.[10] The other studies have also reported potential effects of AHCC on the side effects of chemotherapy, which was to reduce the severity of neutropenia and the use of granulocyte colony-stimulating factor,[5] to get a sense of well-being, to maintain general condition by improving intake,[8] and to improve mean survival time with better QOL.[6,9] From these investigations, it was considered that an administration of conventional dose of AHCC (3 – 6 g/day) to the patients with cancer undergoing chemotherapy have no harmful effect, may maintain the QOL, and have some beneficial effects on chemotherapy-induced adverse effects.

Pancreatic ductal adenocarcinoma (PDAC) is the fifth most common cancer worldwide, and the prognosis of patients with this type of cancer is dismal. For patients with unresectable PDAC, the chemotherapy treatment options are limited. Gemcitabine (GEM) was the current standard therapy until FOLFIRINOX and the combination therapy of GEM and nanoparticle albumin-bound pacritaxel (GEM + nab TPX) became available.[12–15] Although recent chemotherapy has made great advances and has exhibited prominent efficacy, concerns are raised for the impairment of the cancer patients' quality of life (QOL) owing to adverse events.

The role of AHCC in supportive care for chemotherapy of unresectable advanced pancreatic cancer patients is described retrospectively in the current study.

Patients and Methods

In the present study, patients with (a) unresectable histologically or cytologically proven adenocarcinoma of the pancreas; (b) Eastern Cooperative Oncology Group (ECOG) performance status of 0 – 1; and (c) aged between 18 and 75 years, having sufficient organ function and chemotherapy (Gemcitabine) is scheduled were considered. Patients were prospectively divided into an AHCC treatment group (AHCC group) and a non-treatment group (control group) according to the patients' wishes.

Gemcitabine was given intravenously at a dose of 1,000 mg/m^2 over 30 minutes once a week for three weeks, followed by a week of rest. Patients in both groups did not take any other functional foods, including vitamin tablets, during the study. The evaluation of the adverse events and clinical responses was carried out using the data until disease progression. The primary endpoint was to estimate the alleviating effect of AHCC for the adverse events caused by gemcitabine in patients with PDAC, while the secondary endpoint was to assess the clinical response rate and overall survival (OS).

Blood samples were collected every week for eight weeks. The assessment of hematological and non-hematological toxicity was performed using the National Cancer Institute Common Terminology Criteria for Adverse Events (CTCAE Ver 3.0) grading[16] every week during the chemotherapy. To evaluate the taste disorder (TD) subjectively, the patients were requested to complete a questionnaire of symptoms related to TD defined in CTCAE 3.0. The modified Glasgow Prognostic Score (mGPS) is a score system based on both C-reactive protein (CRP) and albumin. Accordingly, patients who had both elevated CRP (>0.5 mg/dl) and hypoalbuminemia (<3.5 g/dl) were assigned a score of 3. While patients with either elevated CRP (>0.5 mg/dl) or hypoalbuminemia (<3.5 g/dl) were assigned scores of 2 and 1, respectively. Finally, patients with neither of these abnormalities were assigned a score of 0.[17] A contrast-enhanced CT scan was done for evaluating the clinical response rate using Response Evaluation Criteria in Solid Tumor (RECIST) every two months until disease progression.[18] A complete written informed consent was obtained from all patients at the time of enrollment in accordance with the provisions of the Declaration of Helsinki.

Results

From December 2007 to July 2009, seventy-five patients were prospectively enrolled in this study and classified as an AHCC group (n = 35) and a control group (n = 40). There were no significant differences in most parameters except the platelet counts at the baseline level between the groups. No differences were found in the albumin level, CRP level, mGPS score, or frequency of taste disorder between the groups.

No occurrences of febrile neutropenia were recorded during the course of the current study. No significant difference was found between the groups for neutropenia, thrombocytopenia, and hepatic dysfunction in grade 3/4. Most of these hematologic toxicities were transient and reversible. Grade 3/4 non-hematologic toxicities were not observed. The lowest hemoglobin (Hb) level during chemotherapy in the AHCC group was significantly higher than in the control group (10.6 g/dL (7.3 – 12.6) vs. 10.3 g/dL (6.7 – 12.6), $p = 0.0360$; see Table 1 on the facing page). In addition, the highest CRP level during chemotherapy in the AHCC group was significantly lower than the control group (0.48 mg/dL (0.02 – 17.53) vs. 1.92 mg/dL (0.05 – 20.20), $p<0.0001$). The lowest serum albumin level during chemotherapy in the AHCC group was significantly higher than the control group (3.8g/dL (2.6 – 4.4) vs. 3.4g/dL (1.9 – 4.7), $p = 0.0074$) (see Table 1 and Figure 1). The occurrence of TD (taste disorder) during chemotherapy in the AHCC group was significantly lower than the control group (n = 6/35 (17%) vs. n = 22/40 (55%), $p = 0.0007$). The mGPS score (0/1/2/3) during chemotherapy in the AHCC group was significantly better than the control group (0/1/2/3: 15/4/11/5 vs. 3/1/15/21, $p = 0.0002$). Significantly lower frequency of grade 3 in mGPS was found in the AHCC group (5/35) relative to the control group (21/40, $p = 0.0005$).

The evaluation for tumor reduction effect will be done by using efficacy, but the response rate according to RECIST 1.0 was 17% in the AHCC group compared with 12% in the control group ($p = 0.571$). The disease control rate (tumor control rate) in the AHCC group was significantly higher than the control group (74% vs. 50%, $p = 0.003$).

The median survival time (MST) was 9.0 months (95% CI: 7.4 – 14.0 months) in the AHCC group and 6.7 months (95% CI: 4.6 – 9.3 months) in the control group ($p = 0.081$). The higher tendency for overall survival was observed in the AHCC group relative to the control group (see Figure 2 on the facing page).

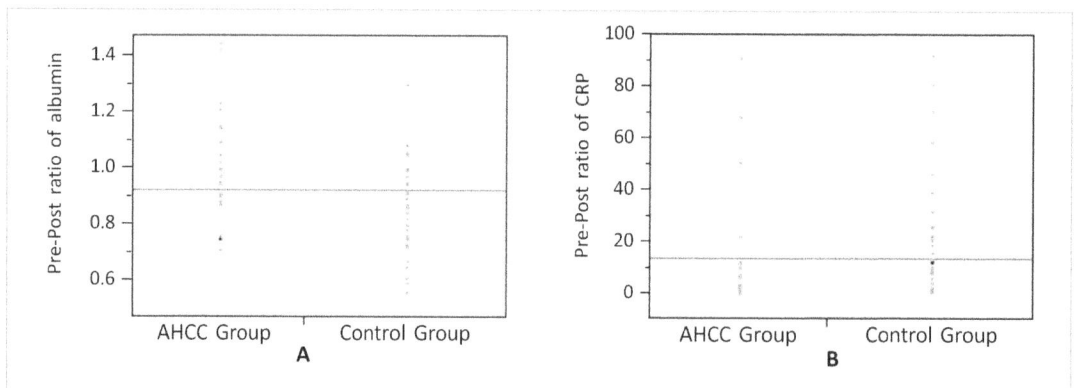

Figure. 1. A: The pre-post ratio of albumin in the AHCC group was significantly higher than in the control group ($P = 0.0007$). **B:** The pre-post ratio of CRP in the AHCC group was significantly lower than in the control group ($P = 0.0012$). (*Nutr. Cancer*, in press, 2016.)

TABLE 1. **COMPARISON OF TOXICITY (PRE- VS. POSTTREATMENT) IN AHCC AND CONTROL GROUP 2**

	AHCC group (n = 35)			Control group (n = 40)		
	Pretreatment	Posttreatment	P	Pretreatment	Posttreatment	P
WBC (x 10^2/μl)	6200 (3912 – 11300)	2600 (1500 – 5300)	<0.0001	6100 (3814 – 21300)	2800 (1700 – 17100)	<0.0001
Hb	12.0 (8.0 – 14.2)	10.6 (7.3 – 12.6)	<0.0001	11.9 (7.6 – 14.1)	10.3 (6.7 – 12.6)	<0.0001
PLT (x 10^4/μl)	27.0 (13.5 – 62.4)	11.0 (6.2 – 34.7)	<0.0001	22.9 (13.3 – 41.6)	10.9 (3.6 – 31.1)	<0.0001
Albumin (g/dl)	3.9 (1.9 – 4.4)	3.8 (2.6 – 4.4)	0.7093	3.8 (2.1 – 4.7)	3.4 (1.9 – 4.7)	<0.0001
CRP (mg/dl)	0.24 (0.01 – 4.38)	0.048 (0.02 – 17.53)	0.1721	0.21 (0.02 – 5.24)	1.92 (0.05 – 20.2)	0.0002
Taste Disorder (%)	4 (11)	6 (17)	0.7113	4 (10)	22 (56)	<0.0001
mGPS (0/1/2/3)	18/8/5/4	15/4/11/5	0.2382	24/6/7/3	3/1/15/21	<0.0001

(*Nutr. Cancer*, in press, 2016.)

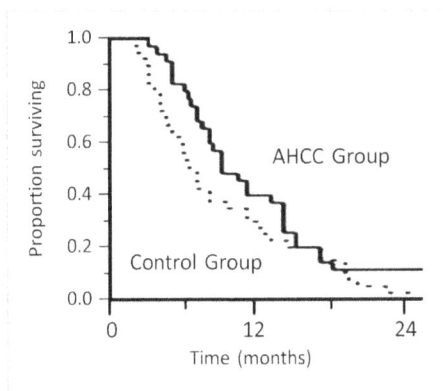

Patient at risk	6m	12m	18m	24m	30m
Control group	21	12	7	2	0
(n = 40)	53%	28	18	5	0
AHCC group	28	13	3	2	1
(n = 35)	80%	37	8.5	5.7	2.8

Figure 2. The overall survival in AHCC group (n = 35, solid line) and the control group (n = 40, broken line). Overall survival in the AHCC group had a higher tendency relative to the control group (*P* = 0.081). (*Nutr. Cancer*, in press, 2016.)

Discussion

Under discussion here is the role of health foods as supportive care for chemotherapy patients with unresectable advanced pancreatic cancer, the most intractable cancer. It is reported that unimaginable pain accompanies pancreatic cancer in patients with rapid progression. The side effects associated with chemotherapy exacerbate the pain, which is also accompanied by emotional distress (spiritual pain) and fear of death and cancer-related pain. Although antiemetics and measures for febrile neutropenia have dramatically improved, measures for anemic progression and dysgeusia have not been developed yet. Dysgeusia is a condition in which the sensation of taste is distorted and unpleasant, regardless of the food eaten. No enjoyment is derived from eating, and this aspect of life cannot be enjoyed. This is a serious Quality-of-Life (QOL) side effect.

Some reports[19-21] mention that there is a reduction in the side effects with the intake of AHCC during chemotherapy for cancer. Hirose et al. indicated that myelosuppression is improved by AHCC with cisplatin using animal models.[21] Further, cell viability is significantly higher in the AHCC-administered group compared to the control group. It can be considered that AHCC improves immunosuppression based on tumor cells in addition to cisplatin. The side effects of chemotherapy based on gemcitabine for pancreatobiliary cancer patients in general are neutropenia 72.7%, anemia 63.3%, thrombocytopenia 54.5%, anorexia 72.7%, and general fatigue 36.4%.[22] In the present study,[11] 90% of patients had hematologic adverse events, and anorexia or general fatigue was observed in 40%. There were no significant changes observed in the onset frequency of side effects with gemcitabine in the present study, but the concentration of hemoglobin in the patients administered with AHCC was relatively maintained when compared to the control group. The onset of dysgeusia during chemotherapy was significantly lower in the AHCC group, and the mGPS score was also good. These findings indicate that AHCC intake can reduce the onset of side effects due to gemcitabine.

Dysgeusia is often observed during chemotherapy and is one of the major side effects along with fatigue, nausea, vomiting, and hair loss.[23] There was progression of dysgeusia due to the occurrence of anorexia, caused by the destruction of the taste buds and related nervous system, in the same way inhibition of saliva secretion and zinc deficiency are caused by chemotherapy. The patients undergoing chemotherapy require more energy than basal metabolism. The malnutrition caused by dysgeusia is a serious problem that interferes with recovery from side effects and healing. Dysgeusia is caused from the start of chemotherapy,[24] and lasts for a few hours to a few weeks, and sometimes over several months.[25] The literature on dysgeusia is scant, although it is a frequent side effect. It has been reported that dysgeusia is caused not only due to chemotherapy but is also caused by the tumors.[26-28] The other factors related to dysgeusia are oral health problems, reflux of digestive fluids, and infection in addition to pharmaceuticals and antibiotics.[29] In the present study, patients with vitamin deficiency, zinc deficiency, and oral candidiasis were not observed. The frequency of anemia and anorexia for the AHCC group during chemotherapy was low, and there is a possibility that this inhibited the occurrence of dysgeusia. The mGPS score,[30,31] which is considered to be closely related to the survival rate of cancer patients, was higher for the AHCC group. Intake increases as a result of improvement in dysgeusia, and this may possibly cause inhibition of albumin in the blood. It is not known why the elevation of CRP is inhibited; it is possible the immunity-enhancing effect of AHCC, which enhances the function of the immune cells for eliminating the cancer cells, has some impact. The fact that there is improvement in mGPS, which is generally used for the prognostic evaluation of various carcinoma, indicates that AHCC may potentially have an antitumor effect or survival advantage.

The present study is within the range of retrospective study, and a simplistic conjecture is risky. In the future, scientific verification is required; at present, double blind randomized controlled trials are in progress.

REFERENCES

1. Matsui Y, et al. "Improved prognosis of postoperative hepatocellular carcinoma patients when treated with functional foods: a prospective cohort study." *J. Hepatol.* 37, 78–86, 2002.

2. Cowawintaweewat S, et al. "Prognostic improvement of patients with advanced liver cancer after active hexose correlated compound (AHCC) treatment." *Asian Pacific J. Allergy Immunol.* 24, 33–45, 2006.

3. Matsui Y, et al. "Retrospective study in breast cancer patients supplemented with AHCC." *Int. J. Integr. Oncol.* 3(2), 12–16, 2009.

4. Kawaguchi Y. "Improved survival of patients with gastric cancer or colon cancer when treated with Active Hexose Correlated Compound (AHCC): Effect of AHCC on digestive system cancer." *Natr. Med. J.* 1(1), 1–6, 2009.

5. Hangai S, et al. "Effect of active hexose-correlated compound in women receiving adjunct chemotherapy for breast cancer: a retrospective study." *J. Altern. Compl. Med.* 19(11), 905–910, 2013.

6. Ishizuka R, et al. "Review of cancer therapy with AHCC and GCP; The long-term follow-up over 12 years for stage IV (M1) cancer of the lung and the breast." *Int. J. Integr. Med.* 2(1), 98–111, 2010.

7. Sumiyoshi Y, et al. "Dietary administration of mushroom mycelium extracts in patients with early stage prostate cancers managed expectantly: A phase II study." *Jpn. J. Clin. Oncol.* 40(10), 967–972, 2010.

8. Parida DK, et al. "Integrating complimentary and alternative medicine in form of active hexose correlated compound (AHCC) in the management of head & neck cancer patients." *Int. J. Clin. Med.* 2, 588–592, 2011.

9. Ishizuka R, et al. "Personalized cancer therapy for stage IV non-small cell lung cancer: Combined use of active hexose correlated compound and genistein concentrated polysaccharide." *Personal. Med. Univ.* 1, 39–44, 2012.

10. Ito T, et al. "Reduction of adverse effects by a mushroom product, active hexose correlated compound (AHCC) in patients with advanced cancer during chemotherapy—The significance of the levels of HHV-6 DNA in saliva as a surrogate biomarker during chemotherapy." *Nutr. Cancer* 66 (3): 377–382, 2014.

11. Yanagimoto H, et al. "Alleviating effect of active hexose correlated compound (AHCC) on chemotherapy-related adverse events in patients with unresectable pancreatic ductal adenocarsinoma." *Nutr. Cancer,* in press, 2016.

12. Rothenberg ML, et al. "A phase II trial of gemcitabine in patients with 5-FU-refractory pancreas cancer." *Ann. Oncol.* 7, 347–353, 1996.

13. Burris III H. A. et al. "Improvements in survival and clinical benefit with gemcitabine as first-line therapy for patients with advanced pancreas cancer: A randomized trial." *J. Clin. Oncol.*15, 2403–2413, 1997.

14. Conroy T. et al. "FOLFIRINOX versus gemcitabine for metastatic pancreatic cancer." *N. Eng. J. Med.* 364, 1817–1825, 2011.

15. Von Hoff DD, et al. "Increased survival in pancreatic cancer with nabpaclitaxel plus gemcitabine." *N. Eng. J. Med.* 369, 1691–1703, 2013.

16. Trotti A, et al. "CTCAE v3.0: Development of a comprehensive grading system for the adverse effects of cancer treatment. *Semin. Radiat. Oncol.*" 13, 176–181, 2003.

17. Toriyama Y, et al. "Evaluation of an inflammation-based prognostic score for the identification of patients requiring postoperative adjuvant chemotherapy for stage II colorectal cancer." *Exp. Ther. Med.* 2, 95–101, 2011.

18. Eisenhauser EA, et al. "New response evaluation criteria in solid tumours: revised RECIST guideline (version 1.1)." *Eur. J. Cancer* 45, 228–247, 2009.

19. Nakamoto D, et al. "Active hexose correlated compound (AHCC) alleviates gemcitabine-induced hematological toxicity in non-tumor-bearing mice." *Int. J. Clin. Med.* 3, 361–367, 2012.

20. Shigama K, et al. "Alleviating effect of active hexose correlated compound (AHCC) for anti-cancer drug-induced side effects in non-tumor-bearing mice." *J. Exp. Therapeut. Oncol.* 8, 43–51, 2009.

21. Hirose A, et al. "The influence of active hexose correlated compound (AHCC) on cisplatin-evoked chemotherapeutic and side effects in tumor-bearing mice." *Toxicol. Appl. Pharmacol.* 222, 152–158, 2007.

22. Okada S, et al. "Phase I trial of gemcitabine in patients with advanced pancreatic cancer." *Jpn. J. Clin. Oncol.* 31, 7–12, 2001.

23. Lindley C, et al. "Perception of chemotherapy side effects cancer versus noncancer patients." *Cancer Pract.* 7, 59–65, 1999.

24. Jensen SB, et al. "Oral mucosal lesions, microbial changes, and taste disturbances induces by adjuvant chemotherapy in breast cancer patients." *Oral Surg. Oral Med. Oral Pathol. Oral Radiol. Endod.* 106, 217–226, 2008.

25. Ravasco P, et al. "Impact of nutrition on outcome: a prospective randomized controlled trial in patients with head and neck cancer undergoing radiotherapy." *Head Neck* 27, 659–668, 2005.

26. Brewin TB. "Can a tumor cause the same appetite perversion or taste change as a pregnancy?" *Lancet* 907–908, 1980.

27. DeWys WD. "Changes in taste sensation and feeding behavior in cancer patients: a review." *J. Hum. Nutr.* 32, 447–453, 1978.

28. Ripamonti C, et al. "A randomized, controlled clinical trial to evaluate the effects of zinc sulfate on cancer patients with taste alterations caused by head and neck irradiation." *Cancer,* 82, 1938–1945.

29. Hong JH, et al. "Taste and odor abnormalities in cancer patients." *J. Support Oncol* 7, 58–65, 2009.

30. McMillan DC, et al. "Evaluation of an inflammation-based prognostic score (GPS) in patients undergoing resection for colon and rectal cancer." *Int. J. Colorect. Dis.* 22, 881–886, 2007.

31. Proctor MJ, et al. "An inflammation-based prognostic score (mGPS) predicts cancer survival independent of tumour site: a Glasgow Inflammation Outcome Study." *Br. J. Cancer* 104, 726–734, 2011.

Chapter 6

INFECTIOUS DISEASE

Prevention of
Infectious Disease by Food

Anil D. Kulkarni

nfectious diseases are afflictions caused by organisms such as bacteria, viruses, fungi, or parasites. The human body has a variety of microflora, which are normally harmless or even beneficial. However, under certain conditions, some organisms cause diseases known as opportunistic infections. Infections can be transmitted person to person, and some are transmitted via vectors by bites from insects or animals. There are others that can be transmitted by ingesting contaminated foods and water or even from exposure to environmental organisms. Depending on the organisms causing infections, symptoms in the hosts vary.

Milder forms of infections may respond to rest with some household remedies while severe life-threatening infections may need hospitalization. Many infections can now be prevented by vaccinations and simple procedures of thorough hand washing and general good hygiene practices. Most common symptoms of infections are fever, diarrhea, coughing, fatigue, and muscle aches. If these symptoms persist, medical intervention is warranted. Clinical impressions, epidemiologic, and histopathologic evidence suggest that nutritional deficiencies may be present, which impair host resistance to infection and results in increased frequency and severity of infections.

Sepsis is still a major threat to critically ill and surgical patients. Over 50% of the patients who develop multiple organ failure will die, despite aggressive antibiotic and supportive therapy. To prevent infections caused by opportunistic pathogens represent major tasks in the management of immunocompromised hosts. Systemic involvement of opportunistic infections such as *Candida albicans* and *Staphylococcus aureus* are disastrous and generally fatal. There is overwhelming evidence that nutritionally compromised individuals are susceptible targets for sepsis and include cardiac and/ or organ transplant patients following surgery, patients following immunosuppressive and cancer therapy, or patients on long-term intravenous hyperalimentation. Mata (1978) reported that low birth weight infants suffered a higher incidence of infections. There are unexplained geographic differences that increase morbidity and mortality, such as kwashiorkor in Africa and marasmus in India. Fetal and neonatal malnutrition reflect the importance of nutrition and immunologic development.

Modern medicine has made giant strides in the treatment of infectious diseases. However, occurrences of resistance and adverse effects have led some people to turn to alternative medicine. In fact, in 1993, a national survey indicated that most Americans were using health-supporting methods that were not taught in any schools and medical colleges. This gave birth to what we now know as complementary and alternative medicine (CAM). The discipline of CAM is currently being applied and practiced in every medical field—especially with regard to cancer treatment and communicable disease prevention.

This methodology is not totally new. Most ancient medicine traditions around the world had some knowledge of what is now considered complementary therapy. India's Ayurvedic medicine had been practicing CAM methodology for thousands of years, and even today, it is the best approach known and available. As a result, many advanced research institutes around the world are embracing the teachings of Ayurveda. Some of the examples of Ayurvedic remedies include the use of turmeric powder (a source of curcumin) in everyday cooking as well as taking turmeric powder in milk before bedtime as a potent preventive method for the common cold, sore throat, and mild flulike symptoms. In addition, a combination of certain herbs and spices (including cloves, ginger, fennel seeds, and black pepper) is known as *Chai masala;* its use is popular, and it is one of the spice mixtures that is exported widely.

The Ayurvedic approach to health follows after determining an individual's constitution—i.e., *Prakriti* in Sanskrit. This type of diagnosis and therapeutic approach is known as *personalized medicine/therapy.* Depending on one's constitution (Kapha, Vata, and Pitta—conditions attributed to functions of organs such as the lungs, liver, and pancreas), a cold medicine prescription might include honey, while for another it might include lemon juice or ginger. Another example is using cranberry juice for urinary infections to keep urine at an acidic level to prevent or heal urinary tract infections.

The use of herbs and spices in Indian cooking not only serves as a preventive and alternative remedy, but it also preserves foods, which maintains the quality of food especially in tropical and subtropical countries where refrigeration is not so common and affordable.

A number of products have been purported to help fend off common illnesses, such cold or flu. While some of these substances appeared promising in early trials, follow-up studies may have had negative or inconclusive results. More research needs to be done. However, some nutritional supplements that have been studied for prevention or alleviation of symptoms and their duration include cranberry, garlic, ginseng, vitamin C, zinc, and Echinacea. Availability and reliability of such products vary from place to place.

Foods such as cabbage, carrots, coconut, curd, garlic, ginger, honey, lemon, onion, pineapple, turmeric, and horseradish are highly recommended and are consumed throughout Asia where they are considered a first line of defense in preventing infections and warding off many physiologic insults to the human body. A description of these foods is as follows:

- **Cabbage:** Cabbage is one of the most highly rated leafy vegetables and a marvelous food that possesses antibacterial powers.

- **Carrot:** The carrot, a popular vegetable, is a highly protective food. It is rich in the antioxidant beta-carotene as well as other beneficial ingredients. This vegetable is one of the most important infection-fighting foods.

- **Coconut:** The coconut is a near-perfect food, as it contains almost all the essential nutrients needed by the human body. The water of the tender green coconut, generally known as mineral water, is an antibacterial food and is especially valuable in fighting cholera infection.

- **Curd:** An ancient wonder food, curd (also called yogurt) is a strong antibacterial. During the curd-making process, bacteria convert the milk into curd by predigesting the milk protein. These bacteria then inhibit the growth of hostile or illness-causing bacteria in the intestinal tract and promote the beneficial bacteria needed for digestion.

- **Garlic:** A garden vegetable of the onion family, garlic has been cultivated from time immemorial. It is one of nature's strongest antibacterial foods. Tests show that garlic kills or cripples at least seventy-two infections spread by bacteria, including diarrhea, dysentery, tuberculosis, and encephalitis. It works as an antibiotic in various forms.

- **Ginger:** Ginger is a root vegetable and a spice. It is an antibiotic and helps fight infection. It has been used for centuries to treat many infectious diseases, including cholera, diarrhea, and chest congestion.

- **Honey:** Honey contains strong antibiotic property. It is very beneficial in the case of many infections. For example, for throat infection, gargling with honey water relieves inflammation.

- **Lemon:** An important citrus fruit, lemon is an excellent antibacterial food. Roasted lemon is a good remedy for throat infections.

- **Onion:** Onion is an exceptionally strong antibiotic and antiseptic food. It was used traditionally to treat wound-related infections.

- **Pineapple:** The pineapple is one of the best tropical fruits. This fruit, and its main constituent, bromelain, possess antibacterial activity.

- **Turmeric:** Turmeric is a common flavoring spice. It has antiseptic properties and is an effective remedy for cold, rhinitis, and throat infection. Half a teaspoon of fresh turmeric powder mixed in 30 milliliters of warm milk is a useful prescription for treating these conditions.

The above is just a sampling of how beneficial these foods are. Each has specific purposes and applications. As mentioned previously, herbs and spices also have significant value in preventive healthcare. Figure 1 at right shows the containers with several spices and herbs from household kitchen pantries in the Indian subcontinent that truly serve as "food as medicine." These are commonly used in Indian cuisine and other traditional dishes.

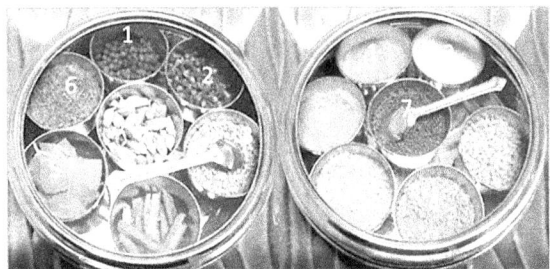

Figure 1. Left panel: 1-Black pepper, 2-Cloves, 3-Fennel seeds, 4-Cinnamon, 5-Bay leaves, 6-Cumin seeds, 7-Cardamum (center)

Right panel: 1-red pepper, 2-turmuric, 3-fenugreek seeds, 4-Cumin seeds, 5-Cumin-crushed, 6-Cumin powder, 7-Black mustard seeds (center)

In addition to the above-mentioned foods, other herbs, spices, fruits, and berries have powerful infection- and disease-fighting effects. According to a study by the U.S. Department of Agriculture, blueberries top the list of antioxidant-rich fruits, followed by cranberries, blackberries, raspberries, and strawberries. Lychees also possess exceptional antioxidant properties that help neutralize cell-damaging molecules called *free radicals,* which may lead to chronic diseases.

REFERENCES AND ADDITIONAL READING MATERIAL

Weil A. "Anti-Inflammatory-Food-Pyramid" http://www.dr.weil.com/drw/u/ART02995/Dr-Weil-Anti-Inflammatory-Food-Pyramid.html

Carlsen MH et al. "The total antioxidant content of more than 3100 foods, beverages, spices, herbs and supplements used worldwide." *Nutrition Journal* 9:3, 2010.

Chandra RK. "The nutrition-immunity-infection nexis: The enumeration and functional assessment of lymphocyte subsets in nutritional deficiency." *Nutr. Res.* ; 3:605-615, 1983.

Mata LJ. "Diseases and Disabilities." In: *Children of Santa Maria Cauque: A prospective field study of health and growth. Int. Nutrition Policy Ser.* No.2, (L.J. Mata, ed.), MIT Press, Cambridge, Massachusetts (1978), pp. 254–292.

Protective Effects of AHCC Against Epidemic Diseases

Shigeru Abe, Shigeru Tansho-Nagakawa, Kazumi Hayama

In 2003, we compiled the results of mice-model studies as a review article in the book "AHCC: Basic and Clinical Practice," showing the systemic preventive efficacy of AHCC against opportunistic infections.[1] In the lethal candida infection murine model, when *Candida albicans* was intravenously injected into mice pre-treated with *cyclophosphamide* to reduce neutrophils, an oral pretreatment of AHCC resulted in significantly extended survival period. In the study, the daily effective dose of AHCC was 1,000 mg/kg, at which the four-day consecutive administration of AHCC prior to the infection obviously showed the prophylactic effect. However, the oral administration of AHCC at 10 or 100 mg/kg, which is the intraperitoneal effective dose, exerted no significant efficacy.[2]

The preventive effect of AHCC was also confirmed against the infection by *Pseudomonas aeruginosa,* which is a representative type of bacteria responsible for opportunistic infections.[2] The oral administration of AHCC at 1,000 mg/kg contributed to the protection from lethal pseudomonal infection in cyclophosphamide-treated neutropenic mice, although there was no statistically significant efficacy at 300 mg/kg.

Using the various models of systemic lethal infection mice, Sonnenfeld's group demonstrated the infection preventive ability of AHCC.[3] In the murine experiment subjected to space stress, the oral administration of 1,000 mg/kg AHCC decreased the mortality from *Klebsiella pneumoniae* infection and increased the survival time. It was found that the mice, which ultimately survived the lethal infection by administering AHCC, recovered the immunity and had a low rate of bacteria detection in blood.[4] Moreover, the research group investigated the effect of oral administration of AHCC in the food-deprivation model used as a surgical-stress model. The result indicated that AHCC increased the 50% lethal infectious dose (LD_{50}) of *Klebsiella pneumoniae* and exhibited the phylactic activity.[5]

The Defense Mechanism of AHCC Against Infections and the Conditions Necessary to Exert the Efficacy in Bacterial and Fungal Systemic Infection Models

Thus far, there have been no reports showing that AHCC can directly inhibit proliferation of microorganisms and possesses bactericidal activities. It is thought that AHCC is able to show protective actions against infection via the host defense mechanism. Corresponding to the consideration, it is evident that the four- to seven-day oral pretreatment with AHCC is necessary to induce the phylactic activity. Furthermore, the efficacy of AHCC might depend on a kind of treatment to suppress the host defense capacity.[6]

Ikeda et al. reported that in the lethal infection model of intravenously injected *C. albicans*, the phylactic activity strength of intraperitoneally administered AHCC

TABLE 1. PROTECTIVE EFFECT OF INTRAPERITONEAL ADMINITRATION OF AHCC ON *CANDIDA ALBICANS* INFECTION IN IMMUNOSUPPRESSED MICE

Survival days[b]	Survival rate (%)	CONTROL		AHCC		Inoculum rate (%)[a]
		Survival Days	Mean Survival (days)	Δ With	Mean Treated size	
—	1×10^6	0/5 (0)	6.20±0.9	0/4 (0)	11.25±1.6	5.1
CY	1×10^5	0/10 (0)	2.80±0.6	10/10(100)	14.00±0	11.2
5-FU	2×10^5	0/8 (0)	3.13±0.1	4/8 (50)	12.00±0	8.9
DXR	2×10^5	0/8 (0)	4.75±1.1	0/8 (0)	7.38±1.5	2.6
PS	5×10^4	0/4 (0)	7.0±0	0/4(0)	6.25±0.8	−0.8

Details of treatment with CY, 5-FU, DXR, or PS, administration of AHCC, and inoculation of *C. albicans* are described in "Materials and Methods."

a : survival mice/tested mice at day 14.

b : mean survival days were calculated from survival days of all tested mice including surviors at day 14. Data represent means ± SD.

Δ : increase of life span by AHCC treatment (days).

was lowered in order of cyclophosphamide-, 5-fluorouracil-, vehicle-, and doxorubicin-treated mice as shown in Table 1. Particularly, an anti-inflammatory steroid, prednisolone, abolished the effect of AHCC. Since AHCC administration simultaneously improved neutropenia caused by cyclophosphamide, it was deduced that the preventive effect on infection might partially be attributable to an amelioration of neutrophil function.[6] Enhancement of leukocyte proliferation and cytokine production was also observed in the AHCC-treated mice.[4] Treatment with anti-inflammatory steroid might diminish the efficacy of AHCC, because the treatment potently suppressed cytokine production. Besides, in the systemic infection models, a clearance ability of infecting bacteria from blood is strongly relevant to the resistance to infection, and it was suggested that the recovery effect for leukocytes, including neutrophils, might be recognized as a main action of AHCC.[4,6]

Effect of AHCC Against Bacterial and Fungal Infections in Local Infection Models

Many people are suffering from microbial local infections as well as lethal systemic infections. The potency of AHCC was evaluated using an experimental model on vaginal candidiasis, which is one of the most common female genital infections. When AHCC and UREX (mixture of *Lactobacillus rhamnosus* GR-1 and *Lactobacillus reuteri* RC-14, from Chr Hansen A/S, Denmark) were mixed with rodent chow and the mixture was given to mice in the vaginal infection model, the result suggested that the combined treatment improved vaginal candidiasis worsened by cyclophosphamide.[7] Further, it was investigated whether the combination of AHCC and UREX was effective against coliform urinary tract infection. Consequently, although UREX alone did not significantly reduce the viable coliform number in the bladder, the combination with AHCC lowered the detection rate of bacteria as shown in Figure 1 on the following page.[8] The interesting thing about this experiment was the natural intake method of AHCC from the mouth by mixing with rodent chow but not by gavage using a tube.

Belay et al. have recently reported the efficacy of AHCC oral administration using a cold stress-induced murine model of genital *Chlamydia trachomatis* infection.[9] After chlamydia intravaginal infection, the fourteen-day administration of AHCC at 700 mg/kg suppressed the reduction of body weight and significantly decreased the viable chlamydia count in genital tracts at day eighteen. They concluded that the increased production of cytokine was associated with the preventive effect because of an enhancement of TNF-α and IFN-γ production in murine abdominal cells. It is

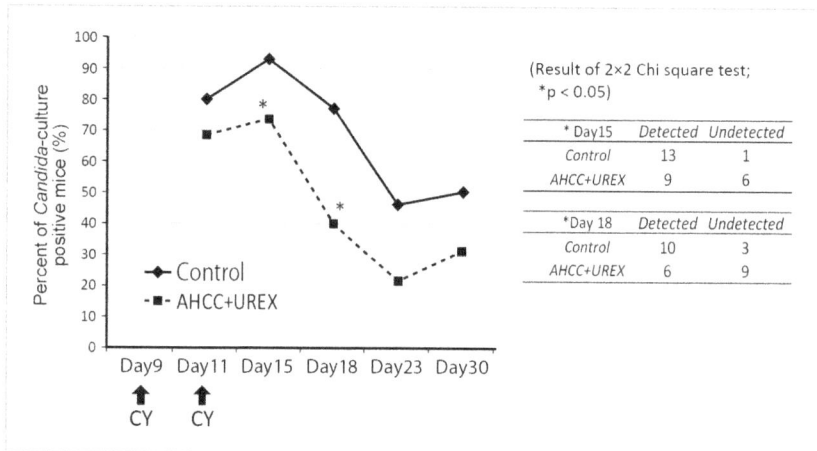

* Day15	Detected	Undetected
Control	13	1
AHCC+UREX	9	6

*Day 18	Detected	Undetected
Control	10	3
AHCC+UREX	6	9

(Result of 2×2 Chi square test; *p < 0.05)

Figure 1. Oral intake of AHCC and UREX facilitated the exclusion of *Candida* cells from vaginal cavities of the mice with vaginal candidiasis.

noteworthy that the protective activity of AHCC oral administration against various local infections contributes to the prevention from mild infection diseases that are commonly experienced.

Preventive Efficacy of AHCC Against Viral Infections

The effects of AHCC on viral infections have been reported not only in murine models,[10,11,12] but also in humans with respect to vaccination-induced enhancement of antibody production.[13] In 2009, Wang et al. reported that AHCC enhanced host resistance to West Nile encephalitis in mice.[11] When 600 mg/kg AHCC was administered to mice for one week prior to infection, the treatment resulted in prolonged survival and elevated production of antibody to virus as well as increased γδ T cells. Interestingly, these benefits were obviously observed in younger mice.

Moreover, Nogusa et al. assessed the effect of AHCC on the immune response in a mouse model of influenza A virus infection.[12] In spite of a low-dose supplementation compared to previous studies, 100 mg/kg of AHCC promoted virus clearance, reduced the loss of body weight, and potentiated the lytic efficacy of natural killer (NK) cells in splenocytes. While 1,000 mg/kg of AHCC had already been found to up-regulate NK cell activity, the similar effect was exerted by lower dosages of AHCC.

Gardner's group conducted a clinical study using a limited number of subjects, based on the underlying results from animal experiments. After healthy subjects received vaccination, intake of 3 g/day AHCC increased CD8+ T cells and significantly augmented blood-protective antibody titers to influenza B virus as shown Figure 2 below.[13] These results suggest that AHCC might potentially show the protective effect against influenza infection in humans as well as in rodents. However, there was no significant difference in antibody titer and production rates of influenza A between the AHCC and control groups. By considering the subjects in the test were older (>60 years old), the subjects might be able to produce good level of influenza A virus antibody so the difference was not significant between AHCC and control groups. The dose of 3 g/day AHCC can be converted to 50 mg/kg in a human with 60 kg body weight. It is at least significant that 3 g/day of AHCC is potent against viral infections. Although there is a discrepancy between rodents and humans in terms of the effective dosage, it is not questionable that a similar trend is found in Chinese traditional medicine containing herbal components.

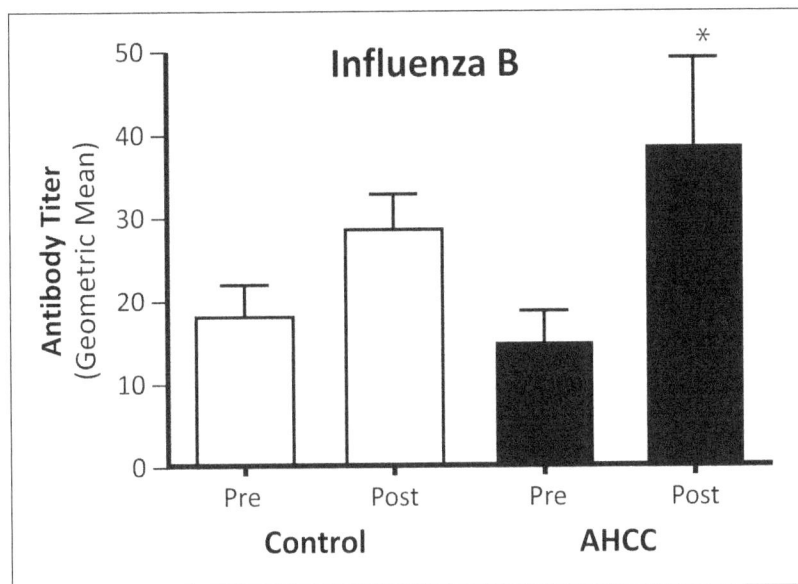

Figure 2. Increase of antibody titer to influenza B virus was significantly enhanced with AHCC administration compared with control group.

Summary

Oral administration of AHCC exerts a protective effect against bacterial and fungal local infections in addition to systemic infections. The preventive ability is particularly enhanced in the immunocompromised host. The protective effect of AHCC is also shown for viral infections. The effective dose for mice in the short-term administration is as high as 1,000 mg/kg; however, for humans, the dosage of 3 g/day is expected to be effective.

REFERENCES

1. Abe S, Ishibashi H, Ikeda T, Tansho S, and Yamaguchi H. "AHCC: basic and clinical practice: preventive efficacy against opportunistic infections." [Article in Japanese] *Life Science* 140–146, 2003.

2. Ishibashi H, Ikeda T, Tansho S, Ono Y, Yamazaki M, Sato A, Yamaoka K, Yamaguchi H, and Abe S. "Prophylactic efficacy of a basidiomycetes preparation AHCC against lethal opportunistic infections in mice." [Article in Japanese] *Yakugaku Zasshi* 120(8): 715–719, 2000.

3. Aviles H, Belay T, Fountain K, Vance M, Sun B, and Sonnenfeld G. "Active hexose correlated compound enhances resistance to *Klebsiella pneumoniae* infection in mice in the hindlimb-unloading model of spaceflight conditions." *J. Appl. Physiol.* 95(2): 491–6, 2003. Epub 2003 Apr 11.

4. Aviles H, Belay T, Vance M, Sun B, and Sonnenfeld G. "Active hexose correlated compound enhances the immune function of mice in the hindlimb-unloading model of spaceflight conditions." *J. Appl. Physiol.* 97(4): 1437–44, 2004. Epub 2004 Jun 11.

5. Aviles H, O'Donnell P, Sun B, and Sonnenfeld G. "Active hexose correlated compound (AHCC) enhances resistance to infection in a mouse model of surgical wound infection." *Surg. Infect.* (Larchmt) 7(6): 527–35, 2006.

6. Ikeda T, Ishibashi H, Fujisaki R, Yamazaki M, Wakame K, Kosuna K, Yamaguchi H, Ono Y, and Abe S. "Prophylactic efficacy of a basidiomycetes preparation AHCC against lethal *Candida albicans* infection in experimental granulocytopenic mice." [Article in Japanese] *Nihon Ishinkin Gakkai Zasshi* 44(2): 127–131, 2003.

7. Hayama K, Yamazaki M, and Abe S. "Protective activity of combination of AHCC and UREX against murine vaginal candidiasis." ICNIM2012 abstract p54.

8. Hayama K, Yamazaki M, and Abe S. "Protective activity of combination of AHCC and UREX against murine urinary tract infection." ICNIM2013 abstract p79.

9. Belay T, Chuh-lung, and Woart A. "Active hexose correlated compound activates immune function to decrease *Chlamydia trachomatis* shedding in a murine stress model." *J. Nutri. Med. Diet Care* 1: 1, 2015.

10. Ritz BW, Nogusa S, Ackerman EA, and Gardner EM. "Supplementation with active hexose correlated compound increases the innate immune response of young mice to primary influenza infection." *J. Nutr.* 136(11): 2868–73, 2006.

11. Wang S, Welte T, Fang H, Chang GJ, Born WK, O'Brien RL, Sun B, Fujii H, Kosuna K, and Wang T. "Oral administration of active hexose correlated compound enhances host resistance to West Nile encephalitis in mice." *J. Nutr.* 139(3): 598–602, 2009. doi:10.3945/jn.108.100297. Epub 2009 Jan 13.

12. Nogusa S, Gerbino J, and Ritz BW. "Low-dose supplementation with active hexose correlated compound improves the immune response to acute influenza infection in C57BL/6 mice." *Nutr. Res.* 29(2): 139–143, 2009. doi:10.1016/j.nutres.2009.01.005.

13. Roman BE, Beli E, Duriancik DM, and Gardner EM. "Short-term supplementation with active hexose correlated compound improves the antibody response to influenza B vaccine." *Nutr. Res.* 33(1): 12–7, 2013. doi:10.1016/j.nutres.2012.11.001. Epub 2012 Dec 4.

An Antisense Transcript-Mediated Mechanism Is Involved in the AHCC-Mediated Suppression of Inducible Nitric Oxide Synthase Expression

Mikio Nishizawa

Inducible nitric oxide synthase (iNOS, also known as NOS2) in hepatocytes and Kupffer cells (resident macrophages) in the liver synthesize the inflammatory mediator nitric oxide (NO), which is involved in the pathophysiology of various hepatic diseases. The prognosis of postoperative hepatocellular carcinoma patients was improved by supplementation with AHCC.[1] From these data, we speculated that AHCC has a certain relationship with the expression of the iNOS gene in the liver. We found that AHCC suppressed iNOS gene expression in rat hepatocytes. In addition, we found natural antisense transcripts transcribed from the iNOS gene and a post-transcriptional regulation mechanism mediated by iNOS asRNAs.

Antisense transcripts (asRNAs) are frequently transcribed from mammalian genes, and each asRNA has the same sequence as that of the complementary (antisense) strand to the mRNA (sense) strand[2,3] (see Figure 1 on the following page). Because most asRNAs do not encode proteins, asRNAs are classified as non-coding RNAs (ncRNAs) or long non-coding RNAs (lncRNAs).[4] Recently, the functional importance of asRNA in the regulation of inducible gene expression has been clarified—for example, asRNAs from the interferon-α1 gene[5] and tumor necrosis factor-α gene.[6] A low-copy-number asRNA hybridizes to *cis*-controlling elements of the mRNA, resulting in the modulation of mRNA stability.[7] As a regulatory RNA, asRNAs may post-transcriptionally regulate gene expression through *cis*-controlling elements on the mRNA.[7,8]

The expression of the iNOS gene is induced in response to interleukin-1β (IL-1β) in rat hepatocytes.[9,10] When AHCC was added to the media used to culture hepatocytes, the iNOS mRNA, iNOS protein, and NO levels all decreased.[11] Then, luciferase assays were performed using two constructs harboring the firefly luciferase (*Luc*) gene driven by the iNOS gene promoter.[11] One construct (iNOS promoter–*Luc*–SVpA) contained the SV40 polyadenylation site (SVpA), which most reporter constructs harbor to terminate transcription. Unexpectedly, AHCC did not reduce luciferase activity when the hepatocytes were transfected with this construct. When we used the other construct (iNOS promoter–*Luc*–3'UTR), in which SVpA was replaced with the 3'-untranslated region (3'UTR) of iNOS mRNA, AHCC decreased the luciferase activity.[11] These results imply that the iNOS 3'UTR may be involved in iNOS mRNA stability and that AHCC may destabilize iNOS mRNA through its 3'UTR. In the iNOS 3'UTR, there are several adenosine and uridine-rich elements (AREs; 5'-AUUUA-3' or 5'-AUUUUA-3'), which are *cis*-controlling elements involved in mRNA stability.[12]

Next, we found that the antisense strand corresponding to the 3'UTR of iNOS mRNA was transcribed from the iNOS gene in IL-1β-treated rat hepatocytes[13] (see Figure 1 below). iNOS asRNA was also detected in the livers of sepsis model rats.[14] Human and mouse iNOS asRNAs harbor sequences complementary to the 3'UTRs

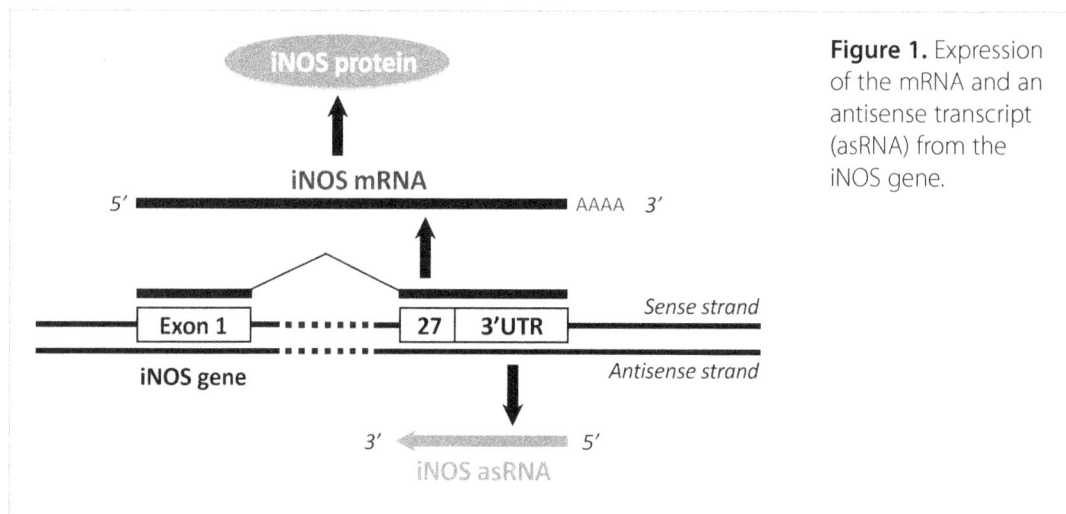

Figure 1. Expression of the mRNA and an antisense transcript (asRNA) from the iNOS gene.

The iNOS gene (human, rat, and mouse) consists of 27 exons. Exon 27 contains the 3'-untranslated region (3'UTR). The mRNA transcribed from the iNOS gene has the same sequence of the sense strand, which encodes the iNOS protein. In contrast, iNOS asRNA has the same sequence of the antisense strand of the gene and does not encode any protein. The 3'UTR of iNOS mRNA overlaps with iNOS asRNA and is the site of the mRNA–asRNA interactions.

of their respective iNOS mRNAs.[15,16] The analysis of these sequences indicated that iNOS asRNAs are conserved among rats, mice, and humans.[16] In humans, iNOS asRNA is expressed in hepatocarcinoma and colon carcinoma tissues.[16]

The expression levels of iNOS asRNA are positively correlated with those of iNOS mRNA, and the stability of iNOS mRNA changes during the stimulation of rat hepatocytes by IL-1β.[13] These results imply that like AHCC, iNOS asRNA may be involved in the stability of iNOS mRNA. Furthermore, many drugs or compounds with anti-inflammatory activities affect the asRNA levels. For example, edaravone, a free radical scavenger,[15] *saireito*, a formula used in Japanese kampo medicine,[17] shisoflavanone A, a constituent of perilla leaves,[18] and flavanol-rich lychee fruit extract (Oligonol), a functional food,[19] decreased the levels of both iNOS mRNA and iNOS asRNA.

To determine how iNOS asRNA affects iNOS gene expression, we performed two experiments in which we overexpressed iNOS asRNA and introduced sense oligonucleotides (*i.e.*, short DNA). To assess the mRNA stability, we used a luciferase construct (*EF* promoter–*Luc*–3′UTR) that was driven by a constitutive promoter (elongation factor-1α [*EF*] gene promoter) and that harbored iNOS 3′UTR.[13] When iNOS asRNA was overexpressed in hepatocytes, it stabilized the mRNA transcribed from this construct, suggesting that iNOS asRNA may stabilize iNOS mRNA through its 3′UTR. In contrast, when the sense oligonucleotides, which had the same sequences as the 3′UTR of iNOS mRNA, were introduced to hepatocytes, these sense oligonucleotides specifically reduced the levels of iNOS mRNA.[13,16] These results implied that the sense oligonucleotides may block the interactions between iNOS mRNA and iNOS asRNA (see Figure 2 on the following page). Taken together, these findings indicate that iNOS asRNA interacts with the 3′UTR of iNOS mRNA to stabilize iNOS mRNA.

This mRNA–asRNA interaction could be a new therapeutic target for diseases involving inflammation by reducing iNOS mRNA levels if AHCC interferes with this interaction in a manner similar to that of sense oligonucleotides. Indeed, the herbal flavonoid epigallocatechin gallate (EGCG) directly binds to RNA,[20] and apigenin (*i.e.*, hydroxylated flavone) can bind RNA with high affinity.[21] Furthermore, acetylpromazine, a phenothiazine derivative that is used as a psychotropic drug, specifically binds to the transactivation-responsive (TAR) RNA and alters its three-dimensional structure, thereby inhibiting the access of Tat protein to the TAR.[22,23] If AHCC or its constituents bind to iNOS mRNA and/or asRNA, this interaction may interfere with the interactions between mRNA and asRNA as well as those between mRNA and microRNA (see Figure 2 on the following page). If so, AHCC or its constituents may

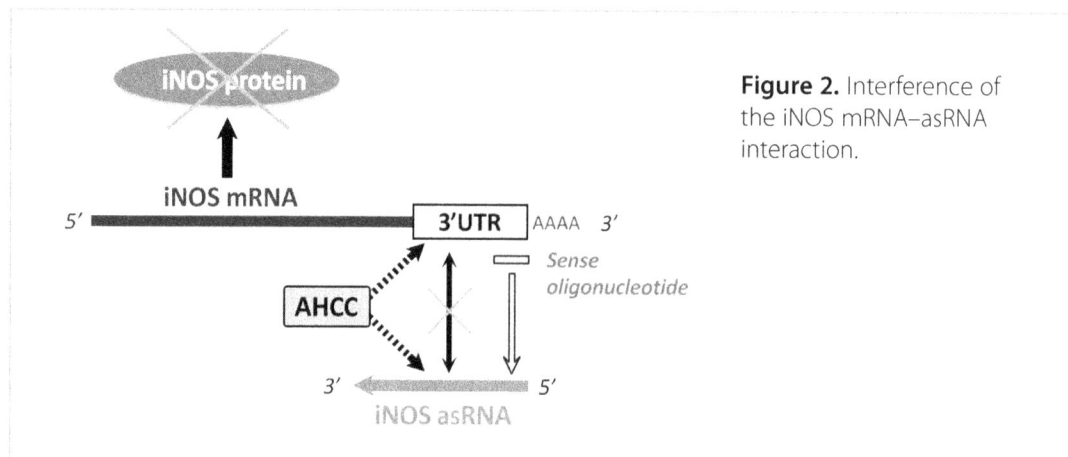

Figure 2. Interference of the iNOS mRNA–asRNA interaction.

A model of mechanisms to reduce the stability of iNOS mRNA is schematically depicted. iNOS asRNA interacts with the 3'-untranslated region (3'UTR) of iNOS mRNA to stabilize the iNOS mRNA (black double-headed arrow). A sense oligonucleotide, which has the same sequence as the mRNA, hybridizes with iNOS asRNA (outlined arrow) to compete with iNOS mRNA. AHCC interferes with the interaction (small cross) by binding to the iNOS mRNA and the asRNA (dashed arrows). The sense oligonucleotide or possibly AHCC interferes with the mRNA-asRNA interaction and then destabilizes the iNOS mRNA, thereby decreasing the iNOS protein (large cross).

reduce iNOS mRNA expression by decreasing mRNA stability. Although adenosine suppresses NO production in IL-1β-treated hepatocytes,[24] adenosine does not seem to bind to RNA. Because it is unknown which constituent is responsible for the interaction between iNOS mRNA and the asRNA, the AHCC–RNA interactions require future investigation. However, AHCC or its constituents could potentially be used to treat human diseases that involve inflammation. Therefore, the bioactive constituents of AHCC should be pharmacologically analyzed and identified in the future.

The author of this section thanks Drs. Yasuo Kamiyama, Tadayoshi Okumura, Tominori Kimura, and Yukinobu Ikeya for their invaluable comments, and Ms. Noriko Kanazawa for her secretarial assistance.

REFERENCES

1. Matsui Y, Uhara J, Satoi S, Kaibori M, Yamada H, Kitade H, Imamura A, Takai S, Kawaguchi Y, Kwon AH, and Kamiyama Y. "Improved prognosis of postoperative hepatocellular carcinoma patients when treated with functional foods: a prospective cohort study." *J. Hepatol.* 37: 78–86, 2002.

2. Katayama S, Tomaru Y, Kasukawa T, Waki K, Nakanishi M, Nakamura M, Nishida H, Yap CC, Suzuki M, Kawai J, Suzuki H, Carninci P, Hayashizaki Y, Wells C, Frith M, Ravasi T, Pang KC, Hallinan J, Mattick J, Hume DA, Lipovich L, Batalov S, Engström PG, Mizuno Y, Faghihi MA, Sandelin A, Chalk AM, Mottagui-Tabar S, Liang Z, Lenhard B, Wahlestedt C; RIKEN Genome Exploration Research Group; Genome Science Group (Genome Network Project Core Group); and FANTOM Consortium. "Antisense transcription in the mammalian transcriptome." *Science* 309: 1564–1566, 2005.

3. Kiyosawa H, Yamanaka I, Osato N, Kondo S, and Hayashizaki Y. "Antisense transcripts with FANTOM2 clone set and their implications for gene regulation." *Genome Res.* 13: 1324–1334, 2003.

4. Kapranov P, Cheng J, Dike S, Nix DA, Duttagupta R, Willingham AT, Stadler PF, Hertel J, Hackermüller J, Hofacker IL, Bell I, Cheung E, Drenkow J, Dumais E, Patel S, Helt G, Ganesh M, Ghosh S, Piccolboni A, Sementchenko V, Tammana H, and Gingeras TR. "RNA maps reveal new RNA classes and a possible function for pervasive transcription." *Science* 316: 1484–1488, 2007.

5. Kimura T, Jiang S, Nishizawa M, Yoshigai E, Hashimoto I, Nishikawa M, Okumura T, and Yamada H. "Stabilization of human interferon-α1 mRNA by its antisense RNA." *Cell. Mol. Life Sci.* 70: 1451–1467, 2013.

6. Yoshigai E, Hara T, Inaba H, Hashimoto I, Tanaka Y, Kaibori M, Kimura T, Okumura T, Kwon AH, and Nishizawa M. "Interleukin-1β induces tumor necrosis factor-α secretion from rat hepatocytes." *Hepatol. Res.* 44: 571–583, 2014.

7. Nishizawa M, Ikeya Y, Okumura T, and Kimura T. "Post-transcriptional inducible gene regulation by natural antisense RNA." *Front. Biosci. (Landmark Ed).* 20: 1–36, 2015.

8. Nishizawa M and Kimura T. "RNA networks that regulate mRNA expression and their potential as drug targets." *RNA & Disease* 3 (1): e864, 2016. doi:10.14800/rd.864.

9. Kitade H, Sakitani K, Inoue K, Masu Y, Kawada N, Hiramatsu Y, Kamiyama Y, Okumura T, and Ito S. "Interleukin 1β markedly stimulates nitric oxide formation in the absence of other cytokines or lipopolysaccharide in primary cultured rat hepatocytes but not in Kupffer cells." *Hepatology* 23: 797–802, 1996.

10. Pautz A, Art J, Hahn S, Nowag S, Voss C, and Kleinert H. "Regulation of the expression of inducible nitric oxide synthase." *Nitric Oxide* 23: 75–93, 2010.

11. Matsui K, Kawaguchi Y, Ozaki T, Tokuhara K, Tanaka H, Kaibori M, Matsui Y, Kamiyama Y, Wakame K, Miura T, Nishizawa M, and Okumura T. "Effect of active hexose correlated compound on the production of nitric oxide in hepatocytes." *JPEN J. Parenter. Enteral Nutr.* 31: 373–380, 2007.

12. Caput D, Beutler B, Hartog K, Thayer R, Brown-Shimer S, and Cerami A. "Identification of a common nucleotide sequence in the 3'-untranslated region of mRNA molecules specifying inflammatory mediators." *Proc. Natl. Acad. Sci. USA.* 83: 1670–1674, 1986.

13. Matsui K, Nishizawa M, Ozaki T, Kimura T, Hashimoto I, Yamada M, Kaibori M, Kamiyama Y, Ito S, and Okumura T. "Natural antisense transcript stabilizes inducible nitric oxide synthase messenger RNA in rat hepatocytes." *Hepatology.* 47: 686–697, 2008.

14. Tanaka H, Uchida Y, Kaibori M, Hijikawa T, Ishizaki M, Yamada M, Matsui K, Ozaki T, Tokuhara K, Kamiyama Y, Nishizawa M, Ito S, and Okumura T. "Na$^+$/H$^+$ exchanger inhibitor, FR183998, has protective effect in lethal acute liver failure and prevents iNOS induction in rats." *J. Hepatol.* 48: 289–299, 2008.

15. Yoshida H, Kwon AH, Habara K, Yamada M, Kaibori M, Kamiyama Y, Nishizawa M, Ito S, and Okumura T. "Edaravone inhibits the induction of iNOS gene expression at transcriptional and posttranscriptional steps in murine macrophages." *Shock* 30: 734–739, 2008.

16. Yoshigai E, Hara T, Araki Y, Tanaka Y, Oishi M, Tokuhara K, Kaibori M, Okumura T, Kwon AH, and Nishizawa M. "Natural antisense transcript-targeted regulation of inducible nitric oxide synthase mRNA levels." *Nitric Oxide* 30: 9–16, 2013.

17. Miki H, Tokuhara K, Oishi M, Nakatake R, Tanaka Y, Kaibori M, Nishizawa M, Okumura T, and Kon M. "Japanese kampo saireito has a liver-protective effect through the inhibition of inducible nitric oxide synthase induction in primary cultured rat hepatocytes." *JPEN J. Parenter. Enteral Nutr.* 40: 1033–1041, 2016.

18. Nakajima A, Yamamoto Y, Yoshinaka N, Namba M, Matsuo H, Okuyama T, Yoshigai E, Okumura T, Nishizawa M, and Ikeya Y. "A new flavanone and other flavonoids from green perilla leaf extract inhibit nitric oxide production in interleukin 1β-treated hepatocytes." *Biosci. Biotechnol. Biochem.* 79: 138–146, 2015.

19. Yamanishi R, Yoshigai E, Okuyama T, Mori M, Murase H, Machida T, Okumura T, and Nishizawa M. "The anti-inflammatory effects of flavanol-rich lychee fruit extract in rat hepatocytes." *PLoS One* 9: e93818, 2014.

20. Kuzuhara T, Sei Y, Yamaguchi K, Suganuma M, and Fujiki H. "DNA and RNA as new binding targets of green tea catechins." *J. Biol. Chem.* 281: 17446–17456, 2006.

21. Nafisi S, Shadaloi A, Feizbakhsh A, and Tajmir-Riahi HA. "RNA binding to antioxidant flavonoids." *J. Photochem. Photobiol. B.* 94: 1–7, 2009.

22. Lind KE, Du Z, Fujinaga K, Peterlin BM, and James TL. "Structure-based computational database screening, in vitro assay, and NMR assessment of compounds that target TAR RNA." *Chem. Biol.* 9: 185–193, 2002.

23. Du Z, Lind KE, and James TL. "Structure of TAR RNA complexed with a Tat-TAR inter-action nanomolar inhibitor that was identified by computational screening." *Chem. Biol.* 9: 707–712, 2002.

24. Tanaka Y, Ohashi S, Ohtsuki A, Kiyono T, Park EY, Nakamura Y, Sato K, Oishi M, Miki H, Tokuhara K, Matsui K, Kaibori M, Nishizawa M, Okumura T, and Kwon AH. "Adenosine, a hepato-protective component in active hexose correlated compound: its identification and iNOS suppression mechanism." *Nitric Oxide* 40: 75–86, 2014.

Interferon Antisense RNA and AHCC

Tominori Kimura

Innate immunity and adaptive immunity work in coordination when the biological defense system is activated by viral infections. Although the innate immunity possesses neither specificity nor memory against infections, the immediate response plays a critical role in the initial defensive capacity against a wide variety of infections. Type I interferon (IFN) is a cytokine that has a central function of antiviral activity in the innate immune system. It is transiently secreted through viral infection and exerts a potent antiviral action interacting with the surrounding cells.[1]

The fact mentioned above, along with the previous reports that the excessive production of IFN causes various autoimmune responses, suggests that it is necessary for mRNA of IFN gene to be transcribed, translated, converted to protein, and decomposed within a very short time following viral infection. Hence, there is a high interest in the control mechanism of the mRNA stability throughout all these fast processes. In our laboratory, we have been studying mRNA of IFN-α1 gene, which is one of the IFN-α group and is a master gene whose expression is induced first just after viral infection, in order to elucidate how the mRNA stability is regulated when the mRNA is translocated from nucleus to cytoplasm where the translation takes place. Consequently, we have reported that endogenous antisense RNA, which is transcribed from the reverse strand of IFN-α1 gene (IFN-α1 AS RNA), is involved in regulation of the mRNA stability.[2,3]

We found that there are two ways of the mechanism to stabilize the target mRNA via the antisense RNA.

1. First, IFN-α1 AS RNA directly stabilizes the mRNA by forming a double-stranded RNA structure with a single-stranded region within a conserved secondary structure element or CSS consisting with a protein code region of the IFN-α1 mRNA.[2]

116

2. Second, the AS RNA shares the microRNA-1270 (miR-1270) response elements (MRE-1270) with IFN-α1 mRNA. Interactions between IFN-α1 AS RNA and miR-1270 through the response elements would, therefore, titrate away miR-1270 from IFN-α1 mRNA, suggesting that the AS RNA acts as an endogenous decoy or competing endogenous RNA (ceRNA) for IFN-α1 mRNA.[3]

Moreover, there are five types of cellular mRNA composed of IFN-α1 AS RNA, other IFN-α mRNAs, other IFN-α AS RNAs, and other cellular mRNAs, which show the ceRNA effect against miR-1270, and then mutually cooperate and form a network to elicit anti-microRNA efficacy (see Figure 1 below).[3] Based on these observations, we proposed to be able to discover RNA target drugs, which are capable of controlling the mRNA expression regulated by ceRNA and the expression of coded protein, resulting from mutually targeting the constituent molecules of ceRNA network to function as decoy RNA.[4]

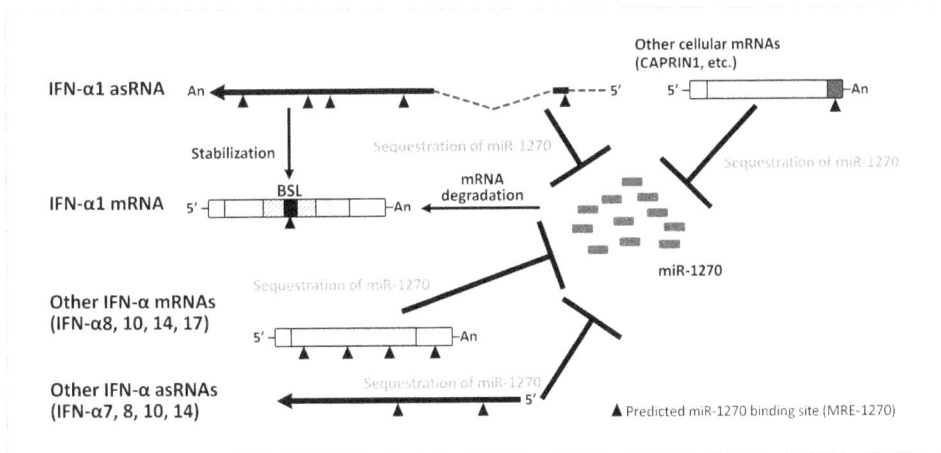

Figure 1. Model for an IFN-a ceRNA network against miR-1270.**Note:** This figure is reproduced from Kimura T., et al., *Cell Mol. Life Sci.*, 2015, 72(14).

AHCC is known to inhibit the expression of cytokine gene mRNA including iNOS mRNA in a post-transcriptional manner.[5,6] Since this inhibition is attributed to suppressing the expression of AS RNA against the mRNA by AHCC (Nisizawa et al., unpublished), we investigated the regulatory effect of AHCC on the expression of IFN-α1 mRNA categorized into early response genes. As a result, in accord with the previous reports from Matsui et al.,[5,6] it was proven that AHCC inhibits the expression of IFN-α1 AS RNA, resulting in reduction of the mRNA and protein expression levels through losing the mRNA stability (see Figure 2 below).[2] Because these results showed that AHCC has the passive ability to exert innate antiviral response in the host, we decided to discontinue these experiments at this stage in our laboratory.

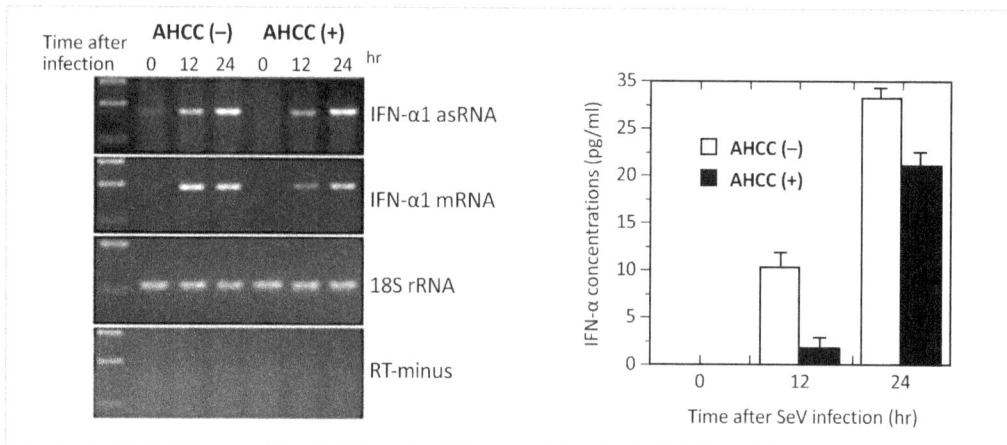

Figure 2. AHCC reduced IFN-α1 asRNA levels, leading to lower IFN-α1 mRNA (left) protein levels (right).Note: This figure is reproduced from Kimura T., et al., *Cell Mol. Life Sci.*, 2013, 70(8).

However, at the 23rd International Congress on Nutrition and Integrative Medicine (ICNIM) in July 2015, the research group of Dr. Smith of the University of Texas presented similar results from the clinical trial using the subjects supplemented with AHCC. Interestingly, when AHCC was treated to investigate the antiviral efficacy against types 16 and 18 of human papillomavirus (HPV) responsible for cervical cancer, the result demonstrated that AHCC inhibited the expression of type I IFN and significantly eradicated HPV16/18 in the patients, showing inverse correlation (Smith et al., AHCC for potential treatment of high risk HPV infections. p16, ICNIM2015 Program & Abstracts). The full publication of the clinical results may give us a better insight for the paradoxical relationship between the suppressive effect of AHCC on the innate antivirus immune response and the anti-HPV efficacy in the clinical setting. However, we cannot rule out the possibility that the effect of AHCC against cancer-causing viruses could be added to the various biological efficacies exerted by AHCC.

REFERENCES

1. He XS, et al. "Differential transcriptional responses to interferon-α and Iiterferon-γ in primary human hepatocytes." *J. Interferon Cytokine Res.* 30(5), 311–320, 2010.

2. Kimura T, et al. "Stabilization of human interferon-α1 mRNA by its antisense RNA." *Cell Mol. Life Sci.* 70(8), 1451–1467, 2013.

3. Kimura T, et al. "Interferon-alpha competing endogenous RNA network antagonizes microRNA-1270." *Cell Mol. Life Sci.* 72(14), 2749–2761, 2015.

4. Nishizawa M, et al. "RNA Networks that Regulate mRNA Expression and their Potential as Drug Targets." *RNA & Disease* 3, e864-e870, 2016.

5. Matsui K, et al. "Effect of active hexose correlated compound on the production of nitric oxide in hepatocytes." *J. Parenter. Enteral Nutr.* 31(5), 373–380, 2007.

6. Matsui K, et al. "Active hexose correlated compound inhibits the expression of proinflammatory biomarker iNOS in hepatocytes." *Eur. Surg. Res.* 47(4), 274–283, 2011.

Pulmonary Non-Tuberculous Mycobacteriosis

Masaki Fujita, Kentaro Wakamatsu

*M*ycobacterium spp. is a human pathogen that proliferates intracellularly in phagocytes and includes *Mycobacterium tuberculosis* complex, *M. leprae,* and nontuberculous mycobacteria. Tuberculosis is a well-known, highly contagious but treatable disease. In contrast, although nontuberculous mycobacteriosis (NTM) is not contagious, it is particularly difficult to treat. *M. avium-intracellulare* complex (MAC) is the most frequent organism among NTM, causing chronic respiratory infection as well as disseminated diseases in immunocompromised hosts, such as HIV patients.[1,2] Therefore, the development of novel treatments for pulmonary NTM is needed.

We examined the role of AHCC as a biological response modifier in attenuating pulmonary NTM and investigated the efficacy of AHCC in treating pulmonary NTM in animals and humans.

Animal Study

C57/BL6 mice were given an intratracheal administration of *M. avium* (10^8 cfu/animal) and then orally treated with 1,000 mg/kg/day of AHCC for twenty-one days until sacrifice. Administration of AHCC attenuated lung inflammation caused by *M. avium* based on histology findings (see Figure 1 on the facing page) and reduced the colony number of *M. avium* in the lungs (Control: 1.0×10^4 cfu/lung vs. AHCC: 2.5×10^3 cfu/lung). No marked differences in colony numbers were noted between control and treated macrophages in vitro. In analysis of lung inflammatory cells, the numbers of γδ T cells and NK cells were unchanged by AHCC administration, but the number of TNFR2 cells was slightly increased. Interestingly, an increased trend was noted in the number of bronchoalveolar lavage fluid differential cells, mainly macrophages, albeit not to a significant degree.[3]

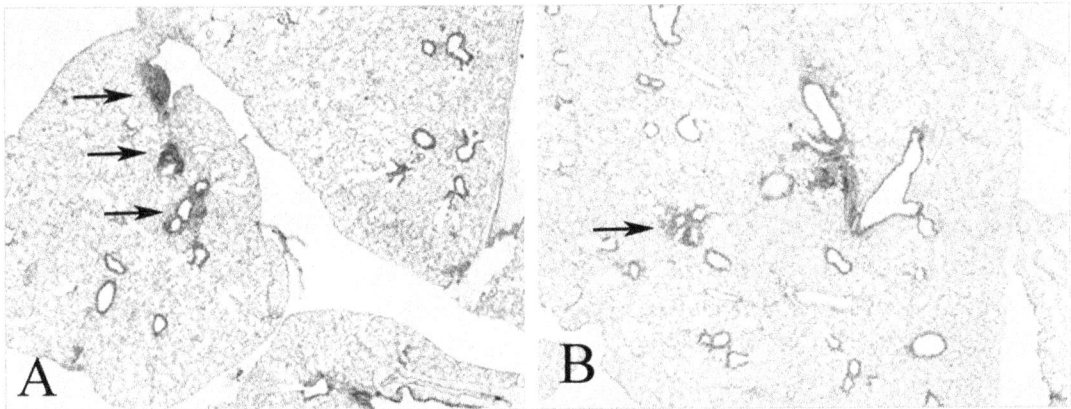

Figure 1. Histological assessment of the lung after *M. avium* **inoculation. (A)** Lung tissue from an *M. avium*-inoculated mouse supplied with water. **(B)** Lung tissue from an *M. avium*-inoculated mouse supplemented with AHCC. Arrows indicate inflammatory processes following NTM infection. AHCC attenuated these inflammatory processes. (H-E staining, original magnification: × 20).

Human Study

The clinical trial involved seven refractory and progressive cases of pulmonary NTM. In addition to conventional therapy for pulmonary NTM, the patients received 3,000 mg/day of AHCC for six months. Clinical courses, including chest imaging and blood test findings, were evaluated. One patient's condition improved and one patient's condition stabilized, but the other five experienced progression. TNF-α and IL-6 levels were unchanged after AHCC treatment, as well as NK cell activity. No serious adverse effects were reported. Since these cases were all refractory and progressive cases, the results appeared to be favorable. Future studies should enroll patients with early-stage pulmonary NTM or reevaluate the administered dose of AHCC.

Discussion

We herein demonstrated the attenuating effect of AHCC against *M. avium* infection in mice. Given that our in vitro study failed to show any bactericidal activity, the effect of AHCC appears to depend on its role as a biological response modifier. In addition to our investigation into the attenuating effect, we also examined the mechanism of the attenuation. AHCC has been reported to increase the number of NK cells in aged mice.[4] α-1,4-Glucans are recognized by C-type lectins, such as Dectin-1 on NK cells, thereby initiating innate immunity.[5] We therefore hypothesized that the mechanism of attenuation resulted from activation of NK cells.[6] However, the number of NK cells was unchanged in both the animal and clinical studies. When TNF signals were investigated, TNF signals and IL-6 levels were also unchanged. The attenuation mechanism should be investigated in future studies.

AHCC played a protective role against pulmonary NTM in the animal model and provided a certain protective effect in the clinical setting. These results suggest that AHCC may be useful as a novel remedy for pulmonary NTM.

REFERENCES

1. Medical Section of the American Lung Association. "Diagnosis and treatment of disease caused by nontuberculous mycobacteria." *Am. J. Respir. Crit. Care Med.* 156, S1–25, 1997.

2. Griffith DE, et al. "An official ATS/IDSA statement: diagnosis, treatment, and prevention of nontuberculous mycobacterial diseases." *Am. J. Respir. Crit. Care Med.* 175, 367–416, 2007.

3. Fujita M, et al., "Attenuation of pulmonary Mycobacterium avium disease by active hexose correlated compound (AHCC) in mice." *J. Nutr. Disorders Ther.* 5, 1000174, 2015.

4. Nguyen KB, et al. "Coordinated and distinct roles for IFN-alpha beta, IL-12, and IL-15 regulation of NK cell responses to viral infection." J. Immunol. 169, 4279–4287, 2002.

5. Mallet JF, et al. "Active Hexose Correlated Compound (AHCC) promotes an intestinal immune response in BALB/c mice and in primary intestinal epithelial cell culture involving toll-like receptors TLR-2 and TLR-4." *Eur. J. Nutr.* 55, 139–146, 2016.

6. Ritz BW. "Supplementation with active hexose correlated compound increases survival following infectious challenge in mice." *Nutr. Rev.* 66, 526–531, 2008.

HPV and Cervical Cancer

Judith A. Smith

Cervical cancer is the second most common cancer among women worldwide. Approximately 80 percent of the cases occur in developing countries, where it is the most common female cancer and the most common cancer-related cause of death. With the exception of childhood cancers and lymphomas, patients with cervical cancer die younger (average, 60 years) than women with any other cancer. The median age of diagnosis for cervical cancer is 47 years old. The association between cervical cancer and sexual activity is well known, and human papilloma virus (HPV) has been identified in over 99 percent cases of cervical cancer and 75 percent of pre-invasive disease. The goal of cervical cytology and HPV testing is to identify and treat cervical dysplasia in order to prevent invasive carcinoma.

The etiology of cervical cancer is well defined. Studies have identified and confirmed the association between HPV and the development of cervical cancer.[1,2] In recent years, cervical cancer research has been focusing on the significance of HPV expression in the pathogenesis of cancer. In the Kaiser study conducted by Sherman et al., which evaluated 20,810 women over a ten-year period, the data demonstrated the relationship between HPV infection and development of neoplastic lesions.[3] Another concern is when multiple HPV types are present; this has been associated with a poor response to treatment and an overall worse prognosis.[4,5] Patients who had a history of multiple HPV infections did not respond as well to radiotherapy and had a shorter duration of response when compared to patients with a history of only one prior infection.[4] The expression of HPV 18 has been determined to be an accurate predictor of early recurrence and overall poor prognosis.[6–8] When HPV infections persist overtime, patients have an increased risk for developing cervical cancer.[9] Thus, there is a need to treat and eradicate HPV infections to reduce the risk of developing cervical cancer.

The HPV is classified as a non-enveloped, double strand DNA virus. It contains circular DNA chromosomes in its nuclear composition, and it generally infects the epithelial layer of cells, including cutaneous and mucosal surfaces.[10] The viral cycle is irrefutably linked to epithelial cell differentiation. HPV infections are associated with benign warts, carcinoma in situ, and ultimately malignant lesions. HPV DNA has been detected in over 99% of cervical cancer patients.[11] Over 230 strains of the papillomavirus have been identified, including one hundred that occur in humans. Fifteen of the HPV types are carcinogenic; the most common types being HPV 16, 18, 31, 39, and 41.[12] Certain HPV types, particularly HPV16 and HPV18, encode proteins that can negate the function of cellular genes that control cellular proliferation. HPV16 encodes a protein (E6) that binds to the p53 tumor suppressor gene product, resulting in accelerated degradation.[13] HPV18 encodes a protein (E7) that binds to the retinoblastoma tumor suppressor gene, resulting in its functional inactivation. When these tumor suppressor genes are inactivated, the HPV-infected cells have a selective growth advantage compared to non-infected cells. It is important to differentiate that although HPV appears to be an important cofactor in the development of cervical dysplasia and cervical cancer, it does not cause either condition by itself. However, if high-risk HPV (HR-HPV) infections could effectively be eradicated, then the incidence of cervical cancer would drastically be reduced.

Hyper Immune Activation and Persistent HPV Infections

HPV, like many viruses, has evolved strategies to counteract interferon (IFN) signaling pathways. Specifically, interferon regulatory factors (IRFs) can promote cell immunity as well as promote oncogenesis pathway in response to a variety of extracellular signals.[14,15] Specifically, IRF-2 has been shown to activate HPV E6/E7 gene expression and promote oncogenesis pathway.[16] However, eventually in persistent infections, IFN α/β also induce IRF-1 that will help sustain persistent viral gene expression.[17] Lace et al. have confirmed that elevated IFN-β levels will induce IRF-1 and IRF-2 promoting HPV16 persistent infections.[18] Recently two independent research teams evaluating lymphocytic choriomeningitis virus (LCMV) persistent infections have demonstrated that suppression of chronic IFN-β signaling can reset the host immunity and enable control and clearance of persistent viral infections.[19,20] Our laboratory is the first to define that it is actually this mechanism of suppression of IFN-β (type I interferon) by AHCC that led to an upregulation of IFN-gamma (IFN-γ; type II interferon) and ultimate clearance of persistent HPV infections.

There are very few effective treatment options for eradicating HR-HPV infections. The objective of current treatment modalities is to alleviate symptoms and remove symptomatic lesions that often reoccur. Often treatment is delayed until the HPV lesions enlarge and the patient becomes symptomatic. This usually involves medical and surgical local treatment interventions, such as topical application of podophyllotoxin, an antimitotic agent that induces tissue necrosis clearing 45 to 88% of local HPV lesions with up to 40% rate of recurrent lesions.[21,22] Another option is the topical application of imiquimod, a derivative of imidazoquinolinamine, which data suggests exerts toxic activity by activating macrophages to secrete cytokines. The response of imiquimod ranges from 33 to 54% with an approximate 15% recurrence. More commonly, ablative or excisional therapies are utilized to treat the abnormal cervical cells. These include cryotherapy, laser ablation, loop electrosurgical excisional procedure (LEEP), or cold knife conization. These procedures have a higher response rate of 80 to 100%. This local treatment removes the lesion but does not clear the systemic HPV infection, and patients will frequently have recurrent lesions. To date, there is no readily available effective systemic treatment of HPV infections.

Prevention of HPV infections with the HPV vaccine before exposure to HPV has demonstrated the best potential for eliminating HPV infections. The functions of particular interest in the HPV arena are AHCC's immunomodulating and potential restorative effects on type II interferon pathway, specifically the natural killer (NK) cells, macrophages, and cellular cytokines. Use of a readily available, nonprescription nutritional supplement like AHCC that has data to support its benefits for immune support and safety is an appealing option for the eradication HPV infections. A phase II study to confirm the efficacy of AHCC for eradiation of HR-HPV infections in women with a history of persistent HR-HPV infections is ongoing at the University of Texas McGovern Medical School in Houston, Texas.

REFERENCES

1. Harris RWC, Brinton LA, Cowdell RH, et al. "Characteristics of women with dysplasia or carcinoma in situ of the cervix uteri." *Br. J. Cancer* 42: 359–369, 1980.

2. Furumoto H and Irahara M. "Human papillomavirus (HPV) and cervical cancer." *J. Med. Invest.* 49(3–4): 124–133, 2002.

3. Sherman ME, Lorincz AT, Scott DR, Wacholder S, Castle PE, and Glass AG. "Baseline cytology, human papillomavirus testing, and risk for cervical Neoplasia: a 10-year cohort analysis." *JNCI* 95(1): 46–52, 2003.

4. Bachtiary BB, Obermair A, Dreier B, et al. "Impact of multiple HPV infection on response to treatment and survival in patients receiving radical radiotherapy for cervical cancer." *Int. J. Cancer* 102: 237–243, 2002.

5. Elfgren K, Jacobs M, Walboomers JMM, Meijer CJLM, and Dillner J. "Rate of human papillomavirus clearance after treatment of cervical intraepithelial neoplasia." *Obstet. Gynecol.* 1000: 965–971, 2002.

6. Rose BR, Thomson CH, Simpson JM, Jarrett CS, Elliott PM, et al. "Human papillomavirus deoxyribonucleic acid as a prognostic indicator in early-stage cervical cancer: a possible role for type 18." *Am. J. Obstet. Gynecol.* 173: 1461–1468, 1995.

7. Lombard I, Vincent-Salomon A, Zafrani B, de la Rochefordiere A, Clough K, Favre M, Pouillart P, and Sastre-Garau X. "Human papillomavirus genotype as a major determinant of the course of cervical cancer." *J. Clin. Oncol.* 16: 2613–2619, 1998.

8. Schwartz SM, Daling JR, Shera KA, Madeleine MM, et al. "Human papillomavirus and prognosis of invasive cervical cancer: a population-based study." *J. Clin. Oncol.* 19: 1906–1915, 2001.

9. Schiffman M, Wheeler CM, and Castle PE. "Human papillomavirus DNA remains detectable longer than related cervical cytologic abnormalities." *J. Infectious Dis.* 186: 1169–1172, 2002.

10. Schiffman M and Castle PE. "Human papillomavirus: epidemiology and public health." *Arch. Pathol. Lab Med.* 127(8): 930–934, 2003.

11. Barnard P, Payne E, and McMillan NAJ. "The human papillomavirus E7 protein is able to inhibit the antiviral and anti-growth functions of interferon-α." *Virology* 277: 411–419, 2000.

12. Wiley DJ, Douglas J, Beutner K, et al. "External genital warts: diagnosis, treatment, and prevention." *CID* 35 (suppl. 2): S210-S224, 2002.

13. Okamoto A, Woodworth CD, Yen K, et al. "Combination therapy with podophyllin and vidarabine for human papillomavirus positive cervical intraepithelial neoplasia." *Oncology Rep* 6:269-276, 1999.

14. Fujita T, Imura Y, Miyamoto M, Barsoumain EI, and Taniguchi T. "Induction of endogenous IFN-α and IFN-β genes by a regulatory transcription factor, IRF-1." *Nature.* 337:270–272, 1989.

15. Honda K and Tanguchi T. "Toll-like receptor signaling and IRF transcription factors." *IUBMB Life.* 58(5-6): 290-295, 2006.

16. Lace MJ, Anson JR, Haugen TH, and Turek LP. "Interferon regulatory factor (IRF)-2 activates the HPV-16 E6-E7 promoter in keratinocytes." *Virology* 399: 270–279, 2010.

17. Goodbourn S, Didcock L, and Randall RE. "Interferons: cell signaling, immune modulation, antiviral responses and virus countermeasures." *J. General Virology* 81: 2341–2364, 2000.

18. Lace MJ, Anson JR, Klingelhutz AJ, Harada H, et al. "Interferon-beta treatment increases human papillomavirus early gene transcription and viral plasmid genome replication by activating regulatory factor (IRF)-1." *Carcinogenesis* 30(8): 1336–1344, 2009.

19. Wilson EB, Yamada DH, Elsaesser H, et al. "Blockage of chronic type I interferon signaling to control persistent LCMV infection." *Science* 340: 202–207, 2013.

20. Teijaro JR, Ng C, Lee AM, et al. "Persistent LCMC infection is controlled by blockade of type I interferon signaling." *Science* 340: 207–211, 2013.

21. Von Krogh G and Heldberg D. "Self treatment using a 0.5% podophyllotoxin cream of external genital condylomata acuminate in women. A placebo controlled, double blind study." *Sex Transm Dis* 19:170-4, 1992.

22. Beutner KR, Conant MA, Friedman-Kien AE, et al. "Patient-applied podofilox for treatment of genital warts." *Lancet* 1 (8642):831–4, 1989.

Wound Infection Models and AHCC

Gerald Sonnenfeld

Infection remains a problem in severely injured individuals. Infection that does not respond well to antibiotic therapy generates extensive medical expenses and deaths in severe trauma patients. It is very difficult to predict which severely injured patients will have difficulties with infection, and several different treatments have been tried without great success.[1–7] These include treatment of patients with muramyl dipeptide and also with interferon-gamma.[1–7] Therefore, development of a treatment for infections in trauma patients that can be started early in the course of the traumatic incident, perhaps before infection commences, could have great value. AHCC has been shown to modulate immune response and to have effects in modulating infections in other mouse models where the immune system is disrupted.[8–9] Immune suppression has been shown to occur in severely injured trauma patients, so AHCC could be a candidate for experiments to determine its effect in models of severe trauma injury infections. Additionally, if the treatment could be included with the nutrition being received, a facile way to present the treatment early in the traumatic incident could be developed.

Several models using rodents for surgical wound infections exist. They include a mouse model with soft tissue infection with *Klebsiella pneumonia*.[8] *Klebsiella pneumoniae* is a gram-negative bacterium that often causes infections in severely injured trauma patients. AHCC has been shown to enhance immune function and is taken orally. Therefore, mice received AHCC orally prior to infection and through the course of infection. Mice that received AHCC slightly enhanced resistance to infection and greater clearance of bacteria. Levels of cytokines that are important in regulating the immune response to infection were increased earlier in infected mice that received AHCC than in control infected mice.[9]

These data suggest that AHCC has a positive effect in enhancing resistance to infection in mice that are maintained in the *Klebsiella pneumoniae* soft tissue wound infection model. The increased resistance to infection is small. In the future, additional experiments will be required to confirm these effects. Additionally, combination of AHCC with other therapies, such as antibiotics and/or immunostimulatory cytokines, could enhance the effects of AHCC that have already been observed. If the mouse studies in the future continue to show a beneficial effect of AHCC for enhancement of resistance to infection, clinical studies in human trauma patients would have to be performed to show that AHCC also has beneficial effects for resistance to infection in humans. AHCC has the benefit of being able to be included with nutrition that is provided for the patients, which would make administration early in the course of the traumatic incident possible.

REFERENCES

1. Hershman MJ, Sonnenfeld G, Mays BW, Fleming F, Trachtenberg L, and Polk HC Jr. "Effects of interferon-gamma on surgically simulated wound infection in mice." *Microbial Pathogenesis* 4: 165–168, 1988.

2. Hershman MJ, Sonnenfeld G, Logan WA, Pietsch JD, Wellhausen SR, and Polk HC, Jr. "Effect of interferon-gamma on the course of a burn wound infection." *J. Interferon Res.* 8: 367–373, 1988.

3. Hershman MJ, Polk HC Jr, Pietsch JD, Kuftinec D, and Sonnenfeld, G. "Modulation of *Klebsiella pneumoniae* infection of mice by interferon-gamma." *Clin. Expt'l. lmmunol.* 72: 406 409, 1988.

4. Hershman MJ, Polk HC Jr, Pietsch JD, Shields RE, Wellhausen SR, and Sonnenfeld G. "Modulation of infection following trauma by interferon-gamma treatment." *Infect. Immun.* 56: 2412–2416, 1988.

5. Livingston DH, Appel SH, Wellhausen SR, Sonnenfeld G, and Polk HC Jr. "Depressed interferon-gamma production and monocyte HLA-DR expression after severe injury." *Arch. Surgery* 123: 1309–1312, 1988.

6. Hershman MJ, Appel SH, Wellhausen SR, Sonnenfeld G, and Polk HC Jr. "Interferon-gamma increases HLA-DR expression on monocytes in severely injured patients." *Clin. Expt'l. lmmunol.* 77: 67–70, 1989.

7. Polk HC Jr, Cheadle WG, Livingston DH, Rodriguez JL, Starko KM, Izu AE, Jaffe HS, and Sonnenfeld G. "A randomized prospective clinical trial to determine the efficacy of interferon-gamma in severely injured patients." *Amer. J. Surgery,* 163: 191–196, 1992.

8. Aviles H, O'Donnell PO, Sun B, and Sonnenfeld G. "Active hexose correlated compound (AHCC) enhances resistance to infection in a mouse model of surgical wound infection." *Surgical Infections,* 7: 527–535, 2006.

9. Aviles H, O'Donnell P, Orshal J, Fujii H, Sun B, and Sonnenfeld G. "Active hexose correlated compound (AHCC) activates immune function to decrease bacterial load in a murine model of intramuscular infection." *Am. J. Surgery,* 195: 537–545, 2008.

Chapter 7

ANTI-INFLAMMATORY EFFECT

Anti-inflammatory Foods

Anil D. Kulkarni

In India's ancient system of medicine, Ayurveda, there is enough knowledge, information, and evidence that all the physiologic diseases arise from *Aahar* (diet) that means diet-induced lifestyle. It is now recognized that lifestyle factors, particularly diet, play a major role in the development or prevention of degenerative diseases, including hypertension, diabetes, cardiovascular disease, and others (see Figure 1 below). Thus, there is growing interest worldwide in the prospect that overall diet as well as particular foods can promote and help maintain a good health.

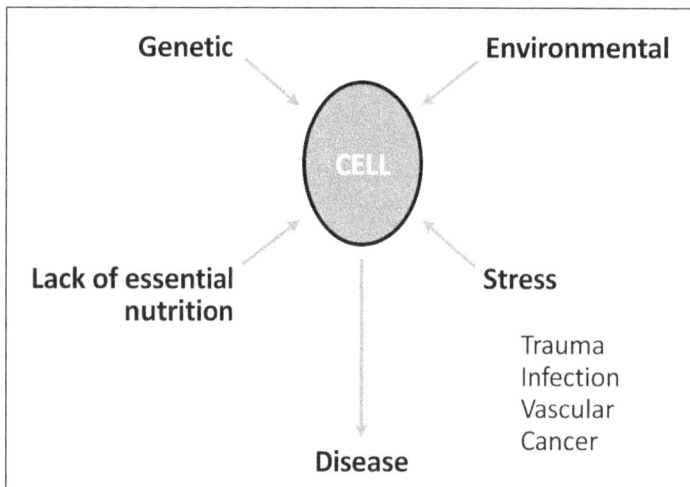

Figure 1A. Adapted from *Ayurveda Revisited* (Dahanukar and Thatte, 1989).

Evidence has been provided suggesting that dietary patterns rich in foods of plant origin, such as fruits and vegetables, play a key role in disease prevention through a multifactorial action involving a modulation of the immune system and the inflammatory response. If the inflammatory response is not properly controlled, excess inflammatory stress may be induced, becoming a key modulator in the breakdown of several physiologic functions, leading to pathogenesis and risk factors for cardiovascular disease, including obesity, hyperglycemia, and dyslipidemia (see Figure 1A and B).

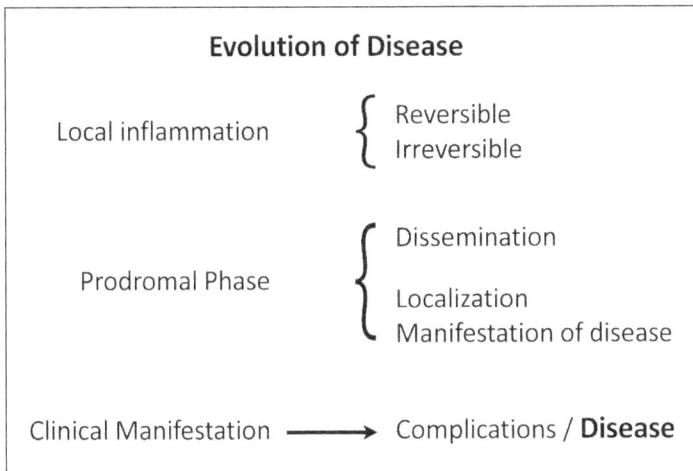

Evolution of Disease

Local inflammation
{ Reversible
  Irreversible

Prodromal Phase
{ Dissemination

  Localization
  Manifestation of disease

Clinical Manifestation ⟶ Complications / **Disease**

Figure 1B.
Adapted from *Ayurveda Revisited* (Dahanukar and Thatte, 1989)

Ayurveda is a holistic science derived from Sanskrit words *Ayu* meaning life and *Veda* meaning knowledge or science. Thus, *Ayurveda* means the science of life. In ancient days, this science was highly advanced in understanding the human body. It includes formulary of entirely plant-based drugs/dietary substances and their modes of action. Ayurvedic principles aim to achieve prophylactic maintenance of health and therapeutically curing illnesses. According to Ayurveda, a person is made of five basic elements: air, water, ether, fire, and earth. These five elements in certain combinations strongly influence the three doshas described as *Vata, Kapha,* and *Pitta*. The Ayurvedic concept of Tridosha is unique in medical science. These constitutions have distinct food and nutrition requirements. There is lot of emphasis on food/nutrition with taste, flavors, and their applications in the daily diet and their impact on health.

Inflammation is a type of immune response. Acute, localized inflammation is a life-saving mechanism to protect a host from pathogens or injury. However, a chronic, low-grade, systemic pro-inflammatory state is a risk factor for a wide range of conditions, such as insulin resistance, metabolic syndrome, atherosclerosis, type II diabetes, cardiovascular disease, cancer, and neurodegenerative disease. One of the major recognized causes of this sustained, underlying pro-inflammatory state is a combination of energy surplus and an imbalanced food intake.

Inflammation is mediated by a variety of molecules, including a group of cell-derived polypeptides, collectively known as *cytokines*, which act both locally and systemically to orchestrate the inflammatory response. The production of pro-inflammatory and anti-inflammatory cytokines is strictly controlled by complex feedback, a mechanism that allows the vulnerable state to continue to cause further damage.

The concept of the role of diet as root cause of pathogenesis slowly reached eastward. As we see today, many of the geographic parts (Far East Asia) of the world have similar cultures and acquired practices related to the use of food and diet to treat illnesses. Of course climatic conditions dictate cultivation, food storage, and preservation, along with adaptation of seasonal food consumption. Major differences are in specific types of foods, such meat and seafood, but plant-based foods are commonalities.

In modern medicine, many drugs were derived from plant-based resources before the age of synthesized recombination drugs. Table 1 below identifies drugs that are still in use.

TABLE 1. **DRUGS IN USE**

NO.	DRUG	PLANT SOURCE	NO.	DRUG	PLANT SOURCE
1	Atropine	*Hyoscyamus muticus*	9	Hyoscine	*Datura metel*
2	Caffeine*	*Thea sinensis*	10	Hyoscyamine	*Hyscyamous muticus*
3	Codeine	*Papaver somniferum*	11	Papaverine*	*Papaver spp.*
4	Colchicine	*Colchinum actumnale*	12	Pilocarpine	*Pilocarpus jaborandi*
5	Digitoxin	*Digitalis purpurea*	13	Quinidine	*Cinchona spp.*
6	Digoxin	*Digitalis lanata*	14	Quinine	*Cinchona spp.*
7	Emetine*	*Cephaelis spp.*	15	Theobromine*	*Theobroma cacao*
8	Ephedrine*	*Ephedra spp.*	16	Theophylline	*Coffea arabica*

* Now mainly synthesized.   Table adapted from *Ayurveda Revisited* (Dahanukar and Thatte, 1989).

A more recently designed and published anti-inflammatory food pyramid shows pictorial information of what foods are considered as beneficial and protective of inflammation. (See Andrew Weil reference below.)

As described earlier, inflammatory response and its mediators serve as a medical alert and warn us of what is to come. Thus, inflammatory response can be beneficial as a warning from the host immune system. Inflammation is a double-edged sword and can be used for therapeutic benefits.

REFERENCES

Dahanukar S and Thatte U. *Ayurveda Revisited* (Popular Prakashan, Bombay, India 1989.)

Weil A. "Dr. Weil's Anti-Inflammatory Food Pyramid." drweil.com. http://www.drweil .com/drw/u/ART02995/Dr-Weil-Anti-Inflammatory-Food-Pyramid.html

Anti-inflammatory Effects of AHCC

Mikio Nishizawa

Noxious stimuli (e.g., chemical irritants and heat) and infection by pathogens (e.g., bacteria and virus) cause damage and injuries to cells and tissues, which provoke the specific response of inflammation. Celsus, a doctor in the Roman Empire, described local inflammation as follows: *"Notae vero inflammationis sunt quattuor, rubor et tumor, cum calore et dolore,"*[1] meaning "The signs of inflammation are four: redness and swelling with heat and pain."

Inflammation is a protective response to remove noxious stimuli, facilitate the processes of damage repair, and/or remove pathogens by producing biologically active substances, such as pain-producing substances (e.g., bradykinin) and inflammatory mediators. Inflammatory cells (e.g., macrophages, neutrophils, and lymphocytes) generate a variety of inflammatory mediators, such as nitric oxide (NO), prostaglandins, pro-inflammatory cytokines, and chemokines. NO, which is produced by stimulated hepatocytes and Kupffer cells (resident macrophages) in the liver, removes pathogens by killing bacteria or inhibiting viral growth.[2] These cells participate in the inflammatory responses involved in innate immunity. The induction levels of the inflammatory mediators nearly correlate with the extent of inflammation.

Systemic inflammation may occur after acute inflammation; one such case is sepsis after bacterial infection. In the liver, bacterial endotoxins (i.e., lipopolysaccharides, LPS) of gram-negative bacteria stimulate Kupffer cells to produce NO and pro-inflammatory cytokines, including interleukin (IL)-1β and tumor necrosis factor-α (TNF-α)[3] (see Figure 1 on the facing page). Then, secreted IL-1β stimulates the hepatocytes, leading to the production of NO and TNF-α. When excess NO is produced, it leads to systemic vasodilation, resulting in septic shock.[4] Excess TNF-α causes the overproduction of many other pro-inflammatory cytokines and chemokines (the so-called *cytokine storm*). The excessive production of both NO and TNF-α provokes multiple organ failure, including fulminant hepatic failure.[5] Therefore, LPS has been experimentally used to prepare an endotoxemia model (also known as hepatic failure model) in mice and rats.[3,6] In addition, IL-1β-treated hepatocytes[2] and LPS-treated macrophages[7,8] have been used to evaluate the anti-inflammatory effects of drugs or functional foods.

Inflammation may cause disease, and vice versa. Chronic inflammation is the basis of many diseases, including autoimmune disease (e.g., rheumatoid arthritis), metabolic disease (e.g., diabetes mellitus), atherosclerosis, chronic obstructive

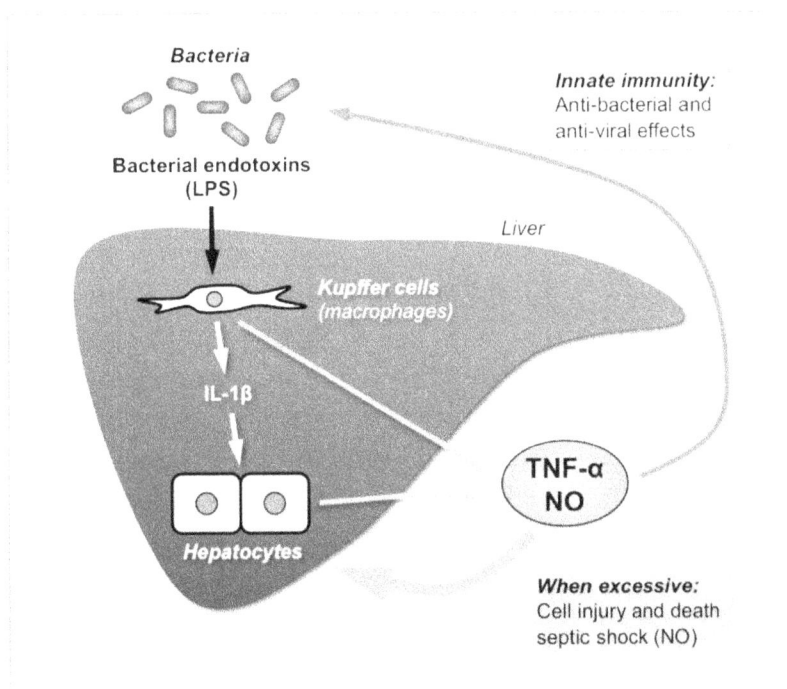

Figure 1. Induction of TNF-α and NO in the liver after bacterial infection. In response to bacterial toxins (LPS), Kupffer cells (resident macrophages) produce inflammatory mediators, including IL-1β, TNF-α, and NO. Then, secreted IL-1β induces adjacent hepatocytes to generate TNF-α and NO. As a part of innate immunity, NO exhibits anti-bacterial and anti-viral effects to kill these pathogens. When NO and TNF-α are produced at high levels, both mediators cause cell injury and death in the liver and other organs. Furthermore, excess NO in the blood provokes vasodilation, thereby causing septic shock.

pulmonary disease (COPD), and cancer. Inflammation is deeply involved in the pathophysiology and sometimes the pathogenesis of these diseases.

Excessive or prolonged inflammatory responses are detrimental; therefore, anti-inflammatory drugs that attenuate unfavorable inflammatory responses are used to facilitate recovery to the healthy state. The levels of inflammatory mediators (e.g., NO, prostaglandins, pro-inflammatory cytokines, and chemokines) are normalized to physiological levels by anti-inflammatory drugs and by some functional foods. Therefore, these mediators are suitable biomarkers for evaluating the anti-inflammatory effects of these drugs and functional foods on cells, animals, and humans.

Anti-inflammatory Effects of AHCC

Bioactive Molecules in AHCC

AHCC is a standardized extract of cultured *Lentinula edodes* mycelia, a Basidiomycetes mushroom species.[9,10] AHCC primarily consists of carbohydrates, of which α-glucan is a major constituent. The α-glucan content is 28.9% (weight) of the freeze-dried AHCC powder, whereas the β-glucan content is very low.[9,11] Oligosaccharides, which include partially acylated α-1,4-glucan, are assumed to confer some of the biological activities of AHCC, such as its antioxidant activity.[12,13] However, the molecules in AHCC that possess anti-inflammatory activities have not been identified.

The pharmacologically active molecules in AHCC have been pursued using an in vitro injury model of hepatocytes.[2] Primary cultured rat hepatocytes have been used to monitor the levels of NO, which is generated by inducible nitric oxide synthase (iNOS, or NOS2) in response to IL-1β. Matsui et al. reported that the addition of AHCC to the media suppressed the IL-1β-induced production of NO and decreased the levels of iNOS at both the protein and mRNA levels.[14]

Next, the sugars in AHCC were investigated. In rat hepatocytes, the sugar fraction of AHCC inhibited NO production and also suppressed iNOS gene expression and IL-1 receptor type I (IL1R1) upregulation.[15] It has been reported that glucose and dextrins do not significantly suppress IL-1β-induced NO production in hepatocytes.[16] Moreover, the sugar fraction of AHCC has no effect on either the activation of nuclear factor κB (NF-κB) or the degradation of NF-κB inhibitor α (IκB-α).[15] NF-κB is a key transcription factor involved in the expression of genes related to inflammation, such as iNOS and pro-inflammatory cytokine genes.[17]

Finally, an active constituent showing NO suppressing activity was purified from AHCC by several chromatography steps.[18] Adenosine, which was recently identified as a constituent of AHCC, suppressed the expression of the iNOS gene and reduced NO production at a 50% inhibitory concentration (IC_{50}) of 56 µM. Similarly to the sugar fraction, adenosine blocked the activation of NF-κB and the upregulation of the IL1R1 pathway, which resulted in the suppression of iNOS production and a subsequent decrease in NO production.[18] Because the content of adenosine in AHCC is estimated to be very low, other bioactive molecules that suppress NO production are expected to be present in AHCC. In addition, molecules that attenuate inflammation in other tissues, such as the intestine, should also be investigated in the future.

Anti-inflammatory Effects of AHCC on the Liver

A ten-year prospective cohort study demonstrated that AHCC supplementation (3 g/day) improved the prognoses of postoperative hepatocellular carcinoma (HCC) patients.[19] The study provided a scientific definition of *functional foods* and proposed that AHCC is a functional food.[20] In addition, NO is considered to be involved in the pathophysiology of various liver diseases as well as in hepatoprotection.[4] As mentioned above, AHCC and its sugar fraction suppressed NO production and iNOS gene expression in IL-1β-treated rat hepatocytes.[14,15] AHCC inhibits the induction of iNOS at a transcriptional level by inhibiting activation of NF-κB.[14] Furthermore, AHCC post-transcriptionally suppresses iNOS gene expression by reducing the stability of iNOS mRNA via the iNOS antisense transcripts[14,21] (see "An Antisense Transcript-mediated Mechanism is Involved in the AHCC-Mediated Suppression of Inducible Nitric Oxide Synthase Expression" by Mikio Nishizawa on page 109). AHCC also decreases the production of pro-inflammatory cytokines and chemokines in rat hepatocytes (T. Okuyama and M. Nishizawa, unpublished data). It is speculated that the suppression of NO by AHCC in hepatocytes may be partly related to a mechanism by which AHCC improved the prognoses of postoperative HCC patients.

Kim et al. reported that AHCC supplementation decreased the levels of hepatic enzymes that are markers of oxidative stress as well as the serum levels of pro-inflammatory cytokines in patients with mild, alcohol-induced elevations in the levels of hepatic enzymes.[22] After twelve weeks of AHCC supplementation (1 or 3 g/day), the serum levels of TNF-α and IL-1β were significantly decreased. The percent change in the serum IL-1β level was positively correlated with that of serum levels of the hepatic enzyme alanine aminotransferase (ALT). In contrast, the adiponectin levels were higher in the AHCC groups than in the placebo group. This human trial suggests the possibility that AHCC has hepatoprotective and anti-inflammatory effects.

Anti-inflammatory Effects of AHCC on the Intestine

The effects of AHCC on the murine intestine were examined. Mallet et al. fed AHCC to BALB/c mice by gavage (0.1, 0.5 or 1.0 g/kg body weight) daily for seven days and prepared intestinal epithelial cells from these animals.[23] AHCC intake resulted in increased numbers of immunoglobulin A (IgA)–positive cells in the intestine and levels of secretory IgA (sIgA), IL-10, and interferon (IFN)-γ in the intestinal fluid. Because IgA functions as the first line of antigen-specific immune defense in the intestinal lumen, sIgA protects against intestinal inflammation.[24] Experiments using primary culture from intestinal epithelial cells showed that toll-like receptor (TLR) 2 and 4 are involved in generating the immune response of the cells to AHCC.[23] Therefore, AHCC may play a role in the maintenance of immune homeostasis at the intestinal epithelium via the signaling pathways involving TLR2 and TLR4.

The intestinal anti-inflammatory effects of AHCC have been estimated using experimental animal models of colitis. These colitis models can be used to represent human inflammatory bowel disease (IBD), including ulcerative colitis and Crohn's disease.[25] Daddaoua et al. investigated the anti-inflammatory effects of AHCC in rats with trinitrobenzene sulfonic acid (TNBS)–induced colitis.[26] AHCC (100 or 500 mg/kg body weight) was administered daily to rats starting two days before colitis induction by TNBS, and the rats were euthanized six days after this induction. The administration of AHCC attenuated inflammation in the intestine. Moreover, AHCC improved the mucosal damage score, extension of necrosis, and colonic weight, and decreased the expression of pro-inflammatory cytokines (IL-1β, IL-1 receptor antagonist, and TNF-α), the chemokine (C-C motif) ligand 2 (CCL2; also known as monocyte chemoattractant protein-1), and trefoil factor 3 (TFF3). The magnitude of the anti-inflammatory effects of AHCC was similar to that of sulfasalazine (salazosulfapyridine), a drug used to treat ulcerative colitis.[26]

In vitro studies using intestinal epithelial cell lines (IEC18 and HT29) treated with AHCC have been recently reported.[27] Unlike IL-1β-treated hepatocytes, AHCC alone induced the secretion of CCL2 and the chemokine (C-X-C motif) ligand 1 (CXCL1) in IEC18 cells as well as the secretion of IL-8 in HT29 cells.[27] These effects depended on the activation of NF-κB and partly on mitogen-activated protein kinases (MAPKs) via TLR4 and myeloid differentiation primary response 88 (MyD88) in IEC18 cells. The authors also examined THP-1, a monocyte line, and showed that AHCC alone induced the secretion of IL-8, IL-1β, and TNF-α via the activation of NF-κB and c-*jun* N-terminal kinase (JNK).[27] These data provide three possibilities regarding the action of AHCC: first, it depends on the cell type as to whether AHCC exerts immunostimulatory and ant-inflammatory effects; second, extracellular stimuli (e.g., cytokines and bacterial endotoxins) determine either the immunostimulatory or anti-inflammatory effects; and finally, both immunostimulatory and anti-inflammatory constituents are included in AHCC. Future studies are required to elucidate the action of AHCC.

Daddaoua et al. analyzed colonic microflora in rats after AHCC was administered.[26] The AHCC-treated rats had higher counts of aerobic bacteria, lactic acid bacteria, and bifidobacteria in addition to lower counts of clostridia compared to the TNBS-treated rats. Furthermore, AHCC synergistically exerted symbiotic effects with *Bifidobacterium longum* BB536 in rats with TNBS-induced colitis.[28] *B. longum* is a genus of beneficial bacteria that is naturally present in the human digestive tract, and the BB536 strain is expected to be a probiotic with potential health-promoting effects. Rats received AHCC (100 or 500 mg/kg body weight) and *B. longum* BB536 (5 × 10[6] cfu/rat) daily for seven days before colitis induction by TNBS and then for another seven days.[28] The administration of both AHCC and *B. longum* BB536 to rats with colitis resulted in the highest anti-inflammatory activity in the intestine as well as suppression of TNBS-induced changes in body weight gain, colonic weight to length ratio, myeloperoxidase (MPO; produced in neutrophils) activity, and iNOS expression. Taken together, these results suggest that AHCC may be used as a prebiotic functional food, and the combination of AHCC (prebiotic) and *B. longum* BB536 (probiotic) may reduce intestinal inflammation in IBD patients.

Another experimental colitis model, T cell–induced colitis, is also used to evaluate the anti-inflammatory effects of AHCC. Mice disrupted in recombination activating gene 1 (*Rag1*), i.e., *Rag1*[−/−] mice, lack mature B and T lymphocytes and have underdeveloped mucosal immune systems.[29] Mascaraque et al. transferred exogenous CD4+ CD62L+ T cells, including naïve T cells and central memory CD4+ cells, to the *Rag1*[−/−] mice, which resulted in chronic colitis that was similar to IBD.[30] AHCC (75 mg/day) was administered by gavage to the *Rag1*[−/−] mice daily for twelve days after the T cell transfer. When primary cultured cells were prepared from the mesenteric lymph nodes of the AHCC-treated mice, the addition of AHCC to the media decreased the activity of MPO and alkaline phosphatase in the intestine and markedly reduced the secretion of TNF-α and IL-1β.[30] These data imply that AHCC improved the T cell–induced colitis by exerting an anti-inflammatory activity in the intestine.

Although many animal experiments have been reported, to date, no bioactive molecules that attenuate intestinal inflammation have been identified. More studies are required to elucidate the anti-inflammatory effects of AHCC on the mucosal immunity of the intestine.

Perspectives

Accumulating data have demonstrated that AHCC has anti-inflammatory effects in several types of cells as well as immunostimulatory effects in certain cell lines (see Figure 2 below). Furthermore, AHCC has a prebiotic effect on intestinal microflora. These effects may be applied using AHCC as a functional food to prevent diseases characterized by chronic inflammation, such as IBD. In this context, AHCC and/or its constituents may be used as complementary and alternative medicine. In addition to adenosine, other pharmacologically active molecules in AHCC should be identified to explain its action. When such bioactive molecules are identified, their anti-inflammatory effects, which suppress the expression of inflammatory genes, would be beneficial as a potential drug for diseases that involve chronic inflammation.

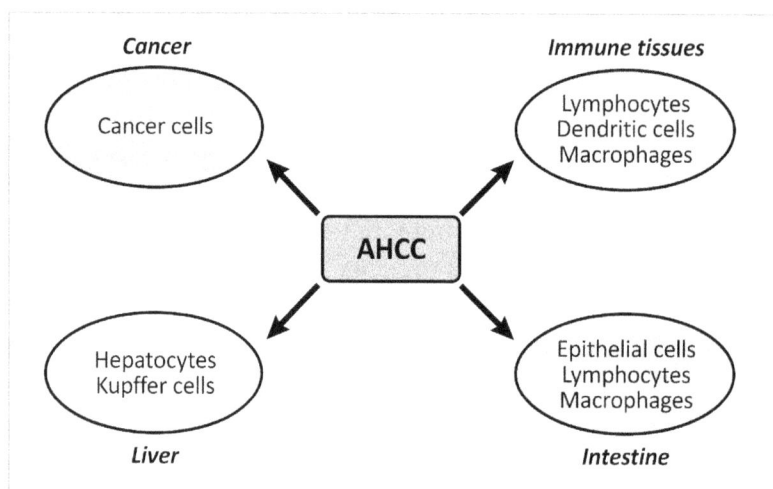

Figure 2. Anti-inflammatory effects of AHCC on various types of cells. The potential target cells of AHCC are shown.

Abbreviations

NO, nitric oxide; IL, interleukin; TNF-α, tumor necrosis factor-α; iNOS, inducible nitric oxide synthase; NF-κB, nuclear factor κB.

The author of this section thanks Drs. Yasuo Kamiyama, Tadayoshi Okumura, and Yukinobu Ikeya for their invaluable comments and Ms. Noriko Kanazawa for her secretarial assistance.

REFERENCES

1. Celsus AC. *De Medicina.* Liber III:10. A Loeb Classical Library. http://penelope.uchicago.edu/Thayer/L/Roman/Texts/Celsus/3*.html

2. Kitade H, Sakitani K, Inoue K, Masu Y, Kawada N, Hiramatsu Y, Kamiyama Y, Okumura T, and Ito S. "Interleukin 1β markedly stimulates nitric oxide formation in the absence of other cytokines or lipopolysaccharide in primary cultured rat hepatocytes but not in Kupffer cells." *Hepatology* 23: 797–802, 1996.

3. Yoshigai E, Hara T, Inaba H, Hashimoto I, Tanaka Y, Kaibori M, Kimura T, Okumura T, Kwon AH, and Nishizawa M. "Interleukin-1β induces tumor necrosis factor-α secretion from rat hepatocytes." *Hepatol. Res.* 44: 571–583, 2014.

4. Colasanti M and Suzuki H. "The dual personality of NO." *Trends Pharmacol. Sci.* 21: 249–252, 2000.

5. Wang H and Ma S. "The cytokine storm and factors determining the sequence and severity of organ dysfunction in multiple organ dysfunction syndrome." *Am. J. Emerg. Med.* 26: 711–715, 2008.

6. Tsuji K, Kwon AH, Yoshida H, Qiu Z, Kaibori M, Okumura T, and Kamiyama Y. "Free radical scavenger (edaravone) prevents endotoxin-induced liver injury after partial hepatectomy in rats." *J. Hepatol.* 42: 94–101, 2005.

7. Yoshida H, Kwon AH, Habara K, Yamada M, Kaibori M, Kamiyama Y, Nishizawa M, Ito S, and Okumura T. "Edaravone inhibits the induction of iNOS gene expression at transcriptional and posttranscriptional steps in murine macrophages." *Shock* 30: 734–739, 2008.

8. Inaba H, Yoshigai E, Okuyama T, Murakoshi M, Sugiyama K, Nishino H, and Nishizawa M. "Antipyretic analgesic drugs have different mechanisms for regulation of the expression of inducible nitric oxide synthase in hepatocytes and macrophages." *Nitric Oxide* 44: 61–70, 2015.

9. Miura T, Kitadate K, Nishioka H, and Wakame K. "Basic and clinical studies on Active Hexose Correlated Compound" in: *Biotechnology in Functional Foods and Nutraceuticals.* Bagchi D, Lau FC, Ghosh DK (eds.). CRC Press Taylor and Francis Group. pp. 51–59, 2010.

10. Shah SK, Walker PA, Moore-Olufemi SD, Sundaresan A, Kulkarni AD, and Andrassy RJ. "An evidence-based review of a *Lentinula edodes* mushroom extract as complementary therapy in the surgical oncology patient." *JPEN J. Parenter. Enteral Nutr.* 35: 449–458, 2011.

11. Okuyama T, Yoshigai E, Ikeya Y, and Nishizawa M. "Active Hexose Correlated Compound extends the lifespan and increases the thermotolerance of nematodes." *Functional Foods in Health and Disease.* 3: 166–182, 2013.

12. Ye SF, Ichimura K, Wakame K, and Ohe M. "Suppressive effects of Active Hexose Correlated Compound on the increased activity of hepatic and renal ornithine decarboxylase induced by oxidative stress." *Life Sci.* 74: 593–602, 2003.

13. Ye SF, Wakame K, Ichimura K, and Matsuzaki S. "Amelioration by active hexose correlated compound of endocrine disturbances induced by oxidative stress in the rat." *Endocr. Regul.* 38: 7–13, 2004.

14. Matsui K, Kawaguchi Y, Ozaki T, Tokuhara K, Tanaka H, Kaibori M, Matsui Y, Kamiyama Y, Wakame K, Miura T, Nishizawa M, and Okumura T. "Effect of active hexose correlated compound on the production of nitric oxide in hepatocytes." *JPEN J. Parenter. Enteral Nutr.* 31: 373–380, 2007.

15. Matsui K, Ozaki T, Oishi M, Tanaka Y, Kaibori M, Nishizawa M, Okumura T, and Kwon AH. "Active hexose correlated compound inhibits the expression of proinflammatory biomarker iNOS in hepatocytes." *Eur. Surg. Res.* 47: 274–283, 2011.

16. Nishizawa M, Kano M, Okuyama T, Okumura T, and Ikeya Y. "Anti-inflammatory effects of enzyme-treated asparagus extract and its constituents in hepatocytes." *Functional Foods in Health and Disease.* 6: 91–109, 2016.

17. Lawrence T. "The nuclear factor NF-κB pathway in inflammation." *Cold Spring Harb. Perspect. Biol.* 1: a001651, 2009.

18. Tanaka Y, Ohashi S, Ohtsuki A, Kiyono T, Park EY, Nakamura Y, Sato K, Oishi M, Miki H, Tokuhara K, Matsui K, Kaibori M, Nishizawa M, Okumura T, and Kwon AH. "Adenosine, a hepato-protective component in active hexose correlated compound: its identification and iNOS suppression mechanism." *Nitric Oxide* 40: 75–86, 2014.

19. Matsui Y, Uhara J, Satoi S, Kaibori M, Yamada H, Kitade H, Imamura A, Takai S, Kawaguchi Y, Kwon AH, and Kamiyama Y. "Improved prognosis of postoperative hepatocellular carcinoma patients when treated with functional foods: a prospective cohort study." *J. Hepatol.* 37: 78–86, 2002.

20. Bass NM. "It could have been something they ate—functional food and the treatment of liver cancer." *J. Hepatol.* 37: 147–150, 2002.

21. Matsui K, Nishizawa M, Ozaki T, Kimura T, Hashimoto I, Yamada M, Kaibori M, Kamiyama Y, Ito S, and Okumura T. "Natural antisense transcript stabilizes inducible nitric oxide synthase messenger RNA in rat hepatocytes." *Hepatology* 47: 686–697, 2008.

22. Kim H, Kim JH, and Im JA. "Effect of Active Hexose Correlated Compound (AHCC) in alcohol-induced liver enzyme elevation." *J. Nutr. Sci. Vitaminol. (Tokyo).* 60: 348–356, 2014.

23. Mallet JF, Graham É, Ritz BW, Homma K, and Matar C. "Active Hexose Correlated Compound (AHCC) promotes an intestinal immune response in BALB/c mice and in primary intestinal epithelial cell culture involving toll-like receptors TLR-2 and TLR-4." *Eur. J. Nutr.* 55: 139–146, 2016.

24. Kaetzel CS. "Cooperativity among secretory IgA, the polymeric immunoglobulin receptor, and the gut microbiota promotes host-microbial mutualism." *Immunol. Lett.* 162: 10–21, 2014.

25. Low D, Nguyen DD, and Mizoguchi E. "Animal models of ulcerative colitis and their application in drug research." *Drug Des. Devel. Ther.* 7: 1341–1357, 2013.

26. Daddaoua A, Martínez-Plata E, López-Posadas R, Vieites JM, González M, Requena P, Zarzuelo A, Suárez MD, de Medina FS, and Martínez-Augustin O. "Active hexose correlated compound acts as a prebiotic and is antiinflammatory in rats with hapten-induced colitis." *J. Nutr.* 137: 1222–1228, 2007.

27. Daddaoua A, Martínez-Plata E, Ortega-González M, Ocón B, Aranda CJ, Zarzuelo A, Suárez MD, de Medina FS, and Martínez-Augustin O. "The nutritional supplement Active Hexose Correlated Compound (AHCC) has direct immunomodulatory actions on intestinal epithelial cells and macrophages involving TLR/MyD88 and NF-κB/MAPK activation." *Food Chem.* 136: 1288–1295, 2013.

28. Ocón B, Anzola A, Ortega-González M, Zarzuelo A, Suárez MD, Sánchez de Medina F, and Martínez-Augustin O. "Active hexose-correlated compound and *Bifidobacterium longum* BB536 exert symbiotic effects in experimental colitis." *Eur. J. Nutr.* 52: 457–466, 2013.

29. Mombaerts P, Iacomini J, Johnson RS, Herrup K, Tonegawa S, and Papaioannou VE. "RAG-1-deficient mice have no mature B and T lymphocytes." *Cell* 68: 869–877, 1992.

30. Mascaraque C, Suárez MD, Zarzuelo A, Sánchez de Medina F, and Martínez-Augustin O. "Active hexose correlated compound exerts therapeutic effects in lymphocyte driven colitis." *Mol. Nutr. Food Res.* 58: 2379–2382, 2014.

Chapter 8

DRUG INTERACTIONS

Drug-Nutrient Interaction

Anil D. Kulkarni

Before the therapeutic drug discoveries of the modern era, the field of medicine was restricted to nutrient-nutrient interaction (NNI) and its beneficial or adverse effects. Beneficial effects were when NNI showed health improvements, and adverse effects were when therapeutic benefits were not observed.

In the modern era, many new discoveries were made, and specific disease-targeted drugs were produced and used. This was very useful in preventing disease and provided cures for years. The use of these modern drugs expanded, leading to important and critical observations and evidence of beneficial and adverse drug-nutrient interaction (DNI).

Interactions between drugs and nutrients can cause an alteration of the pharmacokinetics of a drug, resulting in compromised nutritional status as a result of their DNI interplay. This can be either harmful or beneficial. Common adverse events include nutritional deficiencies, drug toxicity, and loss of therapeutic efficacy or disease control. The working definition of *drug-nutrient interactions* in the excellent *Handbook of Drug-Nutrient Reaction,* Second Edition, by Boullata and Armenti (Humana Press, 2010) is broader than the definition provided elsewhere. It is defined as an interaction resulting from a physical, chemical, physiological, or pathophysiological relationship between a drug and a nutrient, multiple nutrients, food in general, or nutritional status. The clinical consequences of an interaction are related to alterations in the disposition and effect of the drug or nutrient.

The unanticipated effect of drug in a person may be different[1] from the one expected because that drug interacts with another drug the person is taking (drug-drug interaction), food, beverages, dietary supplements the person is consuming (drug-nutrient/food interaction), or presence of other disease the patient has (drug-disease interaction). In many cases, patients are always using dietary supplements for their overall well-being. A drug interaction is a situation in which a substance affects the activity of a drug (i.e. the effects are increased or decreased) or they produce a new effect that neither produces on its own. These interactions may occur out of accidental misuse or due to lack of knowledge about the active ingredients involved in the relevant substances.

Regarding food-drug interactions, physicians and pharmacists recognize that some foods and drugs, when taken simultaneously, can alter the body's ability to utilize a particular food or drug, or cause serious side effects. Clinically significant drug interactions, which pose potential harm to the patient, may result from changes in formulations and their properties. Some may be taken advantage of, to the benefit of patients, but more commonly drug interactions result in adverse drug events. Therefore, it is advisable for patients to follow the medical practitioner's instructions to obtain maximum benefits with least food-drug interactions.

The literature survey was conducted by extracting data from different review and original articles on general or specific drug interactions with food. This review gives information about various interactions between different foods and drugs and will help physicians and pharmacists prescribe drugs cautiously with only suitable food supplement to get maximum benefit for the patient.

A large number of drugs are introduced every year. Food-drug interactions can produce negative effects in safety and efficacy of drug therapy, as well in the nutritional status of the patient. Generally speaking, drug interactions are to be avoided, due to the possibility of poor or unexpected outcomes. Like food, drugs taken by mouth must be absorbed through the lining of the stomach or the small intestine. Consequently, the presence of food in the digestive tract may reduce absorption of a drug. Often, such interactions can be avoided by taking the drug one hour before or two hours after eating. Like drugs, foods are not tested as comprehensively so they may interact with prescription or over-the-counter drugs. Patients should tell their doctors and pharmacists about their food intake and dietary supplements so that interactions can be avoided.

A mini review on drug-nutrient interactions defines those as physical, chemical, physiologic, or pathophysiologic relationships between a drug and a nutrient.[2] The causes of most clinically significant drug-nutrient interactions are usually multifactorial. Failure to identify and properly manage drug-nutrient interactions can lead to very serious consequences and have a negative impact on patient outcomes. Nevertheless, with thorough review and assessment of the patient's history and treatment regimens, as well as a carefully executed management strategy, adverse events associated with drug-nutrient interactions can be prevented. Based on the physiologic sequence of events after a drug or a nutrient has entered the body and the mechanism of interactions, drug-nutrient interactions can be categorized into four main types. Each type of interaction can be managed using similar strategies. The existing data that guide the clinical management of most drug-nutrient interactions are mostly anecdotal experience, uncontrolled observations, and opinions, whereas the science in understanding the mechanism of drug-nutrient interactions remains limited.

The challenge for researchers and clinicians is to increase both basic and higher level clinical research in this field to bridge the gap between the science and practice. The research should aim to establish a better understanding of the function, regulation, and substrate specificity of the nutrient-related enzymes and transport proteins present in the gastrointestinal tract, as well as assess how the incidence and management of drug-nutrient interactions can be affected by gender, ethnicity, environmental factors, and genetic polymorphisms. This knowledge can help us develop a true personalized medicine approach in the prevention and management of drug-nutrient interactions.

Summary

The impact of food on the absorption of drugs significantly complicates the treatment of any chronic disease. Increases in absorption may result in adverse reactions. Importantly, the impact on those with chronic infections differs from conditions such as hypertension and diabetes. Obviously, infections can be transmitted from one individual to another. So a decrease in absorption in treating an infection can lead to the development of a resistant infection. Subsequent spread of a resistant infection has significant public health ramifications. Although many unanswered questions regarding drug-food interactions still exist, the information provided in this chapter should be used to educate healthcare professionals and patients to optimize patient outcome and minimize the development of drug-resistant infections. Older agents still in use were not subject to the more current, rigorous requirements of labeling and should be further investigated for interactions with food. Future studies are also needed to answer remaining questions about interactions between drugs used for chronic infections and food, alternative therapies, or illicit drugs.

Mechanism-Based Classification System for Interactions

The classifications fall into three categories: 1) pharmaceutical, 2) pharmacokinetics and 3) pharmacodynamics. Together these lead to physiological outcomes, which then lead to patient outcomes. These outcomes are either negative or no difference or they are positive. Mechanisms of interaction are based on the site of interaction; such as 1) drug/nutrient delivery device or gastrointestinal GI lumen, 2) GI mucosa, 3) systemic circulation reaching tissues, and the organs of excretion.[1]

Examples of such drug-food interactions and some contraindications are listed in Table 1 below:

TABLE 1. **EXAMPLES OF INTERACTIONS BETWEEN MOST COMMON DRUGS AND FOOD**

acarbose	Maximum effectiveness at start of each meal
ace inhibitors	Grapefruit juice, empty stomach absorption is increased
acetaminophen	Pectin delays absorption and onset
antibiotics	Some foods prevent their absorption, reduce bioavailability
cimetidine	With food (any type) increases bioavailability
cycloserine	High-fat meals decrease serum concentration
esomeprazole	High-fat meal bioavailability was reduced
glimepiride	With breakfast absolute bioavailability
isoniazid	Plants, medicinal herbs, oleanolic acid exert synergistic effect
levothyroxine	Grapefruit juice delays absorption[3]
mercaptopurine	Cow's milk* reduces bioavailability[3]
NSAIDs	Alcohol can increase risk of liver damage or stomach bleeding
tamoxifen	Sesame seeds negatively interferes with this drug.
theophylline	High-fat meal and grape fruit juice increase bioavailability, caffeine increases the risk of drug toxicity
warfarin	High-protein diet, vitamin K, leafy green vegetables, charbroiled foods adverse

Practitioner's Role

There are many common over-the-counter drugs and specific prescriptive medications physicians should discuss with patients regarding their interactions with certain food/drink items so that patients are aware. To optimize a patient's clinical outcomes, it is important to recognize DNIs systematically as part of the patient assessment with the patient's drug regimen review. This requires broader awareness of the DNI framework beyond a handful of isolated examples. By broadening the understanding of the potential mechanisms of interaction, the practitioner can become more proactive in anticipating potential interactions.

Clinicians should have access to interaction information that allows for safe treatment approaches. DNI resources are varied and continually evolving in terms of depth, breadth, and accessibility. Because of limited clinical DNI data generated as part of the drug-development process, much is explored in post-marketing observational studies, or from individual case reports generated by clinicians, with subsequent mechanistic investigations and descriptions when novel interactions are identified.

Recommended Reading

Handbook of Drug-Nutrient Interactions, 2nd Edition, by Jospeph I. Boullata and Vincent T. Armenti, Eds. Humana Press, 2010.

REFERENCES

1. Boullata JI and Hudson LM. "Drug–Nutrient Interactions: A Broad View with implications for practice." *J Acad Nutr Diet.* 112:506–517, 2012.

2. Chan L-N. "Drug-Nutrient Interactions" JPEN *J Parenter Enteral Nutr.* 37: 450–459, 2013.

3. Bushara R, Aslam N, and Khan AY. "Food-Drug Interactions" *Oman Medical Journal* 26(2), 77–83, 2011.

4. De Boer A, van Hunsel F, and Bast A. "Adverse food-drug interactions" *Regulatory Toxicology and Pharmacology* 73 (2015) 859-865

5. Kordas K, Lorrerdal B, and Stoltzfus RJ. "Interactions between nutrition and environmental exposures: Effects on health outcomes in women and children." *J Nutr.* 137(12):2794–2797, 2007.

6. Manoj Kumar P, Kulkarni SS, and Wadkar SD. "Review on interaction of herbal medicines with allopathic medicines." *J. of Ayurveda and Holistic Medicine* 2, 38–43, 2014.

7. Silva RF and Garbi Novaes MRC. "Interactions between drugs and drug-nutrient in enteral nutrition: A review based on evidences" *Nutricion Hospitalaria* 30:514–518, 2014.

Drug Interactions with AHCC

Judith A. Smith

There are many therapeutic agents, including cancer therapeutics, that undergo extensive hepatic metabolism. The liver is the primary route of elimination as well. (See Figure 1 below.) The majority of drug-supplement interactions that are reported focus on phase I metabolism interactions, which involve the cytochrome P450 (CYP450) metabolism pathways. The CYP450 isoenzymes most often associated with drug metabolism include 1A2, 2C8, 2C9, 2D6, and 3A4. For instance, paclitaxel and docetaxel are commonly used in ovarian cancer treatments. Paclitaxel is metabolized through CYP450 2C8 and 3A4 pathways, while docetaxel goes through

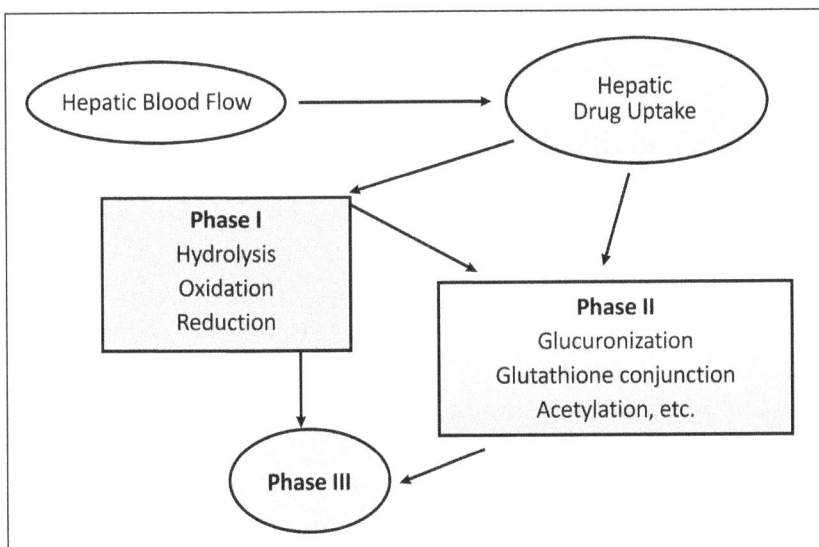

Figure 1.
Illustration of phase I and phase II drug metabolism.

CYP450 3A4 pathway only. Usually the inhibition of CYP3A4 pathway will lead to increase of standard drug concentration and decrease in drug clearance rate, which may cause toxicity of standard drugs. However, depending on specific drugs, induction of the same pathway can cause an increase or decrease in drug clearance, which contributes to an expected drug efficacy or other adverse effects. The intake of phytoestrogens may cause clinically significant drug-drug interaction through hepatic metabolism pathways.

Recently pharmacology studies have also been focused on the induction of phase II metabolism pathways to specifically find out whether xenobiotics induce the detoxification of chemo-agents, which leads to low drug efficacy. The phase II metabolism pathways most often associated with drug/compound interactions are glutathione S-transferase (GST), quinone oxidoreductase (QOR), catechol-O-methyltransferase (COMT), and uridine diphosphate (UDP)-glucuronosyltransferase (UGT).[1-5] QOR is a phase II detoxification enzyme that plays an important role in quinone detoxification and antioxidant function maintenance of the cell. In breast cancer cells, QOR can be upregulated by anti-estrogens, and phytoestrogens biochanin A, genistein, and resveratrol. Therefore, the activity of QOR is associated with estrogen and agents with estrogenic effect. Another critical phase II enzyme GST was also proved to be affected by many natural/plant derived compounds. UGT is responsible for drug glucuronidation in phase II metabolism, which is a major pathway of detoxification for agents such as irinotecan. The study on hepatic metabolism mediated–drug interaction is very critical because, in current clinical settings, many patients are using AHCC products without knowing that there can be potential effect on drug efficacy and safety.

Understanding Metabolism Inhibition and Induction

Drug and supplements that undergo hepatic metabolism can be classified as either a substrate, inhibitor, or inducer of metabolism. A substrate is a compound that undergoes hepatic phase I (cytochrome P450) or phase II (UGT, COMT, QOR, or GST) metabolism. It is possible to impact or alter hepatic metabolism pathways that results in "drug interactions" and not be a substrate.

Inhibition of the hepatic metabolism pathway results in a decreased and almost ceased function of the hepatic enzyme; thus there is no breakdown or elimination of the parent compound. This will result in an accumulation of the "parent compound" in systemic circulation (see Figure 2 on the facing page). Depending on the drug/

compound, this may lead to an increased chance of toxicity, especially with drug/compound "narrow therapeutic" window such as cytotoxic chemotherapy agents. However, with other compounds such as serotonin reuptake inhibitors (5-HT3s) that have a wide therapeutic window, inhibition would be less of a concern. In some cases, inhibition of the metabolism pathway that results in higher plasma concentrations may result in an increase in therapeutic activity.

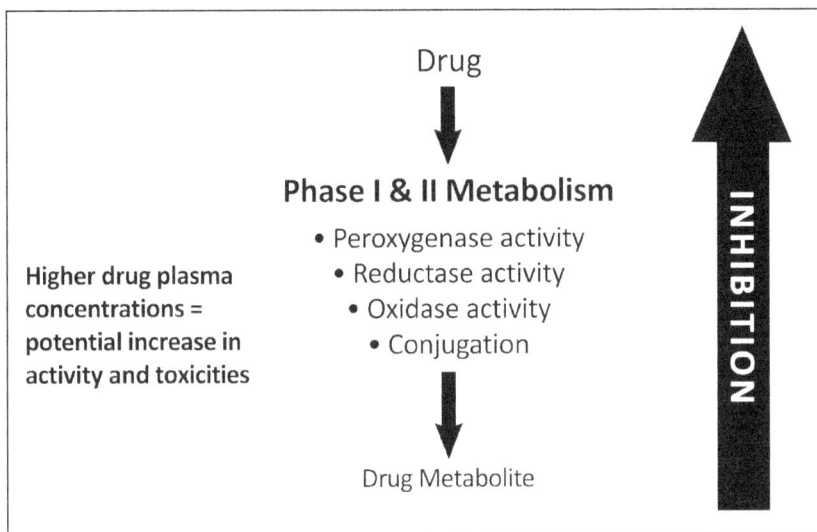

Figure 2. Inhibition of Metabolism.

Induction of the hepatic metabolism pathway results in increased (and can almost double or triple) function of the hepatic enzyme, thus leading to faster elimination of the parent compound to the respective drug metabolite(s). This will result in a decrease of the "parent compound" and an increase in the drug metabolite in systemic circulation (see Figure 3 on the following page). Most often, the decrease in parent compound concentrations is associated with a potential decrease in therapeutic activity as well as a decrease in toxicity. However, in some cases such as doxorubicin or cyclophosphamide that are "pro-drugs," which means that metabolism is necessary to convert to active metabolite, induction of hepatic metabolism leads to higher plasma concentrations of the active metabolite. The higher plasma concentration again may result in an increase in therapeutic activity, but this might be associated with an increase in toxicity as well.

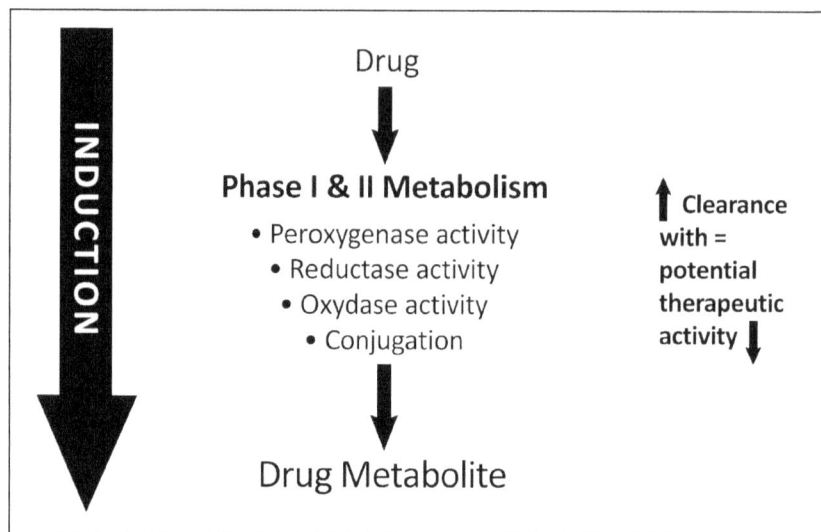

Figure 3. Induction of Metabolism

Screening for Drug-Supplement Interactions

There are multiple approaches for pre-clinical screening for hepatic metabolism–mediated interactions such as in vitro isoenzyme inhibition assays or ex vivo human hepatocyte models.[6] The critical aspect of these studies, regardless of approach, is to be sure there are clinically relevant or achievable systemic concentrations. Often this is information is not available for most nutritional supplements, such as AHCC.[7]

One approach we have used is estimating the highest possible concentration that could be achieved since this would be "worst-case scenario"; hence, from a safety perspective, if no reaction occurs, there is more assurance there will not be an interaction in vivo. If an interaction is observed, it provides guidance that patients should be monitored for a potential interaction. Using a control inhibitor or inducer helps provide guidance on the potential magnitude of the interaction as well. The concern is that a potential interaction would be missed if the supplement concentrations used in the screening studies are too low. In the majority of cases, supplements such as AHCC are being used to augment or improve outcomes, so avoiding the potential for drug-supplement interactions that may increase toxicity and/or decrease therapeutic efficacy is desirable.

AHCC and Hepatic Phase I Metabolism

To identify the potential for AHCC to interact with drugs metabolized via the CYP450 hepatic metabolism pathway, we conducted both in vitro isoenzyme inhibition assays and ex vivo human hepatocyte models.[8] The objective of this study was to describe AHCC hepatic metabolism, particularly involving the possibility for drug interactions with select chemotherapy agents. In brief, high-throughput cytochrome P450 (CYP450) metabolism inhibition and substrate experiments were completed in vitro evaluating CYP450 3A4, 2C8, 2C9, and 2D6. The ex vivo model of cryopreserved human hepatocytes was used to evaluate CYP450 metabolism induction potential of AHCC for CYP P450 3A4, 2C8/2C9, and 2D6.

No inhibition of CYP450 activity was detected in the presence of AHCC; however, AHCC was a substrate of CYP450 2D6 (see Table 1 on the following page). The CYP450 induction metabolism assays suggest that AHCC is an inducer of CYP450 2D6 (see Table 1). AHCC does have the potential for drug-supplement interactions with drugs that are substrates of the CYP450 2D6 pathway such as doxorubicin or ondansetron. Generally, the data indicated that AHCC would be safe to administer with most other chemotherapy agents that are not metabolized via the CYP450 2D6 pathway.[8]

AHCC and Hepatic Phase II Metabolism

To further elucidate the potential drug-supplement interactions, we proceeded to embark on completion of evaluation of the primary four primary hepatic metabolism phase II pathways that are associated with drug-supplement metabolism: glutathione S-transferase (GST), quinone oxidoreductase (QOR), catechol-O-methyltransferases (COMT), and uridine diphosphate (UDP)-glucuronosyltransferase (UGT). Again, this study has been published in full with detailed information.[9] Briefly, we employed in vitro GST, QOR, and UGT metabolism inhibition assays, then utilized the ex vivo human liver hepatocytes model to determine if there was potential induction of UGT and COMT metabolism.

Data demonstrated that AHCC is not an inhibitor of GST or UGT pathways, but may be a potential inhibitor of QOR pathway (see Table 1). Evaluation of induction of the phase II pathways demonstrated that AHCC showed potential induction of the UGT 1A3 and 1A6 pathways. There was no induction of the COMT pathway (see Table 1). Traditionally, drug interaction studies have only concentrated on phase I metabolism pathways, so presently, there is very inadequate information regarding the phase II metabolism of most drugs. In conclusion, additional studies are necessary to determine potential of any phase II hepatic interactions with AHCC when administered with other medications or supplements that are substrates of these pathways.

TABLE 1. **SUMMARY OF AHCC AND HEPATIC METABOLISM PATHWAYS**

METABOLISM SUBSTRATE	INHIBITOR	INDUCER	NO INTERACTIONS	PATHWAY
Phase I Metabolism Pathways[7]				
CYP450 3A4				✗
CYP450 2C8				✗
CYP450 2C9				✗
CYP450 2D6	✓		✓	
Phase II Metabolism Pathways				
GST				✗
COMT				✗
QOR		✓		
UGT 2B17				✗
UGT1A3			✓	
UGT1A6			✓	

Monitoring Patient for Drug-Supplement Interactions

Whenever initiating new nutritional supplements such as AHCC, herbal products or medications, it is always advisable to go through to document and review all supplements, herbals, over-the-counter (OTC), and prescription. If there is any potential for a drug-supplement interaction, then clinically evaluate the likelihood of interaction and whether patient should be monitored closer during the initiation phase- first three months after starting the new supplement. It is important to educate the patient what adverse effect/side effects to watch out for if there is potential for increase toxicity associated with the potential interaction. On the other hand, patients also need to know what is purpose of medication, for example "to help control blood pressure" and associated symptoms "headaches, dizziness, irregular heartbeat" if therapeutic concentrations might be altered.

Fortunately, for AHCC overall it appears to have very limited, if any, potential for drug-supplement interactions. The CYP450 2D6 pathway, QOR and UGT1A3/UGT1A6 pathways have the only observed potential for drug-supplement interactions (see Table 1). While current references should be checked and verified, Table 2 below provides some brief examples of common medications that are substrates of the respective pathways with the potential to interact with AHCC. Since there is continuously new information emerging on pharmacology and metabolism, current references should always be cross-referenced when reviewing a patient's nutritional supplements, herbal products, over-the-counter medicines, and prescription medication profiles.

TABLE 2. COMMON SUBSTRATES OF HEPATIC METABOLISM POTENTIALLY IMPACTED BY AHCC

CYP450 2D6	UGT 1A3	UGT 1A6	QOR
ondansetron	amitriptyline	acetaminophen	acetaminophen
prochlorperazine	buprenorphine	morphine	phenobarbital
promethazine	clozapine	raloxifene	phenolphthalein
fluoxetine	dapsone	troglitazone	olitpraz
amitriptyline	diclofenac	valproate	
haloperidol	estrogen	oltipraz	
risperidone	flurbiprofen		
doxorubicin			

(This is *not* an all-inclusive list.)

Conclusion

Based on the in vitro and ex vivo metabolism data from this study and our previous phase I metabolism studies, AHCC does not have possibilities for potential drug-supplement interaction with drugs/agents that function as substrates of CYP450 3A4, 2C8, or 2C9, GST, UGT 2B17, or COMT pathways.[8,9] AHCC may have potential for drug-supplement interactions with drugs/agents that are substrates of the CYP450 2D6, UGT1A3, UGT1A6, or QOR pathways (refer back to Table 1). However, additional studies are needed to determine the clinical significance of potential interactions. To date, in clinical trials, there have been no documented drug-supplement interactions observed. Overall, AHCC appears to be safe to coadminister with most medications, including chemotherapy with a narrow therapeutic window. The advantageous interactions between AHCC and chemotherapy will be discussed elsewhere in this book.

REFERENCES

1. Mannervik B and Guthenberg C. "Glutathione transferase (human placenta)." *Methods Enzymol.* 77: 231–235, 1981.

2. Ploemen JH, van Ommen B, Bogaards JJ, and van Bladeren PJ. "Ethacryic acid and its glutathione conjugate as inhibitors of glutathione S-transferases." *Xenobiotica* 23(8): 913–923, 1993.

3. Liu Z and Franklin MR. "Separation of four glucuronides in a single sample by high pressure liquid chromatography and its use in the determination of UDP-glucuronosyltransferase activity toward four aglycones." *Anal Biochemo.* 142: 340–346, 1984.

4. Benson AM, Hunkeler MJ, and Talalay P. "Increase of NAD(P)H:quinone reductase by dietary antioxidants: possible role in protection against carcinogenesis and toxicity." *Proc. Natl. Acad. Sci.* 77: 5216–5220, 1980.

5. Kapiszewska M, Kalemba M, Wojciech U, and Cierniak A. "The COMT-mediated metabolism of flavonoids and estrogen and its relevance to cancer risk." *Pol. J. Food Nutri. Sci.* 12(53): 141–146, 2003.

6. "Guidance for Industry Bioanalytical Method Assay Validation," May 2001. www.fda.gov/downloads/Drugs/Guidances/ucm070107.pdf, verified access on 5/9/2014.

7. Spierings ELH, Fujii H, and Walshe T. "A phase I study of the safety and nutritional supplement, active hexose correlated compound, AHCC, in health volunteers." *J. Nutritional Science and Vitaminology* 53(6): 536–539, 2007.

8. Mach CM, Fujii H, Wakame K, and Smith JA. "Evaluation of Active Hexose Correlated Compound (AHCC) hepatic metabolism and potential for drug interactions with chemotherapy agents." *J. Soc. Integr. Oncol.* 6(3): 105–109, 2008.

9. Coffer L, Mathew L, Zhang X, Owiti N, Cegelski J, Myers AL, Faro J, Lucci JA, and Smith JA. "Evaluation of active hexose correlated compound (AHCC) on phase II drug metabolism pathways and the implications for supplement-drug interactions." *J. Integr. Oncol.* 4: 142, 2009. doi:10.4172/2329–6771.1000142.

Comprehensive Analysis
of Liver Metabolism Enzyme Gene

Koji Wakame

Recently, DNA-focused microarray analysis has become a powerful and important tool to elucidate the roles of the modurators of DNA and RNA expressions. In this chapter, we present the investigation of the alteration of metabolic enzymes and anti-inflammatory pathways in AHCC-treated mice liver DNA microarray. The results of the study revealed that AHCC does not affect the drug-metabolizing enzymes, and additionally, suppressed the expression of genes relating to oxidative stress, inflammation, and apoptosis.

Food and Drug Metabolizing Enzymes

When food and drugs are orally consumed, the ingredients in them are digested and absorbed from the intestines, passed through the portal vein, and all the absorbed ingredients are metabolized by the liver. This is part of the important parameter that must be considered as *Absorption, Distribution, Metabolism, and Excretion* (ADME) even when examined pharmacologically. Specifically, metabolizing enzyme group that takes charge of phase I (oxidation and reduction), and phase II (conjugation) are known to exist in the liver. Some of these enzymes are known to be present even in the intestine. If these metabolizing enzymes are induced or suppressed excessively by the food ingredients, the drug absorption and concentration in the blood are significantly affected during medical treatment, and various adverse events may be triggered. Therefore, accurate information based on scientific evidence has to be collected on the effect of food on the drug-metabolizing enzyme and brought to the attention of consumers from the perspective of safety, specifically in clinical practice.

AHCC and Drug Metabolizing Enzymes

AHCC is a standardized extract of cultured *Lentinula edodes* mycelia, and there are many papers indicating the impact and safety of AHCC on the drug-metabolizing enzymes. These reports are the studies conducted on the metabolism (CYP family) of phase I, primarily using in vitro experimental systems. The induction of CYP2D6 has been reported based on these studies.[1]

There are no detailed reports on the ADME of active ingredients with oral intake of AHCC. If polysaccharides are considered to be one of the ingredients in AHCC, then it can be considered that most of the polysaccharides are digested in the intestines. However, this suggests that some of the polysaccharides are absorbed in units of small saccharides that can pass through the intestines and reach the liver. We comprehensively analyzed the gene expressions using a DNA array for the possibility that some kind of AHCC ingredients are metabolized in the liver by the oral intake and, at the same time, has an effect on the liver metabolism enzyme in the in vivo testing system.[2]

DNA-Focused Microarray

DNA-focused microarray was developed around 2000. It has found wide application in genetic diagnosis of various diseases, detection of bacteria and viruses, and analysis of polymorphism (individual differences). There is a growing expectation that these will be put into practice by new industries. At the same time, for example, there are approximately 22,000 types of known genes in mice when application to animal experiments is considered. It is difficult to analyze all these genes and the association between the gene expression and biological functions.

We attempted to perform the genetic analysis by narrowing down the target genes using DNA-focused microarray, Genopal® (Mitsubishi Rayon. Co., Ltd., Tokyo, Japan). The chip for analysis used in Genopal® is equipped with approximately 200 gene probes according to the purpose on one chip. The major feature of this chip is that it can measure three-dimensional fluorescence intensity and obtain gene expression data with higher reliability.[3]

Genetic Analysis of Mice Liver Using DNA-Focused Array

Effect on the Drug Metabolizing Enzyme Group

The ICR mice (male, 7 weeks) were allowed to feed freely for five days on AHCC that was dissolved to 3%. The liver was then removed, and the total RNA was extracted. cDNA was prepared from the RNA, and biotin-labeled RNA was transcribed and amplified. The fluorescence intensity of the color spots on the chip due to hybridization using Genopal® was measured. The special chips used for the DNA array were the METABOLIC CHIP (equipped with 195 types of genes), and the ANTI-AGING CHIP (equipped with 219 types of genes). The probe on the chip was equipped with the well-known types of genes associated with drug metabolism, cytochrome P450 (CYP) for phase I, and glutathione S-transferase (GST) for phase II. Thirty-six types that were closely involved in drug metabolism from the gene group in the chip, which were measured, are shown in Table 1 below.

TABLE 1. GENES RELATED TO DRUG METABOLIZING ENZYME IN THE LIVER THAT WERE ANALYZED WITH THE DNA ARRAY.

CYP (cytochrome P450)	CYP1A2, CYP2E1, CYP2C29 CYP2D22, CYP3A11, CYP4A10 CYP4A12A, CYP7A1, CYP27A1
GSS (glutathlone synthetase)	GSS
GSTA (glutathione S-transferase)	GSTA1, GSTA2, GSTA3 GSTA4
GSR (glutathione reductase)	GSR
GSTK (glutathione S-transferase kappa)	GSTK1
GPX (glutathione peroxidase)	GPX1, GPX2, GPX3
COMT (catechol-O-methytransferase)	COMT1
GSTO (glutathione S-transferase omega)	GST01, GST02
GSTM (glutathione S-transferase, mu)	GSTM1, GSTM2, GSTM3 GSTM4, G$TM5, GSTM6
GSTP(glutathione S-transferase, pi)	GSTP1
GSTT (glutathlone S-transferase, theta)	GSTT1, GSTT2, GSTT3
GSTZ (glutathione transferase zeta)	GSTZ1
MGST (microsomal glutathione S-transferase)	MGST2, MGST3
NDUFS (NADH dehydrogenase [ubiquinone] Fe-S protein 8)	NDUFS8

In the present analysis, signal intensity ratio ($\log_2$; Sample Signal intensity/ Control Signal intensity) fluctuating by +1 or more, or –1 or less were interpreted as differential expression genes (DEG). CYP3A11, and CYP7A1 were detected as DEG among the thirty-six genes listed in Table 1 (see Table 2 below). Moreover, significant changes were not observed in the gene expression of the other thirty-four types. Also, although AHCC induces CYP3A11, CYP7A1 genes, its action was not powerful since the signal intensity ratio did not cross +1 significantly. CYP3A11 is known to be homologous to the liver-metabolizing enzyme CYP3A5, and immunosuppressive agents such as tacrolimus forms its substrate.[4] CYP7A1 is known to be the rate-limiting enzyme for catabolism from cholesterol to the bile acid.[5] From the results so far, it cannot be asserted that by drinking AHCC, adverse events are caused by the combination with the drugs, due to the reasons given above.

TABLE 2. **GENES RELATED TO DRUG METABOLIZING ENZYME IN THE LIVER THAT WERE INDUCED BY AHCC.**

GENE BANK ACCESSION NO.	GENE SYMBOL	GENE NAME	SIGNAL INTENSITY RATIO
NM_007818	CYP3A11	Mus musculus cytochrome P450, family 3, subfamily a, polypeptide 11 (Cyp3a11), mRNA	1.15 + 0.48
NM_007824	CYP7A1	Mus musculus cytochrome P450, family 7, subfamily a, polypeptide 1 (Cyp7a1), mRNA	1.02 + 0.62

Signal intensity ratio = +1 <

Effect on Other Gene Expressions

DEG was confirmed for 23 out of the 414 types of genes, excluding the genes involved with the drug-metabolizing enzyme. The suppression of gene expression was especially observed in five types (Bcl10, Bcl6, Icam1, Map3k5 [ASK1], and Caspase9) among these, with a signal intensity ratio of –10 or less (see Figure 1 opposite).

Of these, Bcl10 (B-Cell CLL/Lymphoma 10) has NF-κB at the downstream of the signaling and is involved in the release of inflammatory cytokines, such as TNF-α and IL-1β. Also, Map3k5 (mitogen-activated protein kinase kinase kinase 5) and ASK1 (apoptosis signal-regulating kinase 1) are known to be closely associated with inflammation, oxidative stress, carcinogenesis, and apoptosis (see Figure 2 opposite).

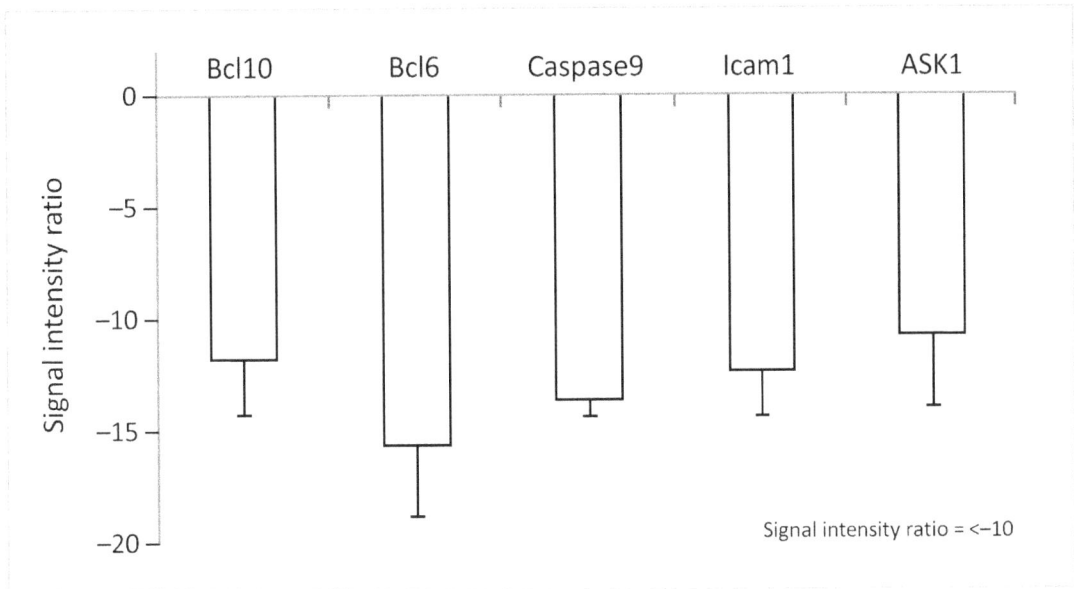

Figure 1. Genes not related to the drug metabolizing enzyme in liver that were suppressed by AHCC.

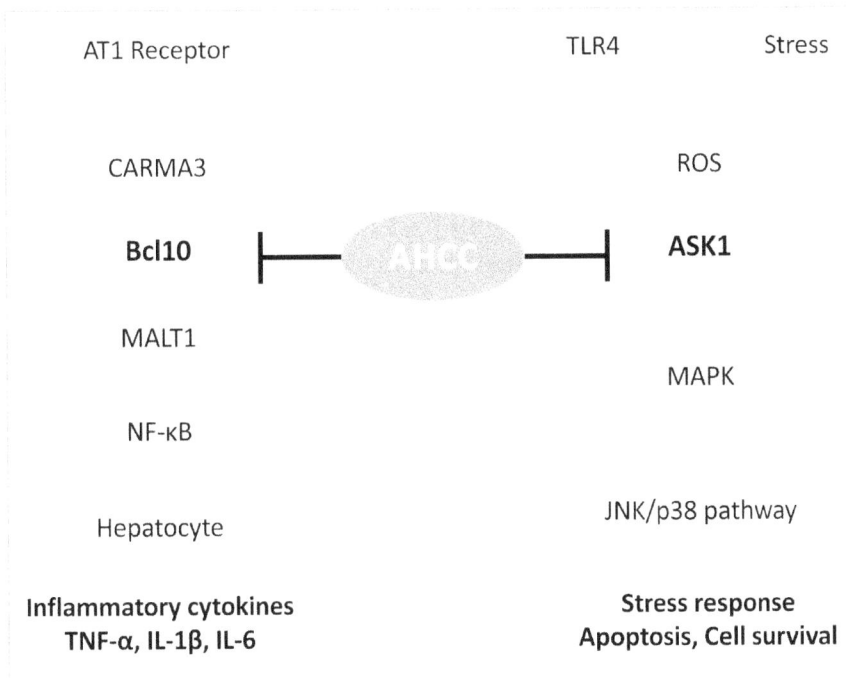

Figure 2. Target genes involved in the anti-inflammation of AHCC.

In relation to apoptosis, AHCC suppresses (Signal intensity ratio = –2.7) Fas (Apo-1/CD95) and strongly inhibits Caspase-9. This suggests that it provides the function of inhibiting the induction of apoptosis in the liver (see Figure 3 below).

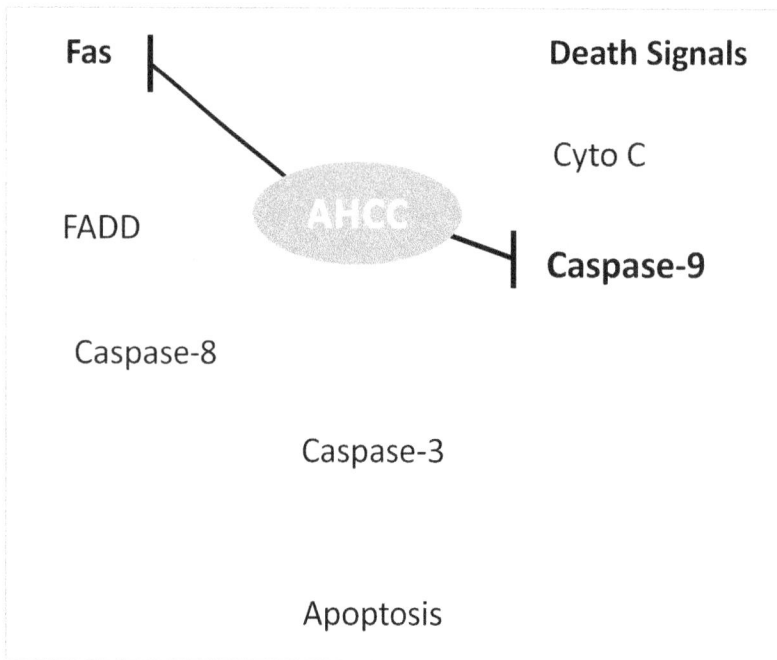

Figure 3. Target genes involved in the apoptosis of AHCC.

Moreover, it is gaining attention as a gene involved in the inflammation of Icam1 (Intercellular Adhesion Molecule 1) vascular endothelium. Furthermore, Bcl6 (B-Cell CLL/Lymphoma 6) is involved in the adhesion and differentiation between the immune cells.

These results suggest that oral intake of AHCC has the ability to protect the cells from inflammation, oxidative stress, and apoptosis in the liver. These findings can strengthen Tanaka's results showing that AHCC suppresses the IL-1 receptor (IL-1R1) up-regulation in liver cells[6] and, as suggested by Ye et al.,[7] is attractive for its antioxidative effects on the liver. In addition, the ASK1, which is located in the down stream of TLR4 pathway, was suppressed by AHCC treatment; however, AHCC was reported as a ligand of TLR2 and TLR 4[8], suggesting that the effectiveness of AHCC may change based on the host conditions. AHCC is also expected to be used as a substance that can balance the immune system.

Conclusion

DNA array can be used for comprehensive analysis of gene expressions, but satisfactory analysis up to the downstream protein expression and signaling was not possible. However, the prediction of the impact and toxicity by conducting comprehensive analysis of the gene action in the liver, based on the oral intake of AHCC that contains many unknown ingredients as in the current study, is of significance even in the field of nutrigenomics. Moreover, AHCC did not have a significant impact on specific drug-metabolizing enzymes in the experiments conducted on normal mice, and it is inferred that AHCC has the function of protecting the cells from oxidative stress, inflammation, and apoptosis.

REFERENCES

1. Mach CM, Fujii H, Wakame K, and Smith J. "Evaluation of active hexose correlated compound hepatic metabolism and potential for drug interactions with chemotherapy agents." *J. Soc. Integr. Oncol.* 6(3): 105–109, 2008.

2. Wakame K, Nakata A, Sato K, et al. "DNA microarray analysis of gene expression changes in ICR mouse liver following treatment with active hexose correlated compound." *Integr. Mol. Med.* 3(3): 739–744, 2016.

3. Okuzaki D, Fukushima T, Tougan T, et al. "Genopal: a novel hollow fibre array for focused microarray analysis." *DNA Research* 17: 369–379, 2010. Advance Access publication on November 8, 2010.

4. Nair SS, Sarasamma S, Gracious N, George J, Anish TS, and Radhakrishnan R. "Polymorphism of the CYP3A5 gene and its effect on tacrolimus blood level." *Exp. Clin. Transplant* 13 Suppl 1: 197–200, 2015.

5. Hebanowska A. "Mechanisms of bile acid biosynthesis regulation—autoregulation by bile acids." *Postepy Biochem.* 57(3): 314–323, 2011.

6. Tanaka Y, Ohashi S, Ohtsuki A, Kiyono T, et al. "Adenosine, a hepato-protective component in active hexose correlated compound: its identification and iNOS suppression mechanism." *Nitric Oxide* 40: 75–86, 2014.

7. Ye SF, Ichimura K, Wakame K, and Ohe M. "Suppressive effects of Active Hexose Correlated Compound on the increased activity of hepatic and renal ornithine decarboxylase induced by oxidative stress." *Life Sci.* 74(5): 593–602, 2003.

8. Mallet JF, Graham É, Ritz BW, Homma K, and Matar C. "Active Hexose Correlated Compound (AHCC) promotes an intestinal immune response in BALB/c mice and in primary intestinal epithelial cell culture involving toll-like receptors TLR-2 and TLR-4." *Eur. J. Nutr.* 55(1): 139–46, 2016.

Chapter 9

APPLICATION IN DISEASE PREVENTION

The Role of Food in Regulating Host Biology

Philip C. Calder

The foods and drinks that make up meals provide the human body with nutrients, many with well-described biological properties (see Figure 1 below). It is now fairly well recognized that many of the chemical constituents of foods and drinks that are not nutrients in the accepted sense of that term also have biological properties; here the term *non-nutrients* is used to describe those constituents.

Any particular food will contain a complex mixture of nutrients and non-nutrients. Certain foods may be characterized by the presence of particular nutrients or non-nutrients. For example, oily fish is richer in long-chain omega-3 fatty acids than most other foods. However, it is important to note that the exact nutrient composition of a specific food may be different in different locations, may change seasonally, and may have changed over time. Thus, the chemical composition of plant foods can differ according to the soil the plant is grown in, while that of animal foods can differ according the diet of

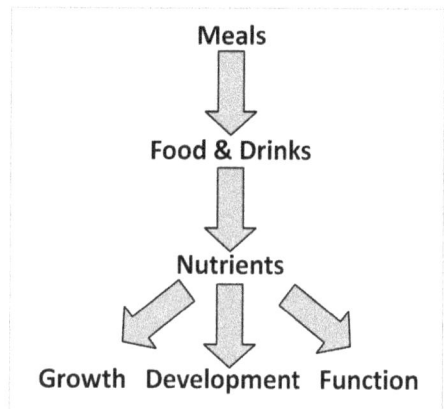

Figure 1. The relationship between meals, foods and nutrients and the generic roles of nutrients.

the animal. For example, the selenium content of wheat used for making flour differs according to the selenium content of the soil on which the wheat is grown, while the fat and fatty acid composition of wild and farmed animals of the same species are often different. Genetics can also play a role in determining nutrient composition and content of both plant and animal foods. Furthermore, processing, storage, and cooking of foods may alter their chemical composition. For these reasons, knowing the precise nutrient composition of a specific food eaten at a specific time is a major challenge, and nutrient composition tables are likely to be inaccurate for many foods. Another challenge to fully understanding nutrient (and non-nutrient) intakes is that no two meals are identical in terms of the types and amounts of foods and drinks consumed.

There are different ways of classifying the chemical constituents in foods and drinks. One is to classify nutrients as macronutrients or micronutrients. Macronu-trients are energy-yielding food components that are consumed daily in grams to hundreds of grams. These include carbohydrates, fats, and proteins. Carbohydrates include complex carbohydrates like starch and simpler carbohydrates like oligo-, di- and monosaccharides; the simplest carbohydrates are termed *sugars*. Dietary fats are mainly in the form of triglycerides (three fatty acid chains linked to a single glycerol) with lesser amounts of other acylglycerols, phospholipids, cholesteryl esters, and cholesterol.

The digestion and absorption of carbohydrates, fats, and proteins are very efficient in healthy people, with limited losses due to maldigestion or malabsorption; how-ever, people with gastrointestinal diseases or dysfunction may have more limited capacity to digest and absorb macronutrients. Alcohol is considered a macronutrient.

All macronutrients are used as energy sources in humans. Any excess intake beyond that used by the body is stored as carbohydrate (glycogen in liver and mus-cle) or fat (triglycerides in adipose tissue). Macronutrients are also vital building blocks for the body; for example, dietary protein is used to provide amino acids for muscle protein synthesis. Many of the components of macronutrients play roles in regulating gene expression and cell function. These include simple sugars and fatty acids that modify the activity of transcription factors like the sterol receptor element binding proteins to control metabolism through alterations in expression of a number of key genes involved.

Micronutrients are necessary food components that are consumed daily in micro-gram to low gram amounts. They include the vitamins and minerals. Vitamins may be water soluble or fat soluble; they typically play roles in regulating metabolism and cell function or as cofactors for enzymes. Some vitamins are regulators of gene expression, either in their own right or after conversion to an active metabolite. Examples of this are vitamin A and vitamin D. Minerals are often found at the active site of enzymes or may be enzyme cofactors; they may also regulate gene expression. Minerals may also have structural roles (e.g., calcium in bones) or roles in signal transduction (e.g., sodium and potassium in nerve transmission). Absorption of vitamins and minerals from the diet can be poor. For example, only 10 to 40% of dietary calcium is absorbed even in healthy people. Thus significant amounts of micronutrients consumed may be lost. In general, bodily stores of micronutrients are low, and for many, excess intakes are excreted.

A second way to classify nutrients is as essential or nonessential. Essential nutrients cannot be produced in the body and so must be obtained from the diet. Essential nutrients include the minerals, most vitamins, nine amino acids (histidine, isoleucine, leucine, lysine, methionine, phenylalanine, threonine, tryptophan, and valine) and two fatty acids (linoleic and α-linolenic). Nonessential nutrients are those that can be produced by the human body as long as essential nutrients are available, and so are not normally required in the diet. Many nonessential nutrients are produced from essential nutrients. Therefore, if an essential nutrient is not consumed in sufficient quantities, a normally nonessential nutrient can become essential. Such nutrients are termed *conditionally essential.* Some clinical states may also produce conditional essentiality.

Malnutrition

Intake of the amounts of energy and essential nutrients needed to meet an individual's requirements will provide that individual with the metabolic basis for growth, development, and achieving optimal function, including defense and repair (refer back to Figure 1). Insufficient intake of energy will mean that the individual cannot support the demands of metabolism for growth, development, and function. Because energy-yielding substrates are macronutrients, insufficient energy intake must, by definition, also involve insufficient intake of one or more of the macronutrient groups. Often, this is protein, and the term *protein-energy malnutrition* is commonly used to describe this situation. Thus, as well as having an insufficient intake of energy, individuals with protein-energy malnutrition will not be able to meet the demands for building blocks or to support many physiological functions, including defense and repair. Such individuals will not thrive, they will lose body weight (both fat and lean mass), they will not function optimally either physically or mentally, they will have immune impairments with increased susceptibility to infection, and they will not be able to repair damaged tissues. Hence protein-energy malnutrition is a major source of morbidity and mortality, especially in children and other vulnerable groups.

A second form of malnutrition is the presence of single or multiple micronutrient deficiencies. In this situation, the individual may consume sufficient energy and macronutrients to meet their demands, but the limiting micronutrient(s) will compromise metabolism, and this will affect development and function. Many micronutrient deficiencies cause such marked physiological abnormalities that they cause a specific disease; examples include thiamine and beriberi, vitamin C and scurvy, and vitamin D and rickets. Protein-energy malnutrition and micronutrient deficiencies can occur together, for example in an individual who is seriously lacking in food intake.

While protein-energy malnutrition and micronutrient deficiencies represent the absence of one or more essential components from an individual's diet, a third type of malnutrition is characterized by an excess of energy (i.e., one or more macronutrients, usually either carbohydrate or fat or both) in the diet (see Figure 2 below). Because mechanisms for digestion and absorption of macronutrients are very efficient

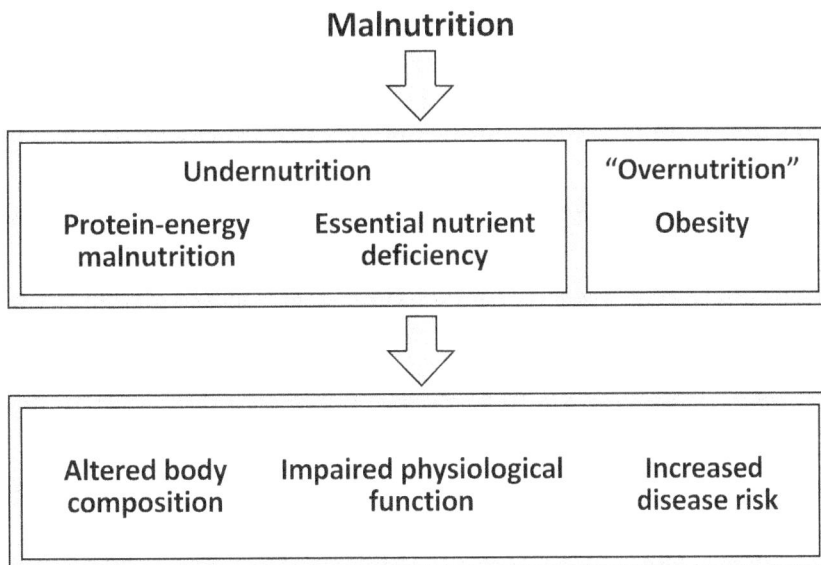

Malnutrition

Undernutrition		"Overnutrition"
Protein-energy malnutrition	Essential nutrient deficiency	Obesity

Altered body composition	Impaired physiological function	Increased disease risk

Figure 2. The classification and consequences of malnutrition.

and because macronutrients consumed in excess of demands are stored, mainly as fat in adipose tissue, the result of energy intake in excess of demand increases body weight, which is mainly the result of increased fat deposition. The situation is clearly explained by the energy balance equation:

Energy stored = Energy intake – Energy expenditure

A phenomenon has arisen in the last few decades with increased consumption of meals out of the home and increased use of prepared meals. The meals, including drinks, consumed in these situations may often be very rich in macronutrients, especially carbohydrates and fat, but relatively poor in micronutrients. These are referred to as "energy dense, nutrient poor" foods or meals. Thus, the individuals may be overweight, perhaps grossly, but also show signs of essential nutrient deficiencies.

The Importance of Dietary Non-Nutrients

Nutritional science has mainly been focused on macro- and micronutrients, as described above. However, in the last few decades, the important role of non-nutrients in physiology and in disease risk has been uncovered. One of the earliest non-nutrients to be considered was dietary fiber, which was found to regulate digestion, improve intestinal tract transit, reduce risk of colorectal cancer, and lower blood cholesterol concentrations.[1] Fiber is mainly of plant origin and represents those components of foods that are not digested in the gastrointestinal tract but instead act to provide bulk to the intestinal contents and are mainly lost from the body in feces. It is now known that some fiber can be metabolized by microbial enzymes within the lower gastrointestinal tract (see "The Role of Gut Microbiota" on the facing page).

Many chemicals of plant origin are now believed to have important roles in human physiology and in lowering disease risk. Collectively, these can be termed *phytochemicals*. They occur naturally in plants, and some are responsible for color and others for organoleptic properties. There are thousands of these compounds, which include carotenoids, phytosterols, polyphenolic compounds (flavonols, flavanones, flavones, flavanols, anthocyanidins), isoflavones, tannins, and aromatic acids. Common sources of these compounds are fruits, berries, vegetables, plant oils (e.g., olive oil), soy, tea, coffee, and cocoa.

The metabolism of many of these compounds is highly complex and poorly understood, and this has limited their identification in biological samples like blood and knowledge of their exact benefits to physiology. However, it seems certain that many of the health properties attributed to eating a diet rich in plant foods and specifically fruits and vegetables are due to the presence of highly bioactive non-nutrients. This is currently an area of huge research activity, and it is likely that significant progress will be made over the next few years.

The Role of Gut Microbiota

Humans have a wide diversity of live organisms in their gut lumen; these are collectively referred to as the *gut microbiota.* The number of organisms varies along the length of the gastrointestinal tract, the greatest number being in the colon (10^{11} to 10^{12} per gram of colonic contents), and varies between individuals, or at least subgroups of individuals.[2] Variation in number and type of organisms within the gut microbiota has been associated with many diseases, including metabolic and immunologic diseases.[3] It is known that the gut microbiota is modified according to diet.[3] This has opened the way to strategies aimed at specifically modifying the gut microbiota in a health-promoting way. Initially the focus of such modifications was improving gut physiology (e.g., transit time) and the immune response.[4] However, it is now recognized that the influence of the gut microbiota is rather widespread. For example, metabolic diseases including obesity, type-2 diabetes, and non-alcoholic fatty liver diseases seem to have a link with an altered gut microbiota.[5–7] Furthermore, there are links between the gut and the brain, with suggestions that gut microbiota may influence mental health and well-being.[8,9]

It is likely that many foods and many dietary components influence the gut microbiota (number and type of organisms present). However, two strategies have been especially explored. The first is simply to provide modest numbers of specific live organisms orally and trust that they will take hold in (colonize) the gastrointestinal tract, particularly the colon. This is the probiotic approach, and favored organisms are typically members of the lactobacillus or bifidobacteria genus. The second approach is to provide substrate that will enable preferential growth of an already existing favored organism; this is the prebiotic approach, and the substrates are usually, though not always, carbohydrates, which are not digestible by mammalian enzymes but which are selectively fermented by gut microbiota (i.e., fermentable fiber). The products of microbial fermentation of fiber are the short chain fatty acids. Of these, butyrate in particular has benefits on the colonic mucosa.[10] Furthermore, acetate, propionate, and butyrate all enter the host's bloodstream and can have systemic effects.[11]

Summary

Foods and drinks provide nutrients and non-nutrients, many with well-described biological properties. Any particular food will contain a complex mixture of nutrients and non-nutrients. Certain foods may be characterized by the presence of particular nutrients or non-nutrients. Nutrients may be macro- or micronutrients and may be essential or nonessential. Nutrients support growth, development, and physiological function. Nutrients act through a variety of mechanisms to affect metabolism and cell and tissue function. A deficiency of energy or one or more essential nutrients impairs growth, development, and function and increases disease risk. Obesity due to intake of energy in excess of requirements is also a form of malnutrition. Non-nutrients are usually of plant origin and possess a range of properties that influence physiological function and disease risk. Many foods and nutrients act to modify gut microbiota. The gut microbiota interacts with the host in a variety of ways, and altered gut microbiota is seen in many metabolic and immunologic conditions. It is now apparent that the gut microbiota also influences the brain and may be important in mental health. It seems likely that nutritional strategies to influence gut microbiota will become an important part of healthy eating in the future. Overall, a balanced diet with variety and a significant content of plant foods seems to be most compatible with human physiology and with health.

REFERENCES

1. Otles S and Ozgoz S. "Health effects of dietary fiber." *Acta Sci Pol Technol Aliment* 13, 191–202, 2014.

2. Wu GD, Chen J, Hoffmann C, Bittinger K, Chen YY, Keilbaugh SA, Bewtra M, Knights D, Walters WA, Knight R, Sinha R, Gilroy E, Gupta K, Baldassano R, Nessel L, Li H, Bushman FD, and Lewis JD. "Linking long-term dietary patterns with gut microbial enterotypes." *Science* 334, 105–108, 2011.

3. Hill C, Guarner F, Reid G, Gibson GR, Merenstein DJ, Pot B, Morelli L, Canani RB, Flint HJ, Salminen S, Calder PC, and Sanders ME. "Expert consensus document: The International Scientific Association for Probiotics and Prebiotics consensus statement on the scope and appropriate use of the term probiotic." *Nat. Rev. Gastroenterol. Hepatol.* 11, 506–514, 2014.

4. Cummings JH, Antoine J-M, Aspiroz F, Bourdet-Sicard R, Brandtzaeg P, Calder PC, Gibson GR, Guarner F, Isolauri E, Pannemans D, Shortt C, Tuijtelaars S, and Watzl B. "PASSCLAIM—Gut health and immunity." *Eur. J. Nutr.* 43 (Suppl. 2) 118–173, 2004.

5. Kobyliak N, Virchenko O, and Falalyeyeva T. "Pathophysiological role of host microbiota in the development of obesity." *Nutr. J.* 15; 43, 2016.

6. Patterson E, Ryan PM, Cryan JF, Dinan TG, Ross RP, Fitzgerald GF, and Stanton C. "Gut microbiota, obesity and diabetes." *Postgrad Med. J.* 92; 286–300, 2016.

7. Machado MV and Cortez-Pinto H. "Diet, microbiota, obesity, and NAFLD: A dangerous quartet." *Int. J. Mol. Sci.* 17; 481, 2016.

8. Yarandi SS, Peterson DA, Treisman GJ, Moran TH, and Pasricha PJ. "Modulatory effects of gut microbiota on the central nervous system: how gut could play a role in neuropsychiatric health and diseases." *J Neurogastroenterol. Motil.* 22, 201–212, 2016.

9. Mu C, Yang Y, and Zhu W. "Gut microbiota: the brain peacekeeper." *Front Microbiol* 7, 345, 2016.

10. Leonel AJ and Alvarez-Leite JI. "Butyrate: implications for intestinal function." *Curr. Opin. Clin. Nutr. Metab. Care* 15, 474–479, 2012.

11. Ríos-Covián D, Ruas-Madiedo P, Margolles A, Gueimonde M, de Los Reyes-Gavilán CG, and Salazar N. "Intestinal short chain fatty acids and their link with diet and human health." *Front Microbiol.* 7, 185, 2016.

Prevention of Cancer and Malformation by AHCC and Dietary Compounds

Taisei Nomura

During embryonic development, the different cell types become determined in their proper places, and the pattern of the body is set up on a small scale and then grows. The appearance of outliers in such processes can be effectively reduced or eliminated by homeostatic surveillance to form a normal body.[1,2] In adults, such non-self outliers can be normalized or eliminated, more likely killing of the altered cells to maintain a healthy body without cancer. Cancer and malformation are induced by environmental, chemical, physical (radiation, etc.), and biological hazards with or without a genetic predisposition. Human ingenuity and careful consideration are required to avoid these hazards and prevent the resulting disorders.

In experimental animals, radiation- and chemical-initiated cancer and malformation are suppressed by error-prone repair inhibitors,[3–10] protease inhibitors,[10,11] vitamins,[10,12–15] and bioresponse modifiers.[2] Error-prone repair inhibitors, such as methylxanthines, can prevent cancer, malformation, and mutation initiated by specific agents such as ultraviolet light (UV), 4-nitroquinoline 1-oxide (4NQO), and ethyl carbamate (urethane),[3–10] but methylxanthines are not effective on mutation and malformation initiated by alkylating agents and ionizing radiations.[3,6,10] "Radioprotector" (sulfhydryl compounds, amifostine, etc.), an agent to protect toxic biological effects of ionizing radiation, are very toxic and cannot be used in healthy humans. A novel radioprotector, an agonist of TLR-5, may be useful in normal animal tissues but not yet in humans.[16] Vitamins (A, C, D, retinoic acid, nicotinamide, etc.) are known to prevent cancer and malformation.[10,12–15] Bioresponse modifiers such as Pyran copolymer (Pyran), Bacillus Calmette-Guérin (BCG), etc., can activate the immunosurveillance system to eliminate altered cells responsible for cancer and malformation, and then prevent these disorders.[2,17,18] The system has to be error-free. Pretreatment of these agents can prevent spontaneous or natural incidence of cancer and malformations.[2,17,18]

It is noted that AHCC from edible mushroom can also prevent spontaneous development of cancer in addition to radiation-initiated leukemia and malformation in mice.[17,18] In cancer patients, AHCC is known to prevent side effects of chemo- and radiotherapy and elevate quality of life (QOL) of the patients[17–19] (see chapters 5 and 10). It is confirmed experimentally that AHCC suppresses the growth of human cancer tissues in specific immunodeficient super-SCID mice.[17,18]

Prevention of Cancer, Malformation, and Mutation by Dietary Compounds

Radiation- and chemical-initiated DNA damage is normalized or eliminated by the homeostatic repair system. In excision repair-less *E. coli*, UV-type DNA damage is repaired by recombination repair, which is error-prone, resulting in mutation. Post-recombination repair inhibitor caffeine (1, 3, 7-methylxanthine) can kill and eliminate damaged cells, possibly in error-free form in survived cells.[3] In fact, caffeine suppressed UV-mimetic compound 4NQO-initiated mutation in excision repair-less *E. coli*, and also suppressed transformation in mouse cells.[4] Furthermore, caffeine killed some of 4NQO-treated mice, but suppressed cancer incidence significantly in surviving mice,[5] supporting a hypothesis, "Mutation Theory of Cancers."[3]

Caffeine also suppressed urethane-initiated cancer and malformation,[6–10] and also spontaneously developing cleft lip and palate in CL/Fr mice.[10] However, caffeine did not suppress, but instead enhanced, cancer and malformation initiated by alkylating agents and ionizing radiation in mice.[6,10] In specific mouse model to detect in vivo embryonic mutation, malformation, and cancer (see Figure 1 on the following page), caffeine did not prevent mutation, but prevented cancer and malformations in this model.[9]

Furthermore, stronger error-prone repair inhibitor, theophylline (1, 3-methylxanthine), never inhibited urethane-initiated cancer and malformation, not supporting the above hypothesis.[3] Theobromine (3, 7-methylxanthine) and 7-methylxanthine prevented cancer and malformation, but 1-and 3-methylxanthine did not prevent cancer[9] (see Table 1 on page 175). "7-methyl-" may play an important role in eliminating altered cells. Selective killing of pre-tumorigenic and pre-teratogenic cells (i.e., elimination of these altered cells) may have resulted in the prevention of can-

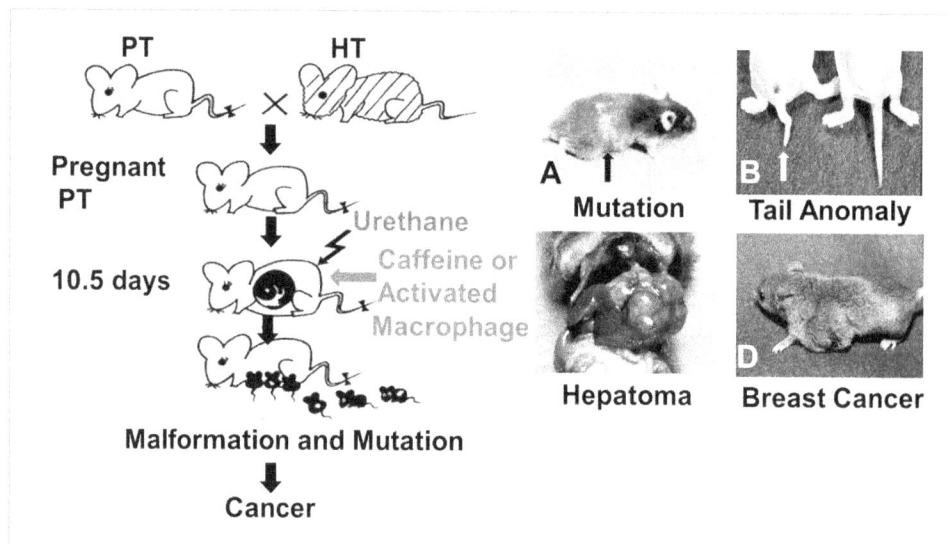

Figure 1. Specific mouse model to detect cancer, malformation, and somatic (embryonic) mutation[9]. Somatic mutation is detected in the form of colored spot on the coat (A: arrow). Tail anomaly (B: arrow) is a common type of radiation- and chemical-initiated malformation, which is prevented by caffeine, theobromine, antipain, nicotinamide, 13 trans-retinoic acid, etc., and also by biodefense modifiers, including AHCC and activated macrophages in ICR, N5, and PT-HTF$_1$ mice. Hepatoma (C) and breast cancer (D) are common types of cancer in C3H/HeJ mice. AHCC prevents spontaneous development of these cancers.

cer and malformation. Protease inhibitor, antipain, which blocks the promoting step in cancer development, also prevented urethane-initiated lung cancer and malformation.[10,11] Among vitamins, nicotinamide most effectively prevented urethane-initiated lung cancer and malformation in mice,[14] and also suppressed growth of murine breast cancer graft in C3H/HeJ mice.[15] 13 trans-retinoic acid, which is known to prevent cancer in mice,[12,13] prevented urethane-initiated malformation at low doses (1–2 µg/g body weight).[10] However, higher dose of 13 trans-retinoic acid (10 µg/g body weight) was very toxic to induce 100% of congenital malformation in mice.[10]

Prevention of Malformation by AHCC and Bioresponse Modifiers

Nonspecific tumoricidal immune cells can prevent malformation by killing precursor (pre-teratogenic) cells destined to cause such defect (see Table 2 on page 178). Pretreatment of pregnant mice with synthetic (Pyran) and biological (BCG) agents significantly prevented X-ray-, urethane- and methylnitrosourea (MNU)–initiated malformation

TABLE 1. **PREVENTION OF CANCER, MALFORMATION, AND MUTATION IN MICE BY DIETARY COMPOUNDS**

	AGENT	CANCER	MALFORMATION	MUTATION	REFERENCE
Caffeine (1, 3, 7-trimethylxanthine)	4NQO	+++ (++++)[a]	—	++++[b]	3–5, 7, 10
Caffeine	Urethane	+++	++++	—	6–10
Caffeine	none	NT	++[c]	NT	9, 10
Theophylline (1, 3-dimethylxanthine)	Urethane	—	—	++++[b]	9
Theobromine (3, 7-dimethylxanthine)	Urethane	++++	++++	NT	9
1-methylxanthine	Urethane	—	+++	NT	9
3-methylxanthine	Urethane	++	++	NT	9
7-methylxanthine	Urethane	+++	++++	NT	9
Antipain	Urethane	+	+++	NT	10, 11
Nicotinamide	Urethane	+++ (++++)[d]	+++	NT	14, 15
13 trans-retinoic acid	Urethane	(+)[e]	+++[f]	NT	10, 12, 13

Caffeine, theophylline, and theobromine are predominantly contained in coffee, tea, and cocoa, respectively.

Prevention level against untreated controls are shown; —; no effect (no significant difference), +; ~25%; ++; 25–50%; +++; 50–75%; ++++; >75%. NT: not tested

a) mouse cell transformation,[4] b) *E. coli*,[3] c) spontaneous cleft lip and palate in CL/Fr mice,[10] d) suppression of tumor-growth of murine breast cancer transplanted to C3H/HeJ mice,[15] e) by Sporn et al.[12] and Konstantin et al.,[1,3] f) prevented at low dose (1~2 µg/g), but instead increased at high dose (10 µg/g).[10]

(cleft palate, digit anomalies, tail anomalies, etc.). Pyran was injected intraperitoneally into pregnant mice on day 3 of gestation, before X-ray or chemical treatment on day 9, when macrophage activation by Pyran becomes maximum. X-ray-initiated malformation was suppressed slightly but significantly (10 to 15%) by the Pyran pretreatment, although caffeine never prevented X-ray-initiated malformation. Dramatic reduction (40 to 100%) was observed with urethane- and MNU-initiated cleft palate, tail anomaly, and digit anomaly. However, Pyran pretreatment reduced neither the average number of living fetuses nor the average body weight of the fetuses.

To examine the association of macrophage activation with antiteratogenic activity by Pyran, peritoneal macrophages that had been activated by Pyran and purified by adherence on tissue culture dishes were injected intravenously into pregnant mice after urethane or X-ray treatment on day 9. Urethane- and X-ray-initiated malformations were significantly prevented by the activated macrophages. Normal macrophages that were elicited by glycogen and purified similarly had no effect on malformation frequency. Such preventive effects of activated macrophages on malformation were lost either after the disruption of activated macrophages by supersonic waves or by inhibition of their lysosomal enzyme activity with trypan blue. These results indicate that a live activated macrophage with active lysosomal enzymes can be an effector cell to suppress maldevelopment. A similar reduction by activated macrophages was observed in strain CL/Fr, which has a high spontaneous frequency of cleft lip and palate. Furthermore, Pyran-activated maternal macrophages could pass through the placenta and enhanced urethane-initiated cell killing but not urethane-initiated mutation in the embryo (refer back to Figure 1 and see Figure 2 below).

It is likely that a maternal immunosurveillance system eliminating pre-teratogenic cells allows for the replacement with normal totipotent blast cells during the pregnancy to prevent abnormal development. Pretreatment with BCG significantly suppressed urethane- and X-ray-initiated malformation even when it was injected fifty-five days before pregnancy. BCG-activated peritoneal macrophages collected forty days after BCG injection also suppressed urethane- and X-ray-initiated malformation. It is likely that chronic BCG infection could continuously activate macrophages to prevent maldevelopment.

Moreover, normal macrophages collected from older mice (12 months of age)

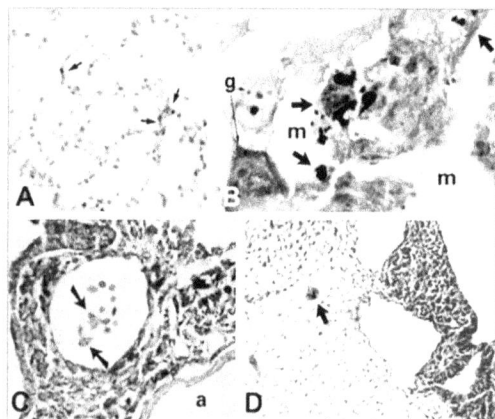

Figure 2. Placental transfer of activated macrophages.[2] Dextran sulfate was injected intraperitoneally 24 hours before the collection of Pyran-activated or normal macrophages, and cells were injected intravenously into pregnant mice. A) Macrophages stained metachromatically by toluidine blue in the capillary of the alveolar wall of the lung. B) Macrophages stained metachromatically in the chorionic villi of the fetal placenta (arrows) bathed in maternal blood = m; giant cells = g. C) Macrophages in the sinus venosus. D) Metachromatic cells in the interstitial tissue of the embryo.[2]

nursed in non-SPF condition did suppress X-ray-initiated malformation, although those collected from two-month-old mice in the SPF condition did not show significant preventive effects[2] (see Table 2 on the following page).

AHCC pretreatment of pregnant mice also prevents X-ray-initiated cleft palate, diaphragmatic hernia, etc. (see Table 2). Preventive effects of AHCC on X-ray-initiated malformation (77% reduction) are much stronger than Pyran (10 to 15%). The immunosurveillance system may have similarly eliminated pre-teratogenic cells, and those cells are replaced by normal blast cells to form normal organs.

Prevention of Radiation-Initiated Leukemia and Natural Incidence of Cancer by AHCC

Bioresponse modifiers are suspected to prevent cancer development. However, there is a scarcity of evidence. We are testing whether AHCC can prevent cancer development in mice.

Some strains of mice such as C57BL/6J are highly sensitive to radiation for leukemia induction. AHCC (2% in water) were given orally starting at 5 weeks after birth until the end of experiment (24 months), and then ^{137}Cs γ-rays were given four times at 6, 7, 8, and 9 weeks after birth. Survival rate of γ-ray-irradiated mice was significantly higher with AHCC, and incidence of γ-ray-initiated leukemia was significantly prevented with AHCC in drinking water (see Table 2).

Spontaneous incidence of leukemia was also suppressed a little. Although leukemia develops early in life, common types of cancer in the lung, breast, liver, etc. develop at older ages in mice and humans. Spontaneous and induced types of cancer in C3H/HeJ mice are very close to those in humans, and spontaneous cancer incidence is also high as is the case in humans. AHCC treatment to young adult C3H/ HeJ mice for two years significantly elevated survival rate and significantly prevented spontaneous development of breast cancer and hepatoma in mice (refer to Table 2 and Figure 1).

The preventive mechanism is not known, but micro-array analysis shows that an increase of gene expression by AHCC in immunoglobulin heavy chain complexes, interferon and adiponectin, guard against non-self. In female mice, AHCC drastically suppressed gene expression of some functional genes in breast gland; casein families, lactotransferrin, estrogen receptor, etc. Suppression of gene expression of breast function and estrogen receptor or estrogen-responding gene by AHCC may prevent spontaneous development of breast cancer in mice.[17,18]

TABLE 2. **PREVENTION OF CANCER, MALFORMATION, AND MUTATION IN MICE BY BIODEFENSE MODIFIERS**[2,17,18]

	AGENT	CANCER	MALFORMATION	MUTATION
Pyran copolymer	X-ray	(—)[a]	++	NT
Pyran copolymer	Urethane	(—)[a]	++++	NT
Pyran copolymer	MNU	NT	++++	NT
Pyran-activated macrophage	Urethane	(—)[a]	+++	—
Pyran-activated macrophage	none	NT	++[b]	NT
Pyran-activated macrophage (disrupted)	Urethane	NT	—	NT
Pyran-activated macrophage (trypan blue-treated)	Urethane	NT	—	NT
Normal macrophage[c]	Urethane	NT	—	NT
Pyran-activate macrophage	X-rays	NT	+++	NT
BCG	Urethane	NT	+++	NT
BCG-activated macrophage	Urethane	NT	++	NT
BCG	X-rays	NT	+++	NT
BCG-activated macrophage	X-rays	NT	++	NT
Macrophage (Non SPF old mice)[d]	X-rays	NT	++	NT
AHCC	**X-rays**	++[e]	++++	**NT**
AHCC	**none**	++++[f] (+++)[g]	**NT**	**NT**

Prevention level against untreated control are shown; —; no effect (no significant difference), +; ~25%; ++; 25–50%; +++; 50–75%; ++++; >75%; NT; not tested.

a) unpublished data,[2] b) spontaneous cleft lip and palate in CL/Fr mice,[2] c) normal macrophage elicited by glycogen,[2] d) normal macrophages collected from older (12 month of age) mice nursed in non-SPF condition,[2] e) leukemia, f) breast cancer and hepatoma, g) suppression of the growth of patient-derived prostate cancer and clear cell renal cell carcinoma xenograft in super-SCID mice.

Prevention of Side Effects of Chemo- and Radiotherapy by AHCC

Among cancer patients, AHCC is known to suppress side effects and elevate QOL in chemo- and radiotherapy (see cancer-related chapters in parts 2 and 3 of this book). In our clinical study in India, 3 g of AHCC were given every morning three days before and seven days after chemotherapy to twenty-five advanced-stage head and neck cancer patients (thirteen cancer in cheek, four in tongue, six in oropharynx, two in nasopharynx).[19] All the patients tolerated AHCC well with no additional symptoms. Twenty patients reported that they were feeling stronger than before at the time of initiation of chemotherapy cycles. Almost all the patients reported to have a better appetite after they started taking AHCC. Patients did not request appetizer with AHCC, diarrhea was also improved, and most patients felt better with AHCC (see Table 3 below). Twelve patients required blood transfusion before chemotherapy

TABLE 3. **COMPARISON OF QUALITY OF LIFE CONCEPTS IN PATIENTS REQUIRING APPETIZER, HAVING LOOSE MOTION, AND BETTER GENERAL CONDITION WITH AND WITHOUT AHCC, AND COMPARISON OF HEMATOLOGICAL PARAMETERS IN PATIENTS WITH AND WITHOUT AHCC[19]**

	NO. OF PATIENTS	AHCC (−)	AHCC (+)
Feeling better	25	—	20
Appetizer[a]	25	18	0
Loose motion	25	6	2
Blood transfusion	25	16	3
Growth factor infusion	25	12	7
Platelet concentrates infusion	25	3	0

a) numbers of patients request appetizer.

This clinical study was carried out at Department of Radiation Oncology, North Eastern Indira Gandhi Regional Institute of Health & Medical Sciences, Shillong, India, on twenty-five advanced-stage (T3:13 and T4:12) head and neck cancer patients (13 cheek cancer, 4 tongue cancer, 6 oropharyngeal cancer, and 2 nasopharynx cancer).

The majority of the patients received taxane-based chemotherapy along with platinum-based antineoplastic (cisplatin/carboplatin). The rest of the patients received platinum-based antineoplastic with 5-fluorouracil combinations. Twelve patients also received targeted monoclonal antibody treatment in the form of epidermal growth factor receptor (EGFR) inhibitor.[19]

cycles, but only three patients required blood transfusion before subsequent chemotherapy cycles. Numbers of growth factor supplement and platelet concentrates infusion were also reduced (see Table 3 on the previous page).

We tested whether AHCC can prevent side effects of radiotherapy. Three grams of AHCC were given daily one hour before radiotherapy to twenty-five head and neck patients. Fifteen patients with advanced-stage (T3N2M0, T4N2M0) head and neck cancer and ten esophageal cancer patients underwent radiotherapy (Curative: 60–70 Gy over 6–7 weeks; Palliative: 20–30 Gy over 2–3 weeks). Twenty patients reported loss of appetite without AHCC, while only one patient reported loss of appetite with AHCC. AHCC not only elevates QOL but also prevents desquamation and mucositis.[17,18] Significant prevention of desquamation ($p < 0.01$) and mucositis ($p < 0.05$) indicates that AHCC protects radiation hazards to radiation-exposed normal skin and mucous membrane.

It is noted that AHCC can suppress not only side effects of chemotherapy and radiotherapy, but also the growth of human cancer xenograft in super-SCID mice (refer back to Table 3; see Figure 3 below). Growth of patient-derived prostate cancer and clear cell renal cell carcinoma xenograft in super-SCID mice[21–25] are suppressed

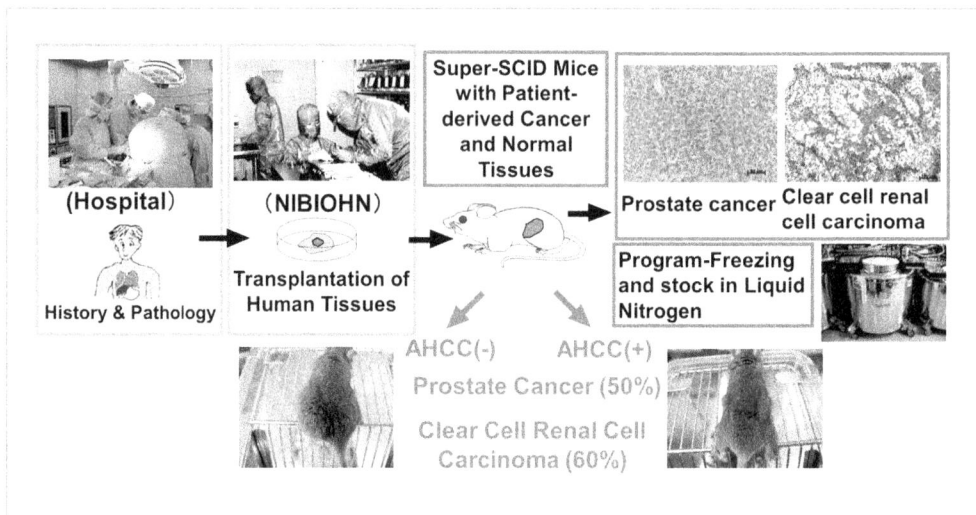

Figure 3. Super-SCID mice with patient-derived cancer and normal tissues for evaluation of chemo- and radiotherapy and their side effects. Mice with patients-derived prostate cancer and clear cell renal cell carcinoma maintained in National Institutes of Biomedical Innovation, Health and Nutrition (NIBIOHN) are treated with or without 2% AHCC in water. Percentage (%) in parentheses indicates the level of tumor growth suppression.

significantly by daily dose (0.5–2% in water) of AHCC (see Figure 3). Suppressive effects of AHCC are stronger than those of typical bioresponse modifier BCG (to be published at ICNIM 2016). SCID mice have normal macrophage and natural killer (NK) cell functions. AHCC may activate these immune cells, suppressing the growth of patient-derived cancer xenograft.

Summary

- Dietary compounds (caffeine, theobromine, 7-methylxanthine, antipain, nicotin-amide, 13 trans-retinoic acid, etc.) prevented radiation- and chemical-initiated cancer and malformation in mice.

- Biodefense modifier, AHCC from edible mushroom prevents radiation-initiated malformation in mice, as another bioresponse modifiers (Pyran copolymer, BCG, etc.) and macrophages activated by these agents prevented radiation- and chemical-initiated and also spontaneously development of malformation.

- AHCC prevents radiation-initiated leukemia in mice. Furthermore, AHCC prevents spontaneous development of breast cancer and hepatoma in mice.

- In cancer patients, AHCC elevates QOL and prevents side effects of radio- and chemotherapy. Radiation injuries on normal skin and mucous membrane in cancer patients are also prevented by AHCC.

- AHCC suppresses growth of patient-derived prostate cancer and clear cell renal cell carcinoma in super-SCID mice.

Note: All data were presented at International Congress of Nutrition and Integrative Medicine (ICNIM), Sapporo, 2007–15. The work is supported by scientific grants from MEXT and MHLW, Japan and Amino Up Co. Ltd.

The author thanks Mrs. Enomoto and Hatanaka for their assistance in preparing the manuscript.

REFERENCES

1. Albert B, Bray D, Lewis J, Raff M, Roberts K, and Watson JD. *Molecular Biology of the Cell.* Garland Publishing Inc., New York, p. 891, 2014.

2. Nomura T, Hata S, and Kusafuka T. "Suppression of developmental anomalies by maternal macrophages in mice." *J. Exp. Med.* 172: 1325–1330, 1990.

3. Kondo S. "Misrepair model for mutagenesis and carcinogenesis." In *Fundamentals in Prevention of Cancer* (edit. by Magee, P. N., Takayama, S., Sugimura, T. and Matsushima, T.) pp. 417–429, University of Tokyo Press, Tokyo, 1976.

4. Kakunaga T. "Caffeine inhibits cell transformation by 4-nitroquinoline 1-oxide." *Nature* 258: 248–250, 1975.

5. Nomura T. "Diminution of tumorigenesis initiated by 4-nitroquinoline 1-oxide by post-treatment with caffeine in mice." *Nature* 260: 547–549, 1976.

6. Nomura T. "Similarity of the mechanism of chemical carcinogen-initiated teratogenesis and carcinogenesis in mice." *Cancer Res.* 37: 969–973, 1977.

7. Nomura T. "Mutagenesis, teratogenesis, and carcinogenesis; evidence obtained by caffeine post treatment after carcinogens." In *Tumours of Early Life in Man and Animals.* (Ed. Severi L.), pp. 821–842, Perugia Univ. Press, Perugia, 1978.

8. Nomura T. "Timing of chemically induced neoplasia in mice revealed by the antineoplastic action of caffeine." *Cancer Res.* 40: 1332–1340, 1980.

9. Nomura T. "Comparative inhibiting effects of methylxanthines of urethane-induced tumors, malformations, and presumed somatic mutations in mice." *Cancer Res.* 43: 1342–1346, 1983.

10. Nomura T, Enomoto T, Shibata K, Kanzaki T, Tanaka H, Hata S, Kimura S, Kusafuka T, Sobue K, Miyamoto S, Nakano H, and Gotoh H. "Antiteratogenic effects of tumor inhibitors, caffeine, antipain, and retinoic acid in mice." *Cancer Res.* 43: 5156–5162, 1983.

11. Nomura T, Hata S, Enomoto T, Tanaka H, and Shibata K. "Inhibiting effects of antipain on urethane-induced lung neoplasia in mice." *Br. J. Cancer* 42: 624–626, 1980.

12. Sporn MB, Dunlop NM, Newton DL, and Smith JM. "Prevention of chemical carcinogenesis by vitamin A and its synthetic analogs (retinoids)." *Fed. Proc.* 35: 1332–8, 1976.

13. Dragnev KH, Rigas JR, and Dmitrovsky E. "The retinoids and cancer prevention mechanisms." *The Oncologist* 5: 361–368, 2000.

14. Gotoh H, Nomura T, Nakajima H, Hasegawa C, and Sakamoto Y. "Inhibiting effects of nicotinamide on urethane-induced malformations and tumors in mice." *Mutat. Res.* 199: 55–63, 1988.

15. Gotoh H, Nomura T, and Hasegawa C. "Growth inhibition of transplanted murine breast cancer by nicotinamide in C3H/HeJ mice." *Cancer Res., Therapy and Control* 3: 121–126, 1993.

16. Burdelya LG, Krivokrysenko VL, Tallant TC, Storm E, Gleiberman AS, Gupta D, Kurnasov OV, Fort FL, Osterman AL, Didonato JA, Feinstein E, and Gudkov AV. "An agonist of toll-like receptor 5 has radioprotective activity in mouse and primate models." *Science* 320: 226–230, 2008.

17. Nomura T. "Dietary modulation to prevent cancer and malformation in mice." 3rd. Asian Pacific Regional Meeting of The International Society for the Study of Xenobiotics. Proceedings 14666, 2009.

18. Nomura T, Adachi S, Ryo H, Hatanaka E, Kikuya R, Tokita Y, Horike N, Nakajima H, Hongyo T, Fujikawa K, Ito T, Ochiai T, Gyotoku J, Wakame K, Parida DK, and Bersimbay RI. "Evaluation of human risk in space environment and its protection: protection of radiation late effects." *Space Utilization Research* 28: 126–129, 2012. (in Japanese)

19. Parida DK, Wakame K, and Nomura T. "Integrating complementary and alternative medicine in form of Active Hexose Co-Related Compound (AHCC) in the management of head & neck cancer patients." *International Journal of Clinical Medicine* 2: 588–592, 2011.

20. Kondo S, Norimura T, and Nomura T. "Programmed cell death for defense against anomaly and tumor formation." *Transactions of the American Nuclear Society* 73: 37–38, 1995.

21. Nomura T, Takahama Y, Hongyo T, Inohara H, Takatera H, Fukushima H, Ishii Y, and Hamaoka T. "SCID (Severe Combined Immunodeficiency) mice as a new system to investigate metastasis of human tumors." *J. Radiat. Res.* 31: 288–292, 1990.

22. Nomura T, Takahama Y, Hongyo T, Takatera H, Inohara H, Fukushima H, Ono S, and Hamaoka T. "Rapid growth and spontaneous metastasis of human germinal tumors ectopically transplanted into SCID (severe combined immunodeficiency) and SCID-nudestreaker mice." *Jpn. J. Cancer Res.* 82: 701–709, 1991.

23. Inohara H, Matsunaga T, and Nomura T. "Growth and metastasis of fresh human benign and malignant tumors in the head and neck regions transplanted into SCID mice." *Carcinogenesis* 13: 845–849, 1992.

24. Nomura T, Hongyo T, Nakajima H, Li Ya Li, Mukh Syaifudin, Adachi S, Ryo H, Baskar R, Fukuda K, Oka Y, Sugiyama H, and Matsuzuka F. "Differential radiation sensitivity to morphological, functional and molecular changes of human thyroid tissues and bone marrow cells maintained in SCID mice." *Mutat. Res.* 657: 68–76, 2008.

25. Adachi S, Ryo H, Hongyo T, Nakajima H, Tsuboi-Kikuya R, Tokita Y, Matsuzuka F, Hiramatsu K, Fujikawa K, Itoh T, and Nomura T. "Effects of fission neutrons on human thyroid tissues maintained in SCID mice." *Mutat. Res.* 696: 107–113, 2010.

AHCC Effects on Psychoneuroimmunological Parameters; Autonomic Nervous Balance, Mood and Immunity

Tatsuya Hisajima

In our daily lives, we are exposed to a variety of mental, social, and physical stressors, including the death of people close to us, unemployment, and loneliness. Stress results in the inhibition of immunoreactivity[1] and tissue damage due to oxidative stress.[2] It also causes psychiatric symptoms, such as sense of anxiety and nervousness,[3,4] as well as physical symptoms, such as insomnia and dizziness, which reduce the ability to concentrate, memorize information, and work.[5] While the abnormalities in the stress response cause a variety of symptoms, it is supposed that even those symptoms worsen the stress response,[6,7] reducing the quality of life for not only the person under the stress but also for other people in their "border zone." The state in which the disease is not exhibited (that is, the body may be on the verge of contracting a disease or suffering from mental problems but doesn't show symptoms) is equivalent to the "pre-disease state," a concept of oriental medicine. The impact of stress in this state is considered high.[8] From the perspective of preventive medicine, support during the pre-disease state, such as stress management, is an essential challenge for extending a healthy life expectancy.

Homeostasis of the human body is maintained by the response of the autonomic nervous system (ANS), immune system, and endocrine system to the stressors. There are two types of stress response: sympathetic-adrenal-medullary (SAM) system and hypothalamic-pituitary-adrenal (HPA) cortex[9–11] (see Figure 1 on the facing page). The SAM system is related to the excitation of the ANS center of the hypothalamus and increases the blood catecholamine concentration by activation of the sympathetic nervous system and by releasing noradrenaline and adrenaline from the adrenal medulla. These result in the increase of blood pressure and heart rate (HR),[9,10] affecting the lowering of the pain threshold.[12] Moreover, the HPA system increases the cortisol level in the blood by stimulating the adrenal cortex of the hypothalamus.[11] Sustained elevation of the cortisol levels in the blood is known to trigger immunosuppression, causing an onset or exacerbation of infection, cancer, and allergy symptoms.[13–15]

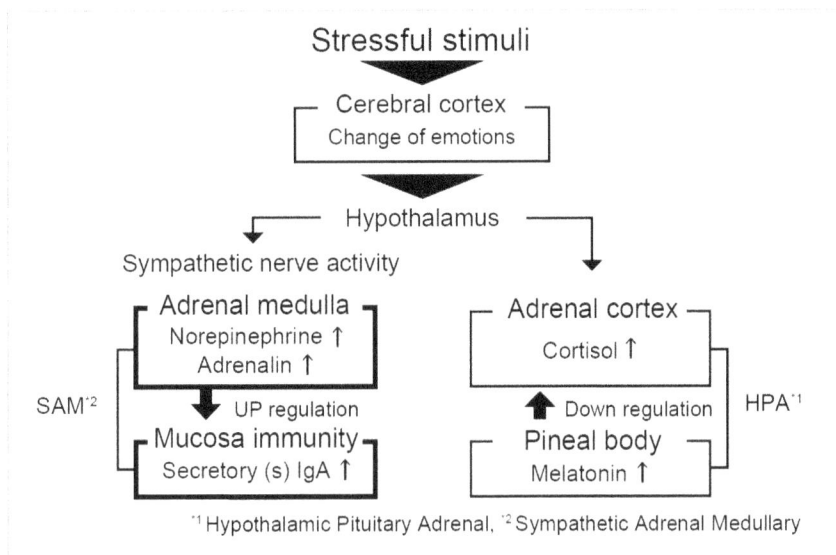

Figure 1. HPA and SAM in stress response.

Excessive or chronic stress stimulates the sympathetic nerves continuously, lowering the quality of sleep[16] and bringing about hyperalgesia.[12] This causes psychiatric symptoms such as depression and melancholia.[17] Psychiatric symptoms and natural killer (NK) cell activation are associated. It is known that NK cell activation reduces in people who are suffering from melancholia.[18,19] In this way, autonomic function also plays an important role in psychoneuroimmunology.

In this section, the effects of AHCC on psychoneuroimmunological parameters are described. There is a possibility that AHCC is effective for the ANS and psychiatric symptoms since it activates cells such as dendritic and NK cells, associated with natural immunity, shown in animal experiments and human clinical trials.[20,21] The effect of AHCC on the ANS function during the stress response is described in the following section.

EFFECTIVENESS OF AHCC ON THE ANS FUNCTION AND RELATED PARAMETERS

Animal Experiments

The oral administration of AHCC inhibited the increase of noradrenaline, adrenaline, dopamine, and glucose levels in the blood after immobilized stress of sixty minutes.[22] This finding shows that AHCC may possibly inhibit the sympathetic nerve activities caused by restraint stress.

Human Clinical Trials

Effectiveness of AHCC for Physical Stress

A randomized double-blind placebo-controlled trial (RCT) was conducted for eight healthy individuals (five males, three females; average age 20.62 ± 0.93 years). The subjects took AHCC (3 g/day) for five days; the washout period for crossover was set to nine days. Physical stress intervention was put by active standing load, autonomic function and HR were measured from heart rate variability (HRV) analysis throughout sitting rest position to active standing, standing, and continuous standing.

Active standing load (see Figure 2 on the facing page) is known as the Schellong standing test.[23,24] Standing after sitting in a rest position causes blood to accumulate in the veins of the lower extremities and trunk. The baroreceptor of aortic arch and carotid sinus facilitates the autonomic responses, which quickly normalizes the blood pressure, enhances the sympathetic nerve activities, and inhibits the parasympathetic nerve activities, increasing HR and contractile force, and maintains the blood pressure by contracting the volume of the blood vessels. Reduced or excessive enhancement of the sympathetic nerve activities and parasympathetic nerve activities may increase or decrease the HR rapidly, or lower the blood pressure without any changes and cause fainting.

Autonomic function evaluation based on the HRV analysis: The electrocardiograph electrode was attached to the side of the chest located above the sternal region and to the left and right nipple line. The ANS activity level was determined with the modified maximum entropy method (MemCalc method), using the HRV analysis software (Crosswell Co., Ltd., Tokyo) for the frequency analysis of the frequency obtained from the HRV of one beat. The low frequency (LF) component of $0.05 - 0.15$ Hz and high frequency (HF) component of $0.15 - 0.4$ Hz were identified. The value

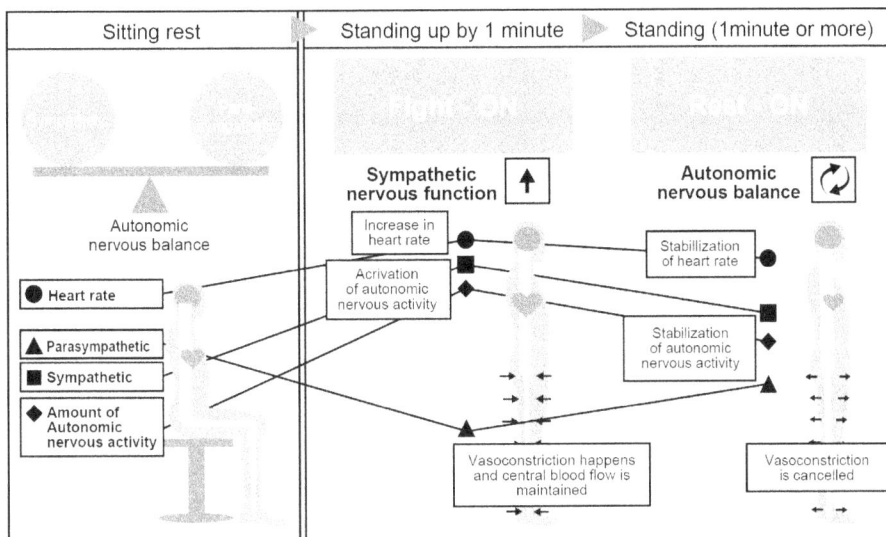

Figure 2. Schellong standing test (Citation: Modified from the information of Crosswell Co., Ltd.)

obtained by dividing the LF component with the HF (LF/HF) component was set as the indicator of the sympathetic nerve activity, and the HF component was set as the indicator of the parasympathetic nerve activity.

The results indicated that there was an increase in the LF/HF component after AHCC intake compared to before intake ($p = 0.08$). Moreover, even five days after AHCC intake, there was increase in the AHCC intake group when compared to the placebo intake group (see Table 1 below). This indicates that AHCC may have a useful action on the sympathetic nerve activities that is required during active standing.

TABLE 1. AUTONOMIC FUNCTION FOR SITTING REST POSITION AND WHILE STANDING * $p < 0.05$

		GROUPS	BEFORE INTAKE	5 DAYS AFTER INTAKE
Standing up / Sitting rest	LF/HF	Placebo	7.95 ± 6.08	2.63 ± 1.65
		AHCC	2.97 ± 1.97	5.62 ± 3.50 *
	HF	Placebo	0.83 ± 0.50	0.82 ± 0.39
		AHCC	0.77 ± 0.24	0.87 ± 0.44

Effectiveness of AHCC When Resting

To examine the effect of AHCC on lifestyle, mood at rest, HR, and autonomic function, five subjects (three male, two female; average age 20.40 ± 0.49 years) who indicated effectiveness with the intake of AHCC for active standing load described above were evaluated. The subjects took AHCC (3 g/day) for seven days, and the autonomic function for the sitting rest position was evaluated using HRV analysis. A questionnaire consisting of seventeen items was used to evaluate the lifestyle and Profile of Mood Scales (POMS) was used to evaluate mood.[25,26]

On Day 1 (pre-intake) and Day 7 (post-intake; final), subjects were asked to fill out a questionnaire by specifying their level of agreement or disagreement on a symmetric agree-disagree scale with five grades (1 = Strongly disagree; 5 = Strongly agree) with the following statements: 1) Feel tired, 2) Hard to get up, 3) Feel heavy, 4) Feel low, 5) Hard to sleep, 6) Awake during the night, 7) Have an appetite 8) Feel good, 9) Have a headache, 10) Feel queasiness in the stomach, 11) Have gastric pain, 12) Have constipation, 13) Have diarrhea, 14) Have a stomachache, 15) Have a sore throat, 16) Have a runny nose, and 17) Have a cough. According to the questionnaire survey for evaluation of lifestyle, the results "Hard to sleep" ($p = 0.080$) and "Feel tired" ($p = 0.099$) showed a trend toward improvement.

A shortened Japanese version of POMS, adapted from the original POMS standard version, was used in this trial. POMS is a self-report measure that allows for the quick assessment of transient, fluctuating feelings and enduring states. The questionnaire consists of thirty items and six factors: Tension-Anxiety (T-A), Depression-Dejection (D-D), Anger-Hostility (A-H), Vigor (V), Fatigue (F), and Confusion (C) in numerical values. Subjects were asked to rate each of the thirty items by choosing as follows: 1 = "not at all"; 2 = "a little"; 3 = "moderately"; 4 = "quite a bit"; and 5 = "extremely." We evaluated each factor at the standardized score using the following equation: T-score = 50 + 10 × [base score – average score]/standard deviation. The item of A-H in POMS was improved significantly ($p < 0.05$).

Regarding the autonomic function, an increase in the HF component was observed, which indicates an increased parasympathetic nerve activity, whereas there was no change in the LF/HF component, which indicates a stable sympathetic nerve activity (see Figure 3A–D on the facing page). AHCC did not increase HR in low stress situations. Overall, it was suggested that AHCC calms down a body when resting.

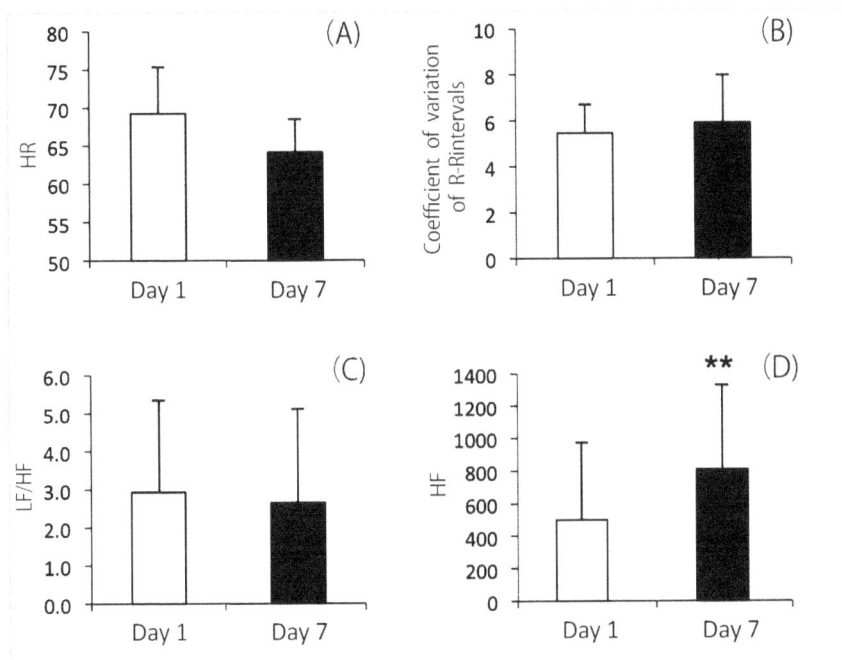

Figure 3. Comparisons of autonomic function before and after AHCC intake (Resting). **$p < 0.01$

Effectiveness of AHCC During Psychological Stress

RCT was conducted for seventeen healthy individuals (nine male, eight female; average age 20.64 ± 0.91 years). The subjects took AHCC (3 g/day) for seven days; the washout period for crossover was set to fourteen days. Uchida-Kraepelin test (U-KT) was used for psychological stress intervention, and HR and autonomic function were evaluated.

U-KT (Nisseiken Inc., Tokyo) is a mental arithmetic test used for psychological stress in which the adjacent numbers are added continuously. It is possible to understand the adaptability to learning activities and job execution ability by determining the calculation speed and accuracy with this test.[27] This test is used as stress during research and is also used for aptitude tests. The validity of using U-KT as an indication of physiological stress was confirmed by the prior evaluation of the effect on the autonomic function of eighty-two subjects (fifty male, thirty-two female; average age 21.23 ± 3.14 years).

As the results showed, the LF/HF component increased while the HF component decreased during the fifteen minutes when U-KT was conducted. It was suggested that the subject raised the sympathetic nerve activity and engaged in mental arithmetic problems, which is considered a stress load (see Figure 4A–B on the next page).

189

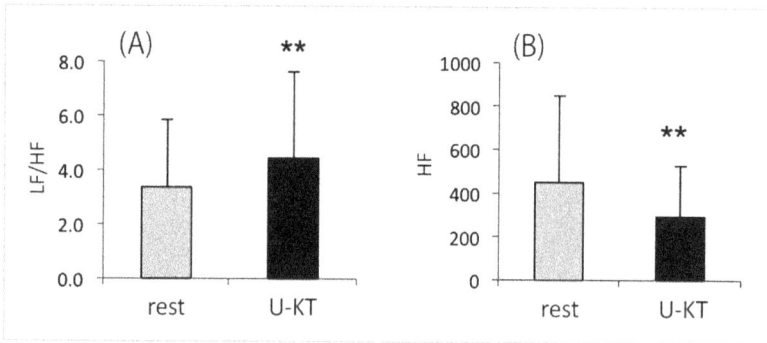

Figure 4.
The impact of U-KT on autonomic function.
$^{**}p < 0.01$

Moreover, there was a significant increase in the LF/HF component during UK-T on Day 7 compared to Day 1 for the AHCC group, and there was no change for the placebo group. A change in the HF component was not observed (see Figure 5A–B below). Overall, it was suggested that AHCC is useful for active tasks that cause stresses.

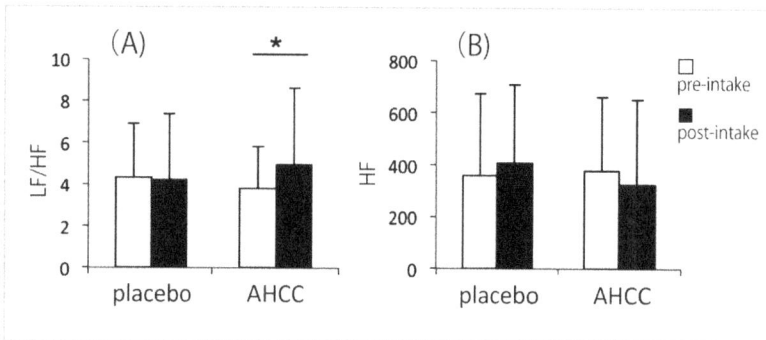

Figure 5.
Comparisons of autonomic function before and after AHCC/Placebo intake (U-KT).
$^{*}p < 0.05$

Effectiveness of AHCC for NK Cells under Chronic Stress

Under excessive or chronic stress, the sympathetic nerve activity is continuously enhanced. This might lead to reduced quality of sleep and subsequent depressive symptoms and depression, resulting in reduction of office work performance.[2,3,4,5] It is known that these mental disorders are related to NK cells activation. It has been reported that NK cells activation are more impaired in patients with chronic stress-associated depression than in healthy people.[18,19] NK cells activation thus reflects mental stress, in addition to its innate immunity function in the prevention of viral and bacterial infections. Therefore, it is considered that maintaining normal NK cells activation would contribute to the maintenance of a healthy immune system and also as a countermeasure to mental stress.

In this trial, subjects with mild depression who were considered to be under chronic stress were selected, and then the effects of AHCC on sleep, on office work performance, and changes in NK cells activation were investigated. RCT was conducted for thirteen healthy male and female subjects (average age 24.07 ± 3.79). To find out if subjects were suffering from chronic stress, the Self-Rating Depression Scale (SDS) questionnaire, which determines the severity of depression, was performed.

The SDS is used to quantitatively determine the severity of depression. It is comprised of twenty items that are based on the results of a factor analysis of depression. If the SDS score is less than 40 points, depression is unlikely. Depression is determined to be mild at an SDS score of 40 to 49 points, and moderate to severe at an SDS score of 50 points or more.[28,29]

Seven subjects were categorized into high SDS group (mean SDS score: 45.0 ± 5.7). Subjects took AHCC (3 g/day) for fourteen days, and after a fourteen-day washout period, they took placebo for fourteen days. Measurements were carried out on the first and fourteenth days.

As the measurements, first, the quality of sleep was investigated using the Oguri-Shirakawa-Azumi sleep inventory MA version (OSA-MA).[30] After five-minute resting, the U-KT was administered for fifteen minutes, and then a blood sample was taken to measure NK cells activation (see Figure 6 below).

The OSA-MA is a self-report questionnaire composed of sixteen items with a four-point scale, which are consolidated into "sleepiness on rising," "initiation and maintenance of sleep," "frequent dreaming," "refreshment," and "sleep length" subscales.

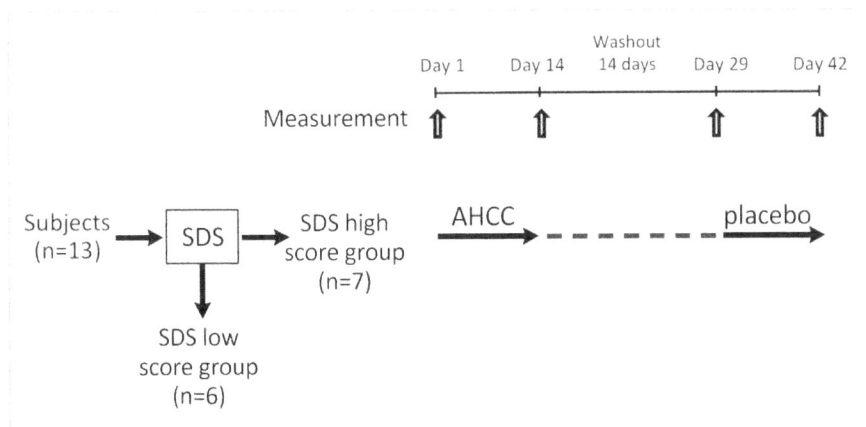

Figure 6. Experimental protocol

Although there were no significant differences in the score for Factor II (initiation and maintenance of sleep) between pre- and post-AHCC intake, the score was significantly greater in the AHCC-intake period than in the placebo-intake period ($p = 0.023$). The score for Factor IV (recovery from fatigue) increased during AHCC intake period ($p = 0.052$) (see Figure 7 below).

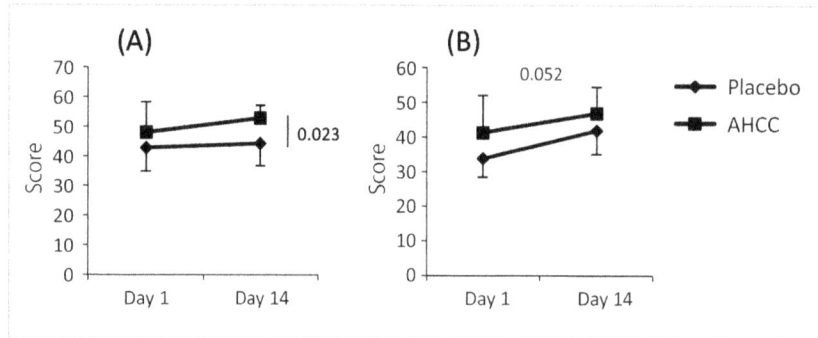

Figure 7. OSA Sleep Study. A: Initiation and maintenance of sleep ($p = 0.023$, Day 14 Placebo vs. AHCC). B: Recovery from fatigue ($p = 0.052$, Pre- vs. Post-AHCC intake).

Because the speed and accuracy of answer in the U-KT are indicative of the capacity to learn and work, the test is used to assess vocational aptitude as well as to administer a mental stress task. In this trial, AHCC increased the number of correct answers in the U-KT ($p = 0.007$) (see Figure 8 below). Depression reduces working memory capacity and thereby impairs concentration, memory, and task performance.[4,31] Therefore, it is expected that AHCC might affect improvement of depression. The results were not definitive. However, considering that anti-stress effects of AHCC were reported in animal experiments,[22] it is expected that AHCC will also show anti-stress effects in patients with depression and thereby will improve concentration, sleep, and fatigue to some extent.

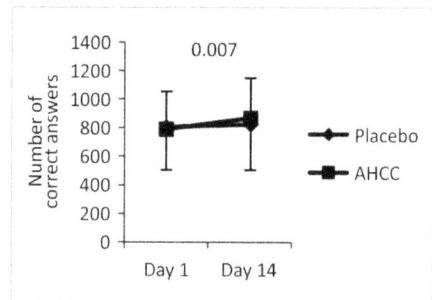

Figure 8. A number of correct answers on U-KT. ($p = 0.007$, Pre- vs. Post-AHCC intake)

After fourteen days of intake by the high SDS score group, the NK cells activation were changed by -2.45 ± 6.58 points (-7.62%) in the placebo and 9.68 ± 5.74 points (34.38%) in the AHCC ($p < 0.05$) as compared to initial NK cells activation. Furthermore, the score on Day 14 was significantly greater in the AHCC-intake period than in the placebo-intake period ($p < 0.05$) (see Table 2 on the facing page). From these results, it can be inferred that AHCC is likely to enhance NK cells activation in subjects with mild depression, which can be considered to be a pre-disease state.

TABLE 2. **HIGH SDS-SCORE GROUP**

	PLACEBO	AHCC
Day 1	32.15 ± 12.64	28.16 ± 10.96
Day 14	29.70 ± 10.73	37.84 ± 15.92
p-value of Day 1 vs Day 14	0.59	0.02
Amount of variation	−2.45 ± 6.58	9.68 ± 5.74*

*$p < 0.05$, p-value of the amount of variation in placebo vs. AHCC.

Conclusion

It was shown by multiple studies that AHCC enhances the activity of the sympathetic nervous system and improves immunity and mental symptoms when a body is stressed physically or psychologically or chronically. On the other hand, it was shown that AHCC calms down a body when resting. Therefore, AHCC can be considered as an effective functional food to improve overall psychoneuroimmunological parameters and maintain and promote mental health.

REFERENCES

1. Bultz BD and Carlson LE. "Emotional distress: the sixth vital sign in cancer care." *J. Clin. Oncol.* 23: 6440–41, 2005.

2. Liu JK, Wang XY, Shigenaga MK, Yeo HC, and Mori A. "Immobilization stress causes oxidative damage to lipid, protein, and DNA in the brain of rats." *FASEB J.* 10(13): 1532–38, 1996.

3. Han KS, Kim L, and Shim I. "Stress and sleep disorder." *Exp. Neurobiol.* 21:141–150, 2012.

4. Kumar A, Rinwa P, Kaur G, and Machawal L. "Stress: neurobiology, consequences and management." *J. Pharm. Bioallied Sci.* 5: 91–97, 2013.

5. Roth T and Ancoli-Israel S. "Daytime consequences and correlates of insomnia in the United States: results of the 1991 National Sleep Foundation Survey. II." *Sleep* 22, 1999.

6. Ader R and Cohen N. "Psychoneuroimmunology: conditioning and stress." *Annu. Rev. Psychol.* 1993;44:53–85.

7. Blazer DG. "Psychiatry and the oldest old." *Am. J. Psychiatry* 157(12): 1915–24, 2000.

8. Konishi T. "Brain oxidative stress as basic target of antioxidant traditional oriental medicines." *Neurochem. Res.* 34(4): 711–716, 2009.

9. Holsboer F. "Stress, hypercortisolism and corticosteroid receptors in depression: implications for therapy." *Journal of Affective Disorders* 62(1–2): 77–91, 2001.

10. Sapolsky RM, Romero LM, and Munck AU. "How do glucocorticoids influence stress responses? Integrating permissive, suppressive, stimulatory, and preparative actions." *Endocrine Reviews* 21(1):55–89, 2002.

11. Natelson BH, Creighton D, McCarty R, Tapp WN, Pitman D, and Ottenweller JE. "Adrenal hormonal indices of stress in laboratory rats." *Physiology & Behavior* 39(1): 117–125, 1987.

12. Imbe H, Iwai-Liao Y, and Senba E. "Stress-induced hyperalgesia: animal models and putative mechanisms." *Front Biosci.* 11: 2179–92, 2006.

13. Rhen T and Cidlowski JA. "Anti-inflammatory action of glucocorticoids new mechanisms for old drugs." *N. Engl. J. Med.* 353(16): 1711–23, 2005.

14. McDonald PG, Antoni MH, Lutgendorf SK, Cole SW, Dhabhar FS, Sephton SE, Stefanek M, and Sood AK. "A biobehavioral perspective of tumor biology." *Discov. Med.* 5(30): 520–526, 2005.

15. Kimata H, Lindley I, and Furusho K. "Effect of hydrocortisone on spontaneous IgE and IgG4 production in atopic patients." *J. Immunol.* 154(7): 3557–66, 1995.

16. Kageyama T, Nishikido N, Kobayashi T, Kurokawa Y, Kaneko T, and Kabuto M. "Self-reported sleep quality, job stress, and daytime autonomic activities assessed in terms of short-term heart rate variability among male white-collar workers." *Ind. Health* 36(3): 263–272, 1998.

17. Miró E, Martínez MP, Sánchez AI, Prados G, and Medina A. "When is pain related to emotional distress and daily functioning in fibromyalgia syndrome? The mediating roles of self-efficacy and sleep quality." *Br. J. Health Psychol.* 16(4): 799–814, 2011.

18. Irwin M, Daniels M, et al. "Life events, depression, and natural killer cell activity." *Psychopharmacol. Bull.* 22(4): 1093–1096, 1986.

19. Locke SE, Kraus L, et al. "Life change stress, psychiatric symptoms, and natural killer cell activity." *Psychosom. Med.* 46(5): 441–453, 1984.

20. Roman BE, Beli E, et al. "Short-term supplementation with active hexose correlated compound improves the antibody response to influenza B vaccine." *Nutr. Res.* 33(1): 12–17, 2013.

21. Terakawa N, Matsui Y, Satoi S, Yanagimoto H, Takahashi K, Yamamoto T, Yamao J, Takai S, Kwon AH, and Kamiyama Y. "Immunological effect of active hexose correlated compound (AHCC) in healthy volunteers: a double-blind, placebo-controlled trial." *Nutr. Cancer* 60(5): 643–651, 2008.

22. Wang S, Wakame K, et al. "Beneficial effects of Active Correlated Compound (AHCC) on immobilization stress in the rat." *Dokkyo Journal Medical Sciences* 28(1): 559–565, 2001.

23. Schellong F and Luderitz B. "Regulationsprtinge des Kreislaufs." Steinkopff, Dmrnstadt, 1954.

24. Nozawa I, Imamura S, Hisamatsu K, and Murakami Y. "The relationship between orthostatic dysregulation and the orthostatic test in dizzy patients." *Eur. Arch. Otorhinolaryngol.* 253(4–5): 268–272, 1996.

25. McNair DM and Lorr M. "An analysis of mood in neurotics." *J. Abnorm. Psychol.* 69:620-627, 1964.

26. Shacham S. "A shortened version of the profile of mood states." *J. Pers. Assess.* 47: 305-306, 1983.

27. Kuraishi S, Kato M, and Tsujioka B. "Development of the Uchida-Krapelin psychodiagnostic test in Japan." *Psycologia* 1: 104–109, 1957.

28. Zung WW. "How normal is depression?" *Psychosomatics* 13(3): 174–8, 1972.

29. Zung WW. "From art to science. The diagnosis and treatment of depression." *Arch. Gen. Psychiatry* 29(3): 328–37, 1973.

30. Yamamoto Y, Tanaka H, Takase M, Yamazaki K, Azumi K, and Shirakawa S. "Standardization of revised version of OSA sleep inventory for middle age and aged." *Brain. Sci. Ment. Disord.* 10: 401-409, 1999 (in Japanese).

31. Fossati P, Amar G, Raoux N, Ergis AM, and Allilaire JF. "Executive functioning and verbal memory in young patients with unipolar depression and schizophrenia." *Psychiatry. Res.* 89(3):171-87, 1999.

Effect of AHCC
on Gastrointestinal Dysfunction

Fermín Sánchez de Medina, Olga Martínez-Augustin

nflammatory bowel disease (IBD) is an immunologically mediated disease that is characterized by chronic inflammation of the gastrointestinal (GI) tract, typically following an irregular clinical course, with phases of activation and remission. It is estimated that globally over 4 million people are affected by IBD, with the highest prevalence in North America and Europe and increasing incidence in non-Western countries.[1,2] Combined prevalence in Western societies is approximately 0.1%.

The two major types of IBD are Crohn's disease (CD), which can affect any part of the GI tract but mostly involves the terminal ileum and proximal colon, and ulcerative colitis (UC), which as the name implies is limited to the colon. These are two separate clinical entities, which differ histologically and immunologically. Thus, Crohn's disease may affect any part of the GI tract as mentioned, and the inflammatory lesions follow a patchy distribution, with fundamentally normal zones interspersed between areas of active inflammation, whereas UC is characterized by a continuous inflamed surface that extends proximally. Inflammation is transmural in CD but affects mainly the mucosal surface in UC. From an immunological point of view, CD is a Th1 lymphocyte driven condition, whereas UC is more akin to a Th2 profile. There are also some differences in pharmacological management. In spite of the above, both diseases present frequently several common symptoms such as abdominal pain, diarrhea, fatigue, and weight loss, and in some patients with colitis, it is virtually impossible to differentiate between CD and UC (hence the name indeterminate colitis).

IBD is a lifelong, remitting-relapsing condition that exerts a heavy toll on the patient's quality of life. There is currently no cure, except for total colectomy when necessary in UC, but IBD can often be managed with anti-inflammatory drugs, such as corticosteroids, aminosalicylates, or immunosuppressants, such as azathioprine or ciclosporin. However, these therapies aim only to control ongoing inflammation of the intestines and do not address the underlying pathophysiologic mechanisms. This is borne out of our limitations in the understanding of IBD etiology and pathophysiology, despite the intense research effort carried out in this area in the past decades. It is clear that IBD is a result of a complex interplay between genetic background and environmental factors, which bring about chronic inflammation in susceptible individuals in certain situations, but not in others. Mucosal immune dysregulation, barrier dysfunction, and *dysbiosis*, a change of the normal gut microbiome, are pivotal in the development of the inflammatory response.[2,3,4] One common view in this regard is that IBD represents a loss of tolerance to the gut microbiota, resulting in an immune and inflammatory response toward bacteria and bacterial antigens. One of the most compelling pieces of evidence to support this hypothesis is the fact that intestinal inflammation is extremely difficult to induce in germ-free animals. The pivotal role of the microbiota opens up a wide array of therapeutic possibilities in IBD by targeting the microbiome imbalance and immune dysregulation, including prebiotics, probiotics, synbiotics, and fecal/microbiota transplantation.

AHCC as a Prebiotic

Prebiotics represent one of the common strategies for promoting a balanced gut microflora. The term *prebiotic* was coined only twenty years ago and defined as "a non-digestible food ingredient that beneficially affects the host by selectively stimulating the growth and/or activity of one or a limited number of bacteria in the colon," thereby improving the host's health.[5] Prebiotics are typically oligosaccharides that reach the colon in significant amounts precisely because they cannot be efficiently absorbed in the small intestine, since they cannot be digested. Once in the colonic lumen, they are selectively fermented, producing short chain fatty acids (SCFAs). SCFAs (acetic, propionic, and butyric acid) are of paramount importance for colonic health, and they exert beneficial effects on gut morphology and function, blood flow, and mucosal cell proliferation.[6,7] In fact, SCFAs are the main energy source for colonic epithelial cells. In addition, SCFAs reduce the intraluminal pH, favoring the growth of good bacteria such as *Bifidobacteria*, *Lactobacilli*, and nonpathogenic *E. coli* while reducing the growth of less acid-resistant pathogenic species. Moreover, butyrate in particular has been shown to have anti-inflammatory properties via multiple pathways, including the inhibition of nuclear factor κB (NF-κB), and the pro-inflammatory cytokines IL-12 and TNF-α,[8,9] all of which have been shown to mediate intestinal inflammation in IBD.[10]

Various types of indigestible oligosaccharides have been shown to have an anti-inflammatory effect in models of intestinal inflammation, associated with beneficial changes in the microbiota, and therefore act presumably as prebiotics.[11,12,13] Since AHCC contains 74% oligosaccharides, we hypothesized that it might also exert therapeutic effects in animal models of IBD. To test this hypothesis, we used the trinitrobenzenesulfonic acid (TNBS) model of colitis in rats. This is one of the most widely used models of IBD and is characterized by semi-chronic transmural colonic inflammation, which can last for several weeks. TNBS acts as a hapten, inducing a strong immune and inflammatory response after reacting with mucosal proteins to generate antigens de novo. In addition, it causes significant oxidative stress.

In this study, AHCC was administered by gavage as a pretreatment, starting two days before colitis induction. Two different doses were assayed, namely 100 and 500 mg/kg. Sulfasalazine (SZ, 200 mg/kg), a drug commonly used in the management of IBD, was used as a reference treatment using the same dosing protocol. Additional groups included a vehicle-treated colitic (TNBS groups) and a noncolitic group, which did not receive the TNBS challenge (control).

Animals were randomly allocated to the different groups, divided into five groups. Six days after colitis induction, the animals were killed, and morphological and biochemical parameters were assessed. In addition, colonic microbiota changes were also determined by studying the bacterial profile of the feces, in order to establish a possible prebiotic mechanism. Morphological assessments showed that AHCC supplementation attenuated colonic inflammation, as measured by macroscopic indices. Thus damage score, extension of necrosis, colonic weight, and colonic weight-to-length ratio were all lower in the AHCC-treated rats than in the TNBS control group, and the values were generally lower than in animals treated with SZ, albeit nonsignificantly so.

Pretreatment of rats with the 500 mg/kg dose of AHCC resulted in less pronounced anorexia and significantly increased relative body weight gain compared to TNBS group. Evaluation of biochemical parameters also revealed the AHCC-treated rats had reduced inflammatory status as indicated by lower levels of pro-inflammatory cytokines and chemokines (IL-1β, IL-1ra, MCP-1, and TNF), reduced myeloperoxidase activity (a marker of neutrophilic infiltration) and alkaline phosphatase (a marker of inflammation and epithelial stress) activity compared to TNBS group. With regard to the microbiota, AHCC normalized aerobic, clostridial and lactic acid bacterial counts compared to the TNBS group and increased *Bifidobacteria* compared to the control group (see Table 1 below).

TABLE 1. EFFECTS OF AHCC TREATMENT ON BACTERIA FECAL LEVELS IN THE DIFFERENT EXPERIMENTAL GROUPS OF RATS WITH TNBS COLITIS[1]

	C	T	SZ	AHCC100	AHCC500
	Log CFU[2]				
Aerobes	7.83 ± 0.21[a]	6.36 ± 0.16[b]	6.79 ± 0.20[b]	8.03 ± 0.21[a]	7.58 ± 0.31[a]
Anaerobes	8.34 ± 0.18	8.76 ± 0.21	8.16 ± 0.13	9.17 ± 0.23	8.58 ± 0.26
Lactic acid bacteria	7.46 ± 0.28[a]	5.90 ± 0.35[b]	5.50 ± 0.27[b]	7.58 ± 0.37[a]	7.00 ± 0.40[a]
Bifidobacteria	5.99 ± 0.37[b]	5.39 ± 0.12[b]	8.21 ± 0.22[a]	6.73 ± 0.48[a]	6.84 ± 0.45[a]
Clostridium	3.06 ± 0.26[b]	4.52 ± 0.19[a]	2.90 ± 0.65[b]	3.46 ± 0.14[b]	2.95 ± 0.14[b]

[1] Values are means ± SEM, n = 6 for all groups. There is a significant difference between a and b of the same row, $p < 0.05$.

[2] Colony-forming units

Lastly, the mucins 2–4 (MUC, proteins protecting the epithelial surface) expression profile and trefoil factor-3 (TFF3, a peptide implicated in the maintenance and healing of intestinal mucosa) were assessed. Colitis induction produced an increase in both TFF3 and MUC expression, but in every case, AHCC administration resulted in a normalization of the values.[14] This study provided evidence for AHCC's intestinal anti-inflammatory activity at the preclinical level, which was accounted for in principle by its prebiotic properties. Furthermore, AHCC effects were largely comparable to those of an established IBD drug used at a clinically relevant dose based on body surface adjustment.

Probiotics are another widely used strategy to modulate the microbiota to induce a beneficial effect in the host. By contrast with prebiotics, probiotics are live bacterial (or yeast) strains whose administration is intended to directly modify the composition of the microbiota. In order to do so, probiotics must reach the colon in substantial amounts, normally requiring large doses and frequently the use of gastric resistant forms. It should be noted, however, that the mechanism whereby these microorganisms may confer a benefit to the host is ill characterized, and may even be more related to the probiotic constituents than to their thriving in the gut, inasmuch as several studies have documented positive results with dead bacteria. This variant of the probiotic angle has been denominated *metabiotics*.

Obviously, probiotic species bear a strong relation to the ones present in a healthy microbiota (i.e., the ones whose growth and/or activity are actually promoted by prebiotics). Therefore, a synergistic effect may be expected for rightly targeted prebiotic/probiotic combinations, called (perhaps somewhat confusedly) *synbiotics*. Based on the prebiotic properties of AHCC, a synbiotic combination was tested in the same TNBS rat model using *Bifidobacterium longum* BB536 as probiotic. Experimental groups included the separate prebiotic (AHCC 100 or 500 mg/kg) and probiotic (*B. longum* BB536 5×10^6 CFU/day) groups, plus the two combined synbiotic groups, and the TNBS and noncolitic control groups as above. The results indicate that while both treatments had significant intestinal anti-inflammatory activity separately, the combination of AHCC and the probiotic had a synergistic effect, as shown by changes in body weight gain, colonic weight-to-length ratio, myeloperoxidase activity, and nitric oxide synthase expression[15] (see Figure 1 below).

Synergism was manifested particularly with the lower dose of AHCC (100 mg/kg). This is consistent with the intricacies of the experimental design and model used, in which a differential therapeutic effect of separate interventions (prebiotic/ probiotic vs. synbiotic) was sought. This aim in turn is hampered by the limited sensitivity of this model of colitis to pharmacological or nutritional modulation. Therefore,

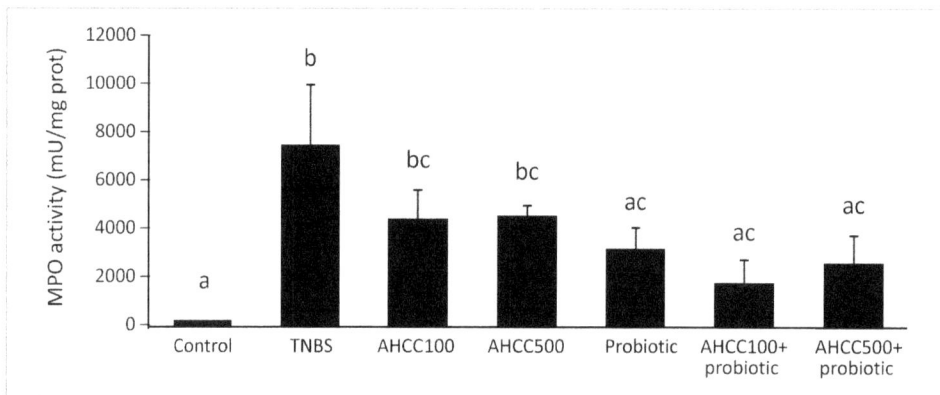

Figure 1. Colonic myeloperoxidase activity in rat TNBS colitis. Rats were treated with AHCC at two different doses with or without *B. longum* BB536 for 7 days (or the corresponding controls) prior to colitis induction and daily thereafter and their MPO activity measured in longitudinal colon samples. Means without a common letter differ ($p < 0.05$)

synergism is best detected using relatively low doses, so that there is sufficient room for added clinical benefit.

The results of both of these studies support the therapeutic activity of AHCC in colonic inflammation using a well-established IBD model. The mechanism of action is consistent with its prebiotic properties (i.e., normalization of intestinal dysbiosis, augmented SCFA production, and so forth).

One limitation of the aforementioned studies is that the TNBS model, while used profusely in the field of intestinal inflammation research and resembling IBD to a large extent, has important differences compared with the human disease. Thus, TNBS colitis is not strictly chronic (i.e., it does not progress indefinitely but rather it heals gradually in a few weeks even if untreated). It is also not lymphocyte driven, since it can be induced normally in the absence of lymphocytes, while lymphocytes are considered to play a central role in the immunopathogenesis of IBD.[16] Therefore, in order to enhance the translational potential of our findings on AHCC, the anti-inflammatory effect of AHCC was also investigated in the CD4+ CD62L+ T cell transfer model of colitis. This is an animal model employed chiefly for immunological research in the field of IBD, based on the parenteral transfer of a lymphocyte pool poor in regulatory T cells to mice devoid of lymphocytes. Over a period of several weeks, the transferred lymphocytes expand and colitis ensues as a reaction toward the colonic microbiota. This model is obviously driven by T cells, is truly chronic, and can be modulated by therapeutic interventions as shown by our group.

Colitis was induced in immunodeficient mice by transfer of naïve CD4+ CD62L+ T cells. After eight weeks, the mice were randomized to receive AHCC (75 mg/day) by gavage or vehicle (control group). In addition, there was a noncolitic control group. AHCC treatment resulted in lower disease activity index, colonic damage score, colonic inflammatory markers (myeloperoxidase and alkaline phosphatase activities), and normalized ex vivo production of inflammatory cytokines compared to the control group. Morphological measurements showed a positive response, as the colonic weight-to-length ratio was not significantly increased in AHCC-treated mice but was doubled in the control animals. Treatment with AHCC generally tended to normalize the mRNA levels of inflammatory markers increased by colitis, particularly TNF and IL-1β. Because of the closer resemblance of this model to "human" IBD, these results provide, by themselves, strong evidence of intestinal anti-inflammatory activity of AHCC. Further, considered together with the results obtained in the rat TNBS model presented above, they conform a strong body of evidence that supports the possible use of AHCC to dampen colonic inflammation in chronic IBD patients, although clinical studies are obviously necessary.[17]

Other Mechanisms

As discussed in previous chapters, AHCC has well-established immunomodulatory activity by enhancing both the innate and adaptive immune response. In addition, AHCC has been described as a biological response modifier for use in cancer immunotherapy. Recently, additional research has provided evidence that AHCC may have immunomodulatory effects in IBD models, independent of its prebiotic properties. To test this theory, the effects of AHCC on intestinal epithelial cells and monocytes/macrophages were investigated in the absence of bacteria. AHCC was added to intestinal epithelial cells and monocytes and the secretion of pro-inflammatory cytokines was measured. AHCC was shown to induce cytokine secretion in epithelial cells (growth regulated oncogene α [GRO α], monocyte chemotactic protein-1 [MCP-1]) via toll-like receptor 4 (TLR4) and the adaptor molecule myeloid differentiation factor 88 (MyD88), based on siRNA analysis (see Figure 2A below). In monocytes, AHCC also stimulated, rather than decreased, the secretion of a number of pro-inflammatory cytokines, including IL-8 (see Figure 2B below), IL-1β, and TNF (data not shown). This effect was highly sensitive to pharmacological inhibition of NF-κB and MAPK.

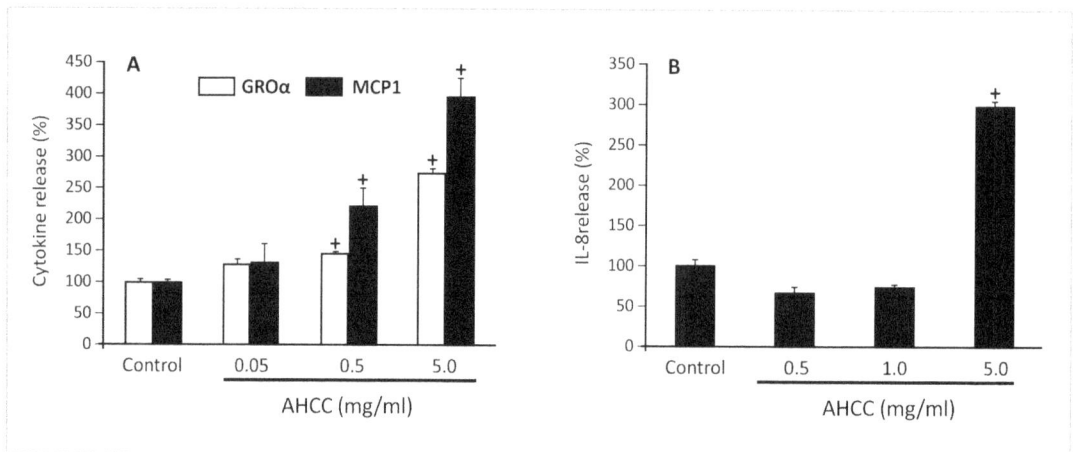

Figure 2. Effect of AHCC on intestinal epithelial cells. **(A)** Effect on the secretion of GROa and MCP-1 by IEC18 cells. **(B)** Effect on IL-8 secretion by HT-29 cells. Different concentrations of AHCC were added to the culture medium, and cytokine concentration in the culture medium was measured by ELISA after a 24-hour incubation. Results are expressed as mean ± SEM of three different experiments (n = 3 in each experiment). +:$p < 0.05$ vs. control (C).

Considered globally, these results suggest that AHCC activates TLR4 in intestinal epithelial cells and monocytes, eliciting the expected downstream signaling steps leading to NF-κB/MAPK activation and the secretion of pro-inflammatory cytokines.[18]

These results appear to be counterintuitive for the treatment of a chronic inflammatory disease. In fact, previous research suggests that TLR dysfunction, particularly TLR4, may play a role in immunopathogenesis of IBD[19] and it has been suggested that the expression of TLR4 is *increased* in IBD patients.[20] Along with other pathogen-associated molecular pattern receptors, TLR4 is involved in the activation of the innate immune system during pathogen recognition in intestinal epithelial cells, monocytes, and other cell types. However, the gut presents a more complex scenario, which is best exemplified by the fact that, almost invariably, mice genetically defective in a TLR or other pattern receptor, or in an involved signaling molecule such as MyD88, are more sensitive to colitis induction. In some cases, colitis actually develops spontaneously. These findings may be related in part to the role played by TLR signaling in many important cytoprotective functions in the intestinal epithelium that support barrier preservation, cell survival, and stability.[21]

Another issue is the fact that barrier function in the gut pertains not only to physical elements but also to the contribution of the mucosal immune system, which may be weakened by a number of factors, including genetic polymorphisms. As one researcher explains, the impact of toll-like receptors on IBD is a "multiple-edged sword" because it is not clear yet whether modulation of TLRs is best accomplished by activating, inhibiting, or rather a combination of both at different stages of mucosal disease.[17] Thus the results of this study with AHCC are compatible with the premise that the primary defect of IBD is in the mucosal barrier defense system and that IBD is not the result of an overactive immune system, but to a relatively weak one. The activation of TLRs may be therapeutic because the engagement of TLR4 in intestinal epithelial cells and macrophages may result in enhanced mucosal barrier function in vivo.[19]

Conclusion

Despite extensive research, the etiology and pathogenesis of IBD still remains unclear. However, the current hypothesis indicates that IBD is a result of either an excessive, abnormal, or an appropriate, but ineffective, immune response to antigens in the intestinal lumen. Dysbiosis of gut microflora in IBD patients is also believed to play an important role in initiating and maintaining the inflammatory response of IBD. In this regard, it is interesting to point out that recent studies correlate alterations in the mucosal barrier function, intestinal dysbiosis, and systemic diseases. In fact, in several systemic diseases, like obesity or fatty liver disease, a subclinical inflammation has been observed possibly related to the intestinal bacterial antigens. Therefore, the use of prebiotics could impact the balance of microbes in the gut, helping to restore the mucosal homeostasis required for balancing the pro- and anti-inflammatory response in IBD and to manage systemic diseases.

AHCC is considered a prebiotic as it contains 74% oligosaccharides. Studies in animal models of colitis are consistent with a prebiotic action of AHCC, normalizing colonic microflora, as well as improving both morphological and biochemical parameters of colonic inflammation. In addition, further studies suggest that AHCC may also contribute immunomodulating activity by TLR4 ligation, resulting in cytokine secretion in intestinal epithelial cells and in macrophages and possibly other effects, which may enhance mucosal barrier function and contribute to better control of inflammation, at least under certain conditions. Globally, these in vivo and in vitro data are supportive of a possible use of AHCC to aid in controlling inflammation in IBD patients, although this will undoubtedly require additional clinical research.

REFERENCES

1. Ananthakrishnan AN. "Epidemilogy and risk factors for IBD." *Nat. Rev. Gastroenterol. Hepatol.* 12(4), 205–217, 2007.

2. Hold GL, et al. "Role of the gut microbiota in inflammatory bowel disease pathogenesis: what have we learnt in the past 10 years?" *World J. Gastroenterol.,* 20(5), 1192–1210, 2014.

3. Ko JK, et al. "Inflammatory bowel disease: etiology, pathogenesis and current therapy." *Curr. Pharm. Des.,* 20(7), 1082–96, 2014.

4. Gyires K, et al. "Gut inflammation: current update on pathophysiology, molecular mechanism and pharmacological treatment modalities." *Curr. Pharm. Des.* 20(7), 1063–81, 2014.

5. Gibson GR, and Roberfroid MB. "Dietary modulation of the human colonic microbiota. Introducing the concept of prebiotics." *J. Nutr.* 125, 1401–12, 1995.

6. Damaskos D, and Kolios G. "Probiotics and prebiotics in inflammatory bowel disease: microflora 'on the scope.'" *Br. J. Clin. Pharmacol.* 65(4), 453–467, 2008.

7. Scheppach W. "Effects of short chain fatty acids on gut morphology and function." *Gut* 35(1 Suppl), S35–S38, 1994.

8. Saemann MD, et al. "Anti-inflammatory effects of sodium butyrate on human monocytes: potent inhibition of IL-12 and up-regulation of IL-10 production." *FASEB J.* 14(15), 2380–2, 2000.

9. Segain JP, et al. "Butyrate inhibits inflammatory responses through NFkappaB inhibition: implications for Crohn's disease." *Gut* 47(3), 397–403, 2000.

10. Strober W and Fuss IJ. "Pro-Inflammatory cytokines in the pathogenesis of IBD." *Gastroenterology* 140(6), 1756–1767, 2011.

11. Daddaoua A, et al. "Goat milk oligosaccharides are anti-inflammatory in rats with hapten-induced colitis." *J. Nutr.* 136, 672–6, 2006.

12. Hoentjen F, et al. "Reduction of colitis by prebiotics in HLA-B27 transgenic rats is associated with microflora changes and immunomodulation." *Inflamm. Bowel Dis.* 11, 977–85, 2005.

13. Koleva PT, et al. "Inulin and fructo-oligosaccharides have divergent effects on colitis and commensal microbiota in HLA-B27 transgenic rats." *Br. J. Nutr.* 108(9), 1633–43, 2012.

14. Daddaoua A, et al. "Active hexose correlated compound acts as a prebiotic and is anti-inflammatory in rats with hapten-induced colitis." *J. Nutr.* 137, 1222–28, 2007.

15. Ocon B, et al. "Active hexose-correlated compound and Bifidiobacterium longum BB536 exert symbiotic effects in experimental colitis." *Eur. J. Nutr.* 52: 457–466, 2013.

16. Ghosh S and Panaccione R. "Anti-adhesion molecule therapy for inflammatory bowel disease." *Therapeutic Advances in Gastroenterology* 3(4), 239–258, 2010.

17. Mascaraque C, et al. "Active hexose correlated compound exerts therapeutic effects in lymphocyte driven colitis." *Mol. Nutr. Food Res.* 11, 1–4, 2014.

18. Daddaoua A, et al. "The nutritional supplement Active Hexose Correlated Compound (AHCC) has direct immunomodulatory actions on intestinal epithelial cells and macrophages involving TLR/MyD88 and NF-κB/MAPK activation." *Food Chemistry* 136, 1288–95, 2013.

19. Cario E. "Therapeutic impact of toll-like receptors on inflammatory bowel diseases: a multiple-edged sword." *Inflamm. Bowel Dis.* 14, 411–421, 2007.

20. Cario E and Podolsky DK. "Differential alteration in intestinal epithelial cell expression of toll-like receptor 3 (TLR3) and TLR4 in inflammatory bowel disease." *Infect. Immun.* 68(12), 7010–17.

21. Cario E. "Toll-like receptors in inflammatory bowel diseases: a decade later." *Inflamm. Bowel Dis.* 16(9), 1583–97, 2010.

22. Sturm A and Dignass AU. "Epithelial restitution and wound healing in inflammatory bowel disease." *World J. Gastroenterol.* 14(3), 348–353, 2008.

23. Rhee SH. "Lipopolysaccharide: basic biochemistry, intracellular signaling, and physiological impacts in the gut." *Intestinal Res.* 12(2), 90–95, 2014.

AHCC and Anti-aging

Tetsuya Okuyama

The functional food AHCC has been shown to have a positive effect on diseases such as cancer and and infectious diseases (see "Cancer" and "Infectious Disease" in part 2 of this book).. A report based on a cohort study suggests that the recurrence rate of cancer in patients with hepatocellular carcinoma after hepatectomy reduced with the oral intake of AHCC, and moreover, there was an improvement in the prognosis such as prolongation of survival time.[1] AHCC also has the effect of activating the immune system (see "Immune Modulation" in part 2 of this book).[2] A good effect can be expected with the intake of AHCC even when healthy from the perspective of prevention. We used the nematode *Caenorhabditis elegans,* which is a model organism suitable for the study of regulating life span, and determined that AHCC has an effect on longevity. Induced HSPs (Heat Shock Proteins) gene expression has gained prominence as an anti-aging factor and was found to be enhanced in *C. elegans* that were given AHCC; this suggests the involvement of AHCC in the longevity of *C. elegans*. This chapter is an introduction to the research on anti-aging in *C. elegans*, and the longevity effect and molecular mechanism of AHCC.

The nematode *C. elegans* is a small animal that belongs to the phylum Nematoda. The length of a nematode *C. elegans* is approximately 1 mm, with a simple system and without any organs in the extremities such as the hands and feet. In the natural world, the nematode *C. elegans* preys on bacteria that live in the soil, and do not depend on other plants and animals as parasites. The nematode *C. elegans* was proposed as a model organism by Dr. S. Brenner of the United Kingdom in the 1960s, and is used for the research of development and nervous systems.[3] The body of *C. elegans* is transparent and can be observed with a microscope while it is alive; all cell lineages of the developmental stages have been elucidated. The concepts of programmed cell death and apoptosis were discovered during the research on development. Also, the research on the nervous system is in progress, and all information on the formation of neural circuits has been ascertained. Memorization and learning have also been ana-lyzed in detail.

The research on aging and life span are relatively new fields of research compared to the above fields. Aging is a process of physiological decline, and life span is considered to be determined by environmental factors. On the other hand, experience has shown that natural death (maximum life) is decided by the animal species when the environment is constant, so that it is easy to understand that genetic factors also significantly impact the deter-mination of life. Based on this concept, studies on regulating life span using model organisms have progressed in recent years. C. elegans has a short life span of approximately twenty days and is a model organism that is appro-priate for the study of regulating life span. The C. elegans mutant with the phenotype that prolongs longevity (age) was discovered and named "age-1."[4] The long-life phenotype of age-1 mutant results from a single gene mutation and the gene encodes a phosphatidylinositol-3-kinase, one of the major fac-tors in intracellular signal cascades.[5] C. elegans grows into a larva that is differ-ent from the normal developmental stage, called the dauer larva, when kept in a poor environment. The dauer larva is covered with a thick cuticle, does not require nutrient intake, tolerates various external stresses, and survives longer compared to C. elegans that undergo normal development.[6] The gene product of age-1 is the configuration factor of insulin/IGF signaling that works such that the transition to this developmental stage is normally inhibited. The gene involved in the formation of dauer larva has been named daf, and many genes have been identified. Furthermore, most of the genes are also shown to be involved in the longevity of C. elegans. Especially, the daf-16 gene encodes the transcription factor of FOXO type that directly controls the transcription for many of the longevity-associated genes. At present, the homologs of daf-16, FOXO type transcription factor, are known to play a key role in controlling the life span even in Drosophila and mice.[7]

We found a reproducible increase of about 10% in the life span of wild-type C. elegans when given the functional food AHCC. The number of off-spring slightly decreased, but noticeable side effects caused by AHCC such as delayed growth and inhibition of development was not observed. The life span in mutants lacking daf-16 was not prolonged by AHCC, this suggests that

AHCC has an effect on the insulin/IGF signaling, which plays a key role in life span control and exhibits life-prolongation effect. On the other hand, AHCC significantly enhanced thermotolerance in wild-type *C. elegans*. The expression of anti-stress gene group named Heat Shock Proteins (HSPs) is induced transiently during heat shock. HSF-1 (Heat Shock Factor-1) is known as the transcription factor that governs the induced expression of these HSP genes, and *hsf-1* gene is reported to enhance thermotolerance and longevity in *C. elegans*.[8] A significant enhancement in thermotolerance with AHCC was invalidated when a mutant lacking HSF-1 was used. Also, on the other hand, AHCC promoted the induction of the HSP genes expression based on heat shock. Moreover, we found the antisense transcript (asRNA) of *hsf-1,* and revealed that the asRNA of *hsf-1* increases due to AHCC.[9] Antisense transcripts (asRNAs) are transcribed with the reverse strand relative to the mRNA from the same gene locus as the template, namely an RNA with a sequence complementary to mRNA. The genes whose expressions are regulated by the stabilization of the mRNA after binding with asRNA are known to be present in mammalian cells.[10] From these, AHCC is implied to enhance the activation of HSF-1 and the induction of HSP genes expression through mechanisms such as post-transcriptional regulation, and this increases the thermotolerance and is also linked to longevity.

The genome project for the nematode *C. elegans* was completed in 1998, ahead of the project for humans.[11] There are many common genes in mammals, including humans; life span–related genes and signaling mechanisms have also been shown to be common. The interaction network formed by longevity related factors, including the above-mentioned insulin-signaling pathway and heat shock transcription factor HSF-1, are saved in many organisms as the key to prevent aging.[7] Specifically, many among the HSPs have the function to act as molecular chaperones that act to fold the nascent proteins. The molecular chaperones control the quality during protein synthesis and also select the refolding and degradation of the denatured proteins; further, they have an important role in mediating apoptosis of the cells when the denatured proteins in the cells are excessive.[12] The aggregation of proteins is said to be the cause for most of the neurodegenerative diseases, including Huntington's, Alzheimer's, and Parkinson's, and age-related diseases such as cataracts, age-related macular degeneration, and arteriosclerosis, and HSPs play a role in preventing abnormal protein aggregation.[8,13] The function as a molecular chaperone is important for the survival of the cells and maintenance of body homeostasis because protein denaturation is not only caused by heat shock but also by diverse factors such as active oxygen or heavy metals, and inflammatory stimuli. HSPs expression is reduced in many of the tissues along with aging, and transcriptional activity of HSF-1 is also inhibited.[14–16]

In the future, further expansion of AHCC as a functional food that combines anti-aging action can be expected by elucidating the molecular mechanism maintaining the activation of the HSF-1 transcription factor and inhibiting the decrease of HSPs expression during the aging process

REFERENCES

1. Matsui Y, Uhara J, Satoi S, Kaibori M, Yamada H, Kitade H, Imamura A, Takai S, Kawaguchi Y, Kwon AH, and Kamiyama Y. "Improved prognosis of postoperative hepatocellular carcinoma patients when treated with functional foods: a prospective cohort study." *J. Hepatol.* 37: 78–86, 2002.

2. Mallet JF, Graham É, Ritz BW, Homma K, and Matar C. "Active Hexose Correlated Compound (AHCC) promotes an intestinal immune response in BALB/c mice and in primary intestinal epithelial cell culture involving toll-like receptors TLR-2 and TLR-4." *Eur. J. Nutr.* 55: 139–146, 2016.

3. Brenner S. "The genetics of *Caenorhabditis elegans*." *Genetics* 77: 71–94, 1974.

4. Johnson TE. "Increased life-span of *age-1* mutants in *Caenorhabditis elegans* and lower gomperz rate of aging." *Science* 249: 908–912, 1990.

5. Morris JZ, Tissenbaum HA, and Ruvkun G. "A phosphatidylinositol-3-OH kinase family member regulating longevity and diapause in *Caenorhabditis elegans*." *Nature* 382: 536–539, 1996.

6. Riddle DL and Albert PS. "Genetic and environmental regulation of dauer larva development." In C. *elegans* II (Riddle DL, Blumenthal T, Meyer BJ, et al., eds), pp. 739–768, Cold Spring Harbor Lab. Press, Plainview, N.Y., 1997.

7. Kenyon C. "The genetics of aging." *Nature* 464: 504–512, 2010.

8. Hsu AL, Murphy CT, and Kenyon C. "Regulation of aging and age-related disease by DAF-16 and heat-shock factor." *Science* 300: 1142–1145, 2003.

9. Okuyama T, Yoshigai E, Ikeya Y, and Nishizawa M. "Active hexose correlated compound extends the lifespan and increases the thermotolerance of nematodes." *Functional Foods in Health and Disease* 3: 166–182, 2013.

10. Matsui K, Nishizawa M, Ozaki T, Kimura T, Hashimoto I, Yamada M, Kaibori M, Kamiyama Y, Ito S, and Okumura T. "Natural antisense transcript stabilizes inducible nitric oxide synthase messenger RNA in rat hepatocytes." *Hepatology* 47: 686–697, 2008.

11. "The *C. elegans* Sequencing Consortium. Genome sequence of the nematode *C. elegans*: A platform for investigating biology." *Science* 282: 2012–18, 1998.

12. Balch WE, Morimoto RI, Dillin A, and Kelly JW. "Adapting proteostasis for disease intervention." *Science* 319: 916–919, 2008.

13. Wyttenbach A, Sauvageot O, Carmichael J, Diaz-Latoud C, Arrigo AP, and Rubinsztein DC. "Heat shock protein 27 prevents cellular polyglutamine toxicity and suppresses the increase of reactive oxygen species caused by huntingtin." *Hum. Mol. Genet.* 11: 1137–51, 2002.

14. Wu B, Gu MJ, Heydari AR, and Richardson A. "The effect of age on the synthesis of two heat shock proteins in the hsp70 family." *J. Gerontol.* 48: B50–56, 1993.

15. Gagliano N, Grizzi F, and Annoni G. "Mechanisms of aging and liver functions." *Dig. Dis.* 25: 118–123, 2007.

16. Kayani AC, Morton JP, and McArdle A. "The exercise-induced stress response in skeletal muscle: failure during aging." *Appl. Physiol. Nutr. Metab.* 33: 1033–41, 2008.

PART 3

CASE REPORTS AND UNPUBLISHED STUDIES

Chapter 10

CANCER

Case Report #1

Yusai Kawaguchi

In the case of patients diagnosed with cancer, the first treatment to be recommended is surgery and/or chemotherapy. However, some patients refuse Western medicine treatments. In this chapter, the cases that resulted in long-term survival, QOL improvement, and eased patients' mental suffering with administration of AHCC in the cancer patients are introduced.

Case A: Long-Term Survival Due to AHCC, Refusing Gastric Surgery

Western medicine treatments are mainstream when treating stomach cancer, with methods such as surgery and chemotherapy. This is because their five-year survival rate is statistically superior to that of other treatment methods. However, it is also a fact that some patients refuse surgery due to a fear of having their body operated on or refuse chemotherapy on the basis of its side effects or doubts about its effectiveness. In this case, a patient diagnosed with early stage stomach cancer for whom surgery and chemotherapy had been recommended began to harbor doubts about Western medicine treatments and desired alternative therapy, which he then underwent. The result of his case, which resulted in long-term survival, is provided below.

Case A Details

Patient: Male, 62 years old

Complaint: Refused surgery

Family history: Nothing particular of note

Medical history: Rectal surgery for rectal cancer, May 6, 1994 (stage unknown)

History of illness: After diagnosis in June 1996 with early stage stomach cancer, the patient underwent endoscopic mucosal resection (EMR). In May 2000, upon observation of recurrence in the identical sites, surgery was recommended to the patient, but he began to harbor misgivings about Western medicine treatment. On June 30th of the same year, the patient visited this hospital seeking alternative therapy. Since coming to the hospital, therapy began with only 3 g/day of AHCC. Chemotherapy was not administered. However, upper gastrointestinal endoscopies were carried out once every one to two months, and once every six months blood tests and abdominal CT were administered.

Upper gastrointestinal endoscopy (GIF): Upon a GIF carried out on July 8, 2000, IIb lesions in the gastric upper rear wall were identified, found to be signet ring cell carcinoma upon tissue diagnosis (see Figure 1, right). Upon a GIF carried out on June 28, 2003, the number of cancerous lesions had increased slightly (see Figure 2, right). Upon a GIF carried out on September 9, 2006, IIb+IIc and ulcerative lesions had come to merge (see Figure 3, right). Upon a GIF carried out on February 17, 2010, IIa+IIb and polypoid lesions had also come to merge (see Figure 4, right). Upon a GIF carried out on June 19, 2014, tumors had increased to stage 1 advanced cancer (see Figure 5, right).

Informed consent: Since coming to this hospital, surgery was offered numerous times but was always refused by the patient. However, in 2014, as tumor markers were normal (CEA: 1.0 ng/ml, CA19–9: 9.9 U/ml), and metastatic disease was also not observed (see Figure 6, right), the patient was told that although the cancer had progressed, it was possible to completely cure with surgery, and the patient accepted surgery.

Surgical findings: Total gastrectomy was carried out on July 23, 2014. Roux-en Y reconstruction in stage IIIc.

Course of treatment: Steady progress post-operation, and at present, March 23, 2016, no recurrence nor metastasis has been observed. Additionally, because the cancer had progressed to stage IIIc, chemotherapy was recommended, but the patient refused this option and, at present, is trying various alternative therapies such as AHCC and Chinese medicine.

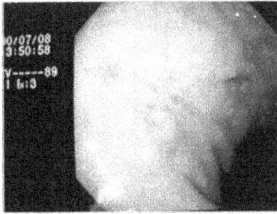
Figure 1. July 8, 2000

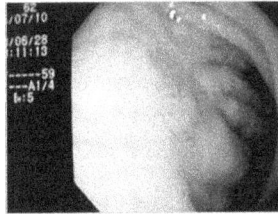
Figure 2. June 28, 2003

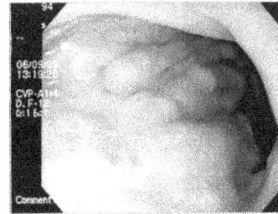
Figure 3. September 9, 2006

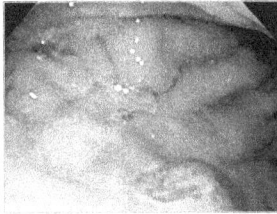
Figure 4. February 17, 2010

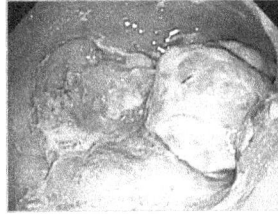
Figure 5. June 19, 2014

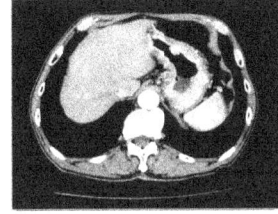
Figure 6. July 8, 2014

Case A Discussion

The post-surgery early stomach cancer five-year survival rate is 95.4%, and five-year recurrence-free survival rate is 93.7%, both quite favorable.[1] This is undoubtedly a result of advances in medical techniques and surgery, but even yet those rates are not quite at 100%. This patient, despite undergoing cutting-edge EMR[2] treatment, began to show misgivings about Western medicine treatment after his cancer reoccurred after only four years and wanted alternative therapy ever since. However, we do not have any reports nor do we have any evidence-based medicine (EBM) to indicate what the five-year survival rate would be if a patient's condition remains stable in early stage stomach cancer without any treatment.

Thus, with this case, in anticipation of the immunomodulatory effect of AHCC,[3] we began a daily dose of 3 g, and while there was no reduction in cancer observed, the patient's life was prolonged by fourteen years. Moreover, despite the fact that the cancer had progressed to an advanced stage, at the time of surgery, the cancer was in stage IIIc with no metastasis, and even at present, there has been no reoccurrence or metastasis observed.

Presently the first treatment for stomach cancer is surgery, but if the patient refuses surgery, it is simply a fact that with our present means of treatment, nothing can be done. However, if there is something that at least modulates the immune system, there may be possible treatment that relies on that. This time, AHCC was validated as an effective functional food that meets those expectations.

CASE A REFERENCES

1. Yajima K and Iwasaki Y. "Greater applications of laparoscopic stomach cancer surgery—Is LAG reasonable for advanced stomach cancer? Greater possibilities to apply laparoscopic gastrectomy as seen from relapse form." *Japanese Journal of Cancer Clinics* 60 (4): 401–409, 2014.

2. Tanabe S. "Current state and future prospects of endoscopic therapy for early stomach cancer (Review)." *The Kitasato Medical Journal* 45 (1): 1–9, 2015.

3. Miura T, Kitadate K, and Nishioka H. "Basics of AHCC and clinical pathology." *Latest Topics: Japanese Society for Complementary and Alternative Medicine* 6 (1): 1–7, 2009.

Case B: Trial Administration of AHCC Due to Intestinal Fistula Resulting from Inoperable Stomach Cancer

There is still no established treatment for inoperable stomach cancer, and in each case, presently symptomatic treatment corresponding to symptoms is carried out. Because of this, doctors recommend ceasing aggressive treatment and shifting focus to palliative and end-of-life care. However, though some patients and families can accept this reality, most cannot and are set adrift. This time, a patient was admitted to the hospital with "desperate hope," and after trying various aggressive treatments, his quality of life (QOL) rose, and we can report that this was a case where he spent his life in a meaningful way.

Case B Details

Patient: Male, 68 years old

Complaint: Heartburn, difficulty swallowing

Family history: Nothing particular of note

Medical history: Nothing particular of note

History of illness: On September 4, 2014, patient was diagnosed with stage 4 stomach cancer, spanning the entire periphery from directly below the esophago-cardiac junction (EC) to the lower gastric corpus (tissue diagnosis of moderately differentiated adenocarcinoma). At this point (at a different hospital), palliative care was recommended, but the patient sought out other treatment methods, visited this hospital, and was admitted September 11 the same year.

Condition when hospitalized: No abnormalities were observed in the systemic and abdominal findings.

Blood test upon hospitalization: WBC 8,100/µl, RBC 4.73×10^6/µl, Hb 15.1 g/dl, Ht 45.9%, PLT 2.21×10^5/µl, were normal, nor were abnormalities observed in biochemical tests. Blood CEA 1.4 ng/ml and CA19–9 10 U/ml were also normal.

Upper endoscopy: GIF did not pass beyond directly below the EC; could not confirm if there were edema tumors present on mucosa (see Figure 1 below).

Abdominal CT examination: The abdominal esophagus was edematous, and the stomach was completely swollen from the EC to the lower body (see Figure 2 below). These aside, lymph node metastasis to the splenic hilum was observed, as well as ascites retention (see Figure 3 below).

Operative findings: Surgery was performed September 22. Tumors had infiltrated the pancreatic area, and furthermore had penetrated into the abdominal esophagus. Additionally, resection was abandoned because of observation of ascites retention and peritoneal dissemination (T4bN3M1, stage IV), and from about 30cm from the Treitz ligament an intestinal fistula was created in the anal jejunum.

Postoperative course: Three days after surgery, patient underwent low-dose chemotherapy with TS-1 (80 mg/day, administered every other day, no break in medicine) and PTX (60 mg/dose administered once a week, with break in treatment after three weeks). Seven days after surgery, administered AHCC 3 g/day through intestinal fistula. AHCC proved to be poorly soluble, and from the beginning, nurses had to administer treatment by hand, but within that time, patient happily agreed to having the medicine dissolved and injected. As cancer advances, stenosis can occur, limiting dietary intake, so a stent was placed at the site of stenosis, but dietary intake

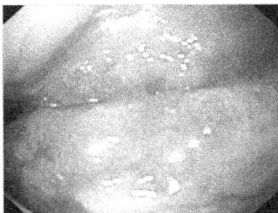

Figure 1. Upper endoscopy below the EC

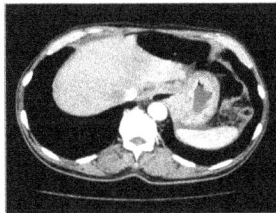

Figure 2. Abdominal CT from the EC to the lower body

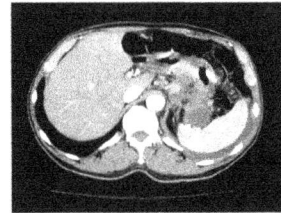

Figure 3. Abdominal CT (metastasis and ascites retention)

was still poor. Thus, nutritional management was carried out via enteral supplement injections from the intestinal fistula. He continued receiving injections of AHCC and enteral supplements and was safely able to enjoy time with his family over the New Year's holiday; the patient then passed away on February 23, 2015.

Case B Discussion

Treatment for those with inoperable stomach cancer is mostly symptomatic therapy, where stomach resection and radiation therapy treat bleeding,[1] and where stenosis is treated by placing stents[2] or bypass surgery.[3] In this way, though current medicine can physically remove the patient's suffering, there is no therapy that can address the patient's strong desire to live.

In this situation, it does not mean we can simply give up doing anything about late-stage cancer. However, I believe there are doctors out there whom, if it is possible, do get attached to patients and wish to treat them. Therefore at our hospital, even if we understand that treatment is futile, if the patient so wishes we will attempt aggressive treatment. With this case, because the tumors had spread so vastly, it was impossible to excise the primary tumor; however, expecting AHCC's immunomodulatory effect[4] and its orexigenic effect,[5] we created an intestinal fistula so as to inject AHCC through that point. As a result, his QOL was quite improved. Additionally, though AHCC is poorly soluble it was successfully injected via the intestinal fistula, and in the future, for cases where nutritional intake is poor, we showed that it is possible to administer nutrition through feeding tube or injections into intestinal fistula.

CASE B REFERENCES

1. Okumura Y, Kawada J, and Fujitani K. "Case of patient undergoing palliative radiation therapy twice and artery embolization for bleeding from inoperable stomach cancer." *Japanese Journal of Cancer and Chemotherapy* 42 (12): 1665–1667, 2015.

2. Takeno A, Tamura S, and Taniguchi H. "Case of long-term oral intake in advanced stomach cancer made possible with stent placement." *Japanese Journal of Cancer and Chemotherapy* 42 (12): 1686–1688, 2015.

3. Nishikawa K, Kawada J, and Fukuda Y. "Study of preoperative prognostic indicators in cases of gastrointestinal bypass surgery." *Japanese Journal of Surgical Metabolism and Nutrition* 49 (2): 95–100, 2015.

4. Miura T, Kitadate K, and Nishioka H. "Basics of AHCC and Clinical Pathology." *Latest Topics: Japanese Society for Complementary and Alternative Medicine* 6 (1): 1–7, 2009.

5. Kawaguchi Y and Kamiyama Y. "[Supplements in Clinical Pathology] Supplements in Clinical Pathology: The Way I Teach, Immunoenhancing Supplements (AHCC, Purple Ipe)." *Progress in Medicine* 24 (6): 1455–1459, 2004.

Case C: Improved QOL in Bile Duct Cancer Due to AHCC

The prognosis for bile duct cancer is poor, as reoccurrence and metastasis rates are high even when surgery is performed.[1] If the cancer reoccurs or metastases, most patients succumb to discouragement, falling into depression and losing the will to live. However, if they do not lose hope and continue searching for reasons to live, they may end up trying alternative therapy. In this case, the cancer reoccurred even after surgery and chemotherapy had no effect, so the patient lost hope for some time, but after overcoming his depression and refusing to lose hope, he came across AHCC in his search, and afterward, we can report that his life turned from pain to enjoyment, and he could pass on meaningfully.

Case C Details

Patient: Male, 73 years old

Complaint: Medical examination showed abnormality in liver function

Family history: Nothing particular of note

Medical history: Nothing particular of note

History of illness: Under a diagnosis of intrahepatic bile duct cancer (tissue diagnosis of moderately differentiated adenocarcinoma), on November 14, 2012, patient underwent surgery for a resection of the left-hand liver in three areas and a hilar lymph node dissection. Patient started chemotherapy in May 2013 due to reoccurrence. However, the tumors gradually expanded, and as the side effects of chemotherapy had intensified, on September 28, 2014, patient was admitted to this hospital for alternative therapy.

Blood test upon hospitalization: WBC 2600/µl, RBC 2.28 × 10⁶/µl, Hb 7.8 g/dl, Ht 22.8%, PLT 28,000/µl, displaying pancytopenia. Did not observe abnormalities in liver function or kidney function. Blood CEA was slightly increased at 5.2 ng/ml, but CA19–9 was normal at 36.9 U/ml.

Abdominal CT scans during visits: Numerous small and large tumors identified in the remaining liver (see Figure 1 below), and observed pleural effusion (see Figure 2 below), and ascites retention (see Figure 3 below).

Course of treatment: From the time of hospital visit, administered 3 g/day of AHCC, and did not administer chemotherapy. After taking AHCC, patient's appetite increased, and he gained 3 kg in weight. Patient was more enthusiastic about life than before and even started traveling, which he had been unable to enjoy due to the effects of chemotherapy, many times with his family; he was also able to enjoy the New Year's holiday with them. QOL for the patient was maintained until he passed January 17, 2015.

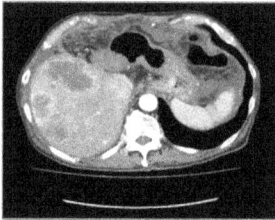

Figure 1. Abdominal CT scans of the remaining liver

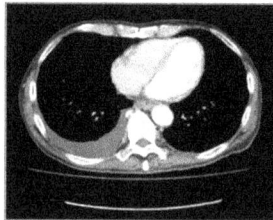

Figure 2. Abdominal CT scans of the remaining liver (pleural effusion)

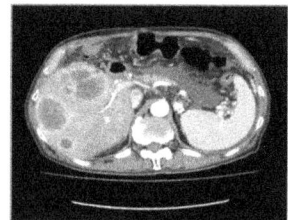

Figure 3. Abdominal CT scans of the remaining liver (ascites retention)

Case C Discussion

Although the mainstream treatments for intrahepatic bile duct cancer are surgery[2] and chemotherapy,[3] it is a reality that Western medicine is at a loss when cancer reoccurs or metastasizes. It is precisely for that reason that patients are recommended palliative treatment and end-of-life treatment. In other words, palliative care, according to the proposed 2002 definition by the WHO, is "an approach that improves the quality of life of patients and their families facing the problem associated with life-threatening illness, through the prevention and relief of suffering by means of early identification and impeccable assessment and treatment of pain and other problems, physical, psychosocial and spiritual." Current medical practice is to attempt to actively prevent suffering and improve QOL through relieving pain. However, with regard to physical therapy, though it is actively being implemented,[4–6] mental therapy is still in its infancy[7] and woefully inadequate.

With that in mind, since AHCC has been previously touted for its immunomodulatory effects,[8] for this case, we used AHCC with the intent of easing the pain caused by the emotional distress of the cancer's reoccurrence and metastasis, and to ease the pain from the side effects of chemotherapy.[9] AHCC met our expectations, and as the patient's mental suffering was eased, his QOL greatly increased. From the above, we can suppose that AHCC is excellently effective as palliative therapy.

CASE C REFERENCES

1. Shirabe K, Yoshizumi T, and Imai D. "[New conventions and treatment strategies for intrahepatic bile duct cancer] Treatment of recurrent intrahepatic bile duct cancer." *Surgery* 78 (2): 168–171, 2016.

2. Ariizumi S, Kodera Y, and Yamamoto M. "[New conventions and treatment strategies for intrahepatic bile duct cancer] Adjuvant chemotherapy after intrahepatic bile duct cancer resection." *Surgery* 78 (2): 163–167, 2016.

3. Shimada K, Miyata Y, and Ezaki M. "[New conventions and treatment strategies for intrahepatic bile duct cancer] Significance of lymph node dissection in intrahepatic bile duct cancer surgery." *Surgery* 78 (2): 155–162, 2016.

4. Sunohara K and Nishiwaki K. "[Aggressive palliative care sought by surgeons—The threshold between survival and symptom relief] Aggressive intervention of palliative care to know: Nerve block therapy for cancer pain." *Clinical Surgery* 70 (13): 1500–08, 2015.

5. Morioka H, Nishimoto K, and Horiuchi K. "[Aggressive palliative care sought by surgeons—The threshold between survival and symptom relief] Aggressive intervention of palliative treatment to know: Drug therapy with surgery and bone modifying agent for bone metastases." *Clinical Surgery* 70 (13): 1493–99, 2015.

6. Ohta K and Matsuzaki K. "[Aggressive palliative care sought by surgeons—The threshold between survival and symptom relief] Aggressive intervention of palliative treatment to know: CART and drug therapy for cancer ascites." *Clinical Surgery* 70 (13): 1487–92, 2015.

7. Hirade M. "Palliative Care and Psycho-oncology Started by a Psychosomatic Medicine Specialist: Aiming for an Air-like Existence: The Role of Psychosomatic Medicine in a Medical Team." *Japanese Journal of Psychosomatic Internal Medicine,* supplemental vol. 19: 56, 2015.

8. Miura T, Kitadate K, and Nishioka H. "Basics of AHCC and Clinical Pathology." *Latest Topics: Japanese Society for Complementary and Alternative Medicine* 6 (1): 1–7, 2009.

9. Urushima H, Hayashi N, and Maeda K. "Clinical trials for alleviating the adverse effects of chemotherapy with AHCC." *Journal of Japanese Society for Medical Use of Functional Foods* 7 (1): 131, 2011.

Case D: Administering AHCC Post-debulking Surgery for Stomach Cancer

While debulking surgery is often carried out for primary peritoneal cancer and ovarian cancer,[1,2] it is not often performed currently for stomach cancer aside from a CY1 procedure.[3] This is because reducing tumors even slightly in cases of primary peritoneal cancer and ovarian cancer is expected to improve survival rates, but conversely, there is no such high expectation in cases of stomach cancer. However, from the perspective of QOL, for those with hope to reduce their tumors with surgery even just slightly, whether reduction is even possible thus becomes a matter of life and death. In this case, the patient wished to have a reduction while in stage IV stomach cancer, and we can report that her post-operative QOL was greatly increased.

Case D Details

Patient: Female, 57 years old

Complaint: Loss of appetite, difficulty swallowing

Family history: Nothing particular of note

Medical history: Nothing particular of note

History of illness: Observed loss of appetite and difficulty swallowing from approximately August 2014, and during the same year in October was diagnosed with stage IV stomach cancer at a local hospital. At this time, though the patient was told that her condition was inoperable and chemotherapy was recommended, she sought out debulking surgery and alternative therapy, and was admitted to this hospital October 31, 2014.

Condition when hospitalized: Abdomen was completely swollen, but superficial lymph nodes, etc. were not palpable.

Blood test upon hospitalization: WBC was normal at 5600/μl, but RBC was 4.33 $\times 10^6$/μl, Hb 9.7 g/dl, and Ht 31.2%, indicating anemia. Liver function and kidney function were normal, but patient had low total protein of 4.8 g/dl and low albumin at 2.2 g/dl. Blood CEA was 3.7 ng/ml, and CA19–9 25.8 U/ml, both normal.

Upper endoscopy: Type 4 tumors identified from the gastric angle to antrum (see Figure 1 on the facing page), with fiber unable to pass. Tissue diagnosis of moderately differentiated adenocarcinoma.

Abdominal CT scan: Stomach was expanded, and a large amount of food reside was observed within the stomach (see Figure 2 below). Identified wall thickening, which spanned the entire circumference from pylorus to gastric antrum (see Figure 3 below). Also identified ascites (see Figure 4 below).

Operative findings: Surgery was performed November 7, 2014. Cancerous lesions had already infiltrated the pancreatic area, but a total gastrectomy was performed so as to debulk tumors (T4aN3M1, stage IV). Roux-en Y reconstruction.

Course of treatment: Ten days after surgery, patient began taking 3 g/day of AHCC. One month after surgery, patient underwent low-dose chemotherapy with TS-1 (80 mg/day, administered every other day, no break in medicine) and PTX (60 mg/dose administered once a week, with break in treatment after three weeks). By combining AHCC with chemotherapy, side effects in general were not observed. From this event, the patient afterward was able to spend meaningful time together with her family. She enjoyed her hobbies with her daughter until one week before she passed away on April 23, 2015.

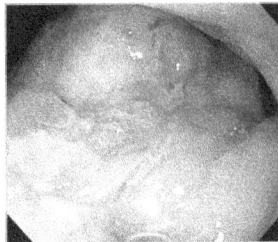

Figure 1. Upper endoscopy from the gastric angle to antrum

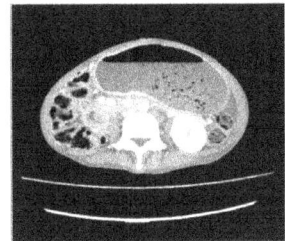

Figure 2. Abdominal CT scan of the gastric region

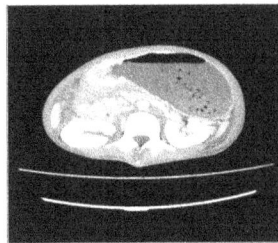

Figure 3. Abdominal CT scan of the gastric region

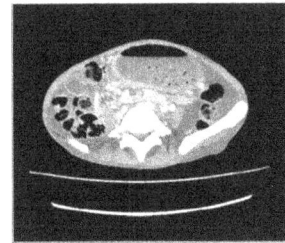

Figure 4. Abdominal CT scan of the gastric region

Case D Discussion

Surgery remains the first choice when treating stomach cancer. Because of this, when a patient is told that the tumors cannot be surgically removed, in many cases, they are often quite discouraged and lose hope. Even so, if there are those who change their minds and put their hopes into chemotherapy, there must be some patients willing to go on a journey to find a surgeon willing to debulk the tumor.

At this time, as a surgeon, even if it is not strictly evidence-based medicine (EBN), I believe it is reasonable to respond to a patient from the perspective of palliative treatment that "improves the quality of life of patients through the prevention and relief of suffering."[4] However, for a surgeon who would perform the debulking surgery, though they may suspect that the cancer would spread and the patient's life would instead be cut even shorter, if there is some way to at least improve their quality of life, then they can wield courage and make an effort to perform the surgery.

We can expect various immunomodulatory effects and more from AHCC.[5] In this case, by combining AHCC with debulking surgery, the patient's postoperative QOL increased, and she could meaningfully live out the rest of her life. Thus AHCC supports not only the hearts of the patient and their families, but the surgeons attending to them as well.

CASE D REFERENCES

1. Yoshikawa H. "[Malignant tumor peritoneum] Diagnosis and treatment of primary peritoneal tumor, primary peritoneal cancer." *Surgery* 77 (10): 1130–33, 2015.

2. Kato K, Nomura H, and Omatsu K. "Case of laparoscopic debulking surgery to recurrent ovarian cancer." *Japan Society of Gynecologic and Obstetric Endoscopy and Minimally Invasive Therapy Journal* 31 (Suppl. I): 271, 2015.

3. Nagata H, Komatsu S, and Ichikawa D. "Treatment Strategies for Stage IV Stomach CancerCY1 Stomach Cancer Reevaluation and Stratification of Prognosis." Japanese Journal of Cancer and Chemotherapy 41 (12): 2235–38, 2014.

4. Definition of Palliative Care. WHO: 2002.

5. Miura T, Kitadate K, and Nishioka H. "Basics of AHCC and Clinical Pathology." *Latest Topics: Japanese Society for Complementary and Alternative Medicine* 6 (1): 1–7, 2009.

Case E: AHCC for Advanced Stomach Cancer in Combination with Low-dose Chemotherapy

In recent years, there have been remarkable advances in chemotherapy, and a variety of cancer chemotherapy drugs and molecular targeted drugs have been developed.[1–3] As a result of those efforts, five-year survival rates have improved, but on the other hand, it is still a reality that many patients are suffering from the side effects of chemotherapy. Because of that, many patients refuse chemotherapy, and even of those who choose to undergo chemotherapy, they are unable to sustain their QOL and stop treatment midway. In this case, to reduce the side effects of chemotherapy, low-dose chemotherapy was administered in combination with AHCC, and we can report that the patient's QOL improved.

Case E Details

Patient: Female, 73 years old

Complaint: Loss of appetite

Family history: Nothing particular of note

Medical history: Nothing particular of note

History of illness: Observed loss of appetite from approximately early March 2015, and after visiting local hospital on March 3 the same year, patient was diagnosed with multiple liver metastases due to stomach cancer. Unwilling to accept her fatal prognosis, she sought out alternative therapy and visited this hospital.

Blood test upon hospitalization: Observed WBC 12700/μl, CRP 1.71 mg/dl and inflammatory response, but no anemia was observed. Observed AST 102U/L, ALT59U/L, ALP 1000U/L, γ-GTP 527U/L, LDH 568U/L, and abnormalities in liver function. Blood CEA 2.4 ng/ml and CA19–9 4.0U/ml were normal.

Upper endoscopy: Observed IIa and IIc lesions from the rear gastric angle (see Figure 1 below). Tissue diagnosis of well-differentiated adenocarcinoma.

Abdominal CT scan: Observed large numbers of metastases in the liver (see Figures 2 and 3 below).

Course of treatment: From March 9, 2015, administered 3 g/day of AHCC, and from March 17 the same year, underwent low-dose chemotherapy with TS-1 (80 mg/day, administered every other day, no break in medicine) and PTX (60 mg/dose administered once a week, with break in treatment after three weeks). After chemotherapy,

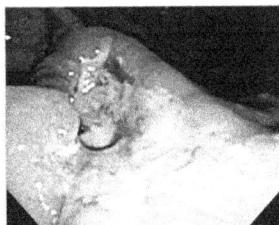

Figure 1. Upper endoscopy from the rear gastric angle

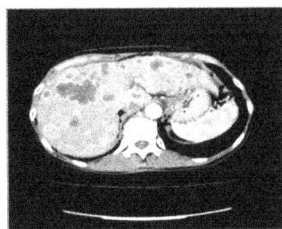

Figure 2. Abdominal CT scan of the liver (March 3, 2015)

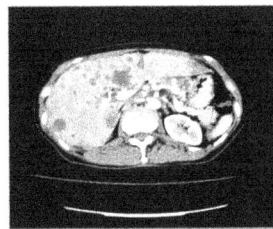

Figure 3. Abdominal CT scan of the liver (March 3, 2015)

an abdominal CT on June 2, 2015, showed that the metastases had gone from no change to a slight increase (see Figures 4 and 5 below), but blood CEA 4.9 ng/ml and CA19–9 3U/ml were normal. Afterward, patient was actively committed to therapy, and though her appetite and vitality were maintained, she passed away August 24, 2015.

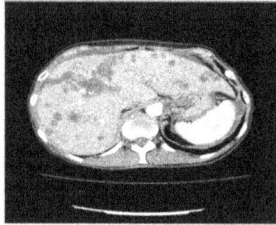

Figure 4. Abdominal CT scan of the liver
(June 2, 2015)

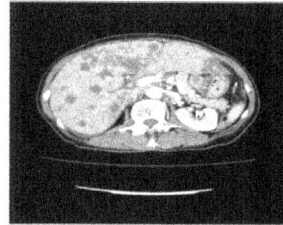

Figure 5. Abdominal CT scan of the liver
(June 2, 2015)

Case E Discussion

In recent years, many attempts have been made to counter the side effects of chemotherapy.[4–6] However, it is still inadequate, and there is currently no end to the great number of patients suffering from the side effects of chemotherapy. This is because the purpose of chemotherapy is aimed at killing off cancer, and as a result, it has the side effect of also killing off normal cells. Because of this, if you switch to thinking that the purpose of chemotherapy is to simply maintain the body's status quo, then you will not have most side effects and will not kill off normal cells. In other words, by lowering the dose of chemotherapy, on a case-by-case basis, to half or a fourth of the usual dosage, the attack on cancer cells will be reduced, but additionally the attack on normal cells will also be reduced. By doing so, there may be some uncertainty of whether the effectiveness of chemotherapy is lowered, but this time, by combining such chemotherapy with AHCC, with its immunomodulatory effect,[7] we were able to reasonably fulfill expectations for low-dose chemotherapy treatment, and the patient's quality of life rose. Because of this, we can suppose that the combination of low-dose chemotherapy and AHCC is effective treatment and is also useful for improving quality of life.

CASE E REFERENCES

1. Kadowaki S and Muro K. "[Surgical treatment for operable stage IV stomach cancer] Effects and limitations of drug therapy: Study of long-term survival in stage IV gastric cancer chemotherapy." *Clinical Surgery* 68 (13): 1410–1415, 2013.

2. Watanabe K and Shirao K. "[Upper gastrointestinal tract disease—All the latest knowledge in transfiguring disease structures for practicing clinicians—] What practicing doctors should know about progress in treatment and usage: Progress in stomach cancer chemotherapy, including molecular target therapy." *Medical Practice* 30 (7): 1241–1243, 2013.

3. Nemoto H, Saito M, and Harada Y. "[Stomach cancer chemotherapy performed by surgeons] Current situation of inoperable stomach cancer chemotherapy performed by surgeons." *Japanese Journal of Cancer Clinics* 57 (1): 47–51, 2011.

4. Nagata N. "[The role of Chinese medicine in team medicine] The current state of cancer chemotherapy and Chinese medicine." *Japanese Journal of Cancer and Chemotherapy* 42 (13): 2423–2429, 2015.

5. Matsuhashi E, Takahashi T, and Yoshida K. "[What Surgeons Need to Know: Cancer Drug Therapy Side Effects and Countermeasures] Cancer Drug Therapy Management and Countermeasures for Side Effects." *Clinical Surgery* 70 (5): 526–531, 2015.

6. Minami H, Yamaguchi K, and Okano S. "Measures against side effects of new molecular target therapies." *Molecular Target Therapy of Cancer* 13 (1): 72–78, 2015.

7. Miura T, Kitadate K, and Nishioka H. "Basics of AHCC and Clinical Pathology." *Latest Topics: Japanese Society for Complementary and Alternative Medicine* 6 (1): 1–7, 2009.

Case Report #2

Norbert Szalus

AHCC is known as a functional ingredient which may support chemotherapy and radiotherapy in cancer patients, but there are not many reports about AHCC supportive effect on rare cancers and autoimmunity diseases. This chapter shows over 10 years of my experience with very rare cancers and autoimmunity disorders.

Case A: AHCC for Treatment of Idiopathic Thrombocytopenic Purpura in 11-Year-Old Girl

Idiopathic thrombocytopenic purpura (ITP), also called immune thrombocytopenic purpura, is a blood-clotting disorder that can lead to easy or excessive bruising and bleeding. ITP results from unusually low levels of platelets—the cells that help the blood clot. ITP affects both children and adults. Children often develop ITP after a viral infection and usually recover fully without treatment. In adults, however, the disorder is often chronic.

Visible symptoms of ITP include the spontaneous formation of purpura (bruises) and petechiae (tiny bruises), especially on the extremities, bleeding from the nostrils, bleeding at the gums, and menorrhagia (excessive menstrual bleeding), any of which may occur if the platelet count is below 20,000 per µl.[1] A very low count (<10,000 per µl) may result in the spontaneous formation of hematomas (blood masses) in the mouth or on other mucous membranes. Bleeding time from minor lacerations or abrasions is usually prolonged. Treatment of ITP depends on the patient's symptoms and platelet count. Treatment is usually initiated with intravenous corticosteroids, such as methylprednisolone or prednisone. Other strategies are immunosuppressants, thrombopoietin receptor agonists, splenectomy (removal of the spleen), and experimental and novel agents (dapsone, rituximab)

We present a case of an 11-year-old girl with ITP. The first symptoms occurred in October 2009. The patient suffered from typical symptoms of ITP (bruises and petechiae, especially on the extremities). The first count of PLT (platelets) in October 2009 was 10,000 per µl (normal range: 150,000 – 400,000 per µl). In the hospital and at home, she was treated by dexamethasone 24 mg/day. The count of PLT rose up to 140,000 per µl. A few months later during therapy of dexamethasone, she suffered from side effects. After reducing the dose of dexamethasone, the count of PLT was decreased. Then she received immunoglobulin for temporary relief. In May 2010, the doctor suggested that she should have a splenectomy, and the parents did not consent. On the first visit in October 2010, the count of PLT was 20,000 per µl. Then I prescribed AHCC 1.5 g/day. After 7 months of continuous AHCC administration, no symptoms were shown, and the level of platelets is 150,000 per µl (normal level). In my opinion, AHCC should be seriously considered for treatment in the patient with ITP.

CASE A REFERENCE

1. Cines DB, McMillan R. "Management of adult idiopathic thrombocytopenic purpura." *Annu. Rev. Med.* 56: 425–442, 2005.

Case B: AHCC's Impact on Immunological System and Adverse Effects on Patients with Disseminated Neuroendocrine Tumors (NETs) Treated with Radioisotope Preparation (^{90}Y-DOTA-TATE)

Neuroendocrine tumors (NETs) are rare tumors which consist of a heterogeneous group of neoplasms with expression of neuroamine uptake mechanisms and/ or specific peptide receptors at the cell membrane. Over expression of somatostatin receptors which is a characteristic feature of NETs occurs in 75 – 90% of cases, and so somatostatin can be used in localization and treatment of these tumors. Conventionally NETs may present with a wide variety of functional or nonfunctional endocrine syndromes. They may be familiar and have other associated tumors, also they have different histology pattern and prognosis. They originate from endocrine glands, such as the pituitary, the parathyroids, and the (neuroendocrine) adrenal, as well as endocrine islets within glandular tissue (thyroid or pancreatic) and cells dispersed between exocrine cells, such as endocrine cells of the digestive system and respiratory tracts. More than 70% of all NETs are gastroenteropancreatic NET (GEP-NET). Typical treatments for NETs are surgery, chemotherapy, somatostatin analogs as an injection form, and new treatment options including somatostatin analogues (DOTA-TATE) labeled with radio isotopes such as ^{90}Y (Yttrium-90).

In our study we assessed influence of AHCC on the immunological profile of NETs patients. We evaluated three patients with histopathologically confirmed NETs, who were included in the study. Those patients were treated with four doses of ^{90}Y-DOTA-TATE ($3.7\ GBq/m^2/dose$) in 8–10 week intervals. Control CT and PET/CT with somatostatin analog ^{68}Ga-DOTA-TATE were conducted three months after the last dose of ^{90}Y-DOTA-TATE. The patients took 6 g of AHCC daily (2 g x 3 times), 40 minutes before meals. The local ethics committee approval was obtained before the study commenced. All results are presented as medium results.

Three months after the last dose of ^{90}Y-DOTA-TATE, the followings were found: T (CD3$^+$) lymphocytes, helper/inducer (CD3$^+$CD4$^+$), NK (CD3$^+$CD16/56$^+$) type cells, and Regulatory T (CD4$^+$CD25^{++}FoxP3$^+$) cells (Tregs) decreased by 4.91%, 36.27%, 14.48%, and 28.2% respectively; Cytotoxic T (CD3$^+$CD8$^+$) and NK (CD3-CD16/56$^+$) type cells increased by 60.43% and 18.84% respectively.

Twelve months after the last dose of ^{90}Y-DOTA-TATE, the followings were found: CD3$^+$, CD3$^+$CD4$^+$, CD3$^+$CD16/56$^+$, and CD4$^+$CD25^{++}FoxP3$^+$ cells (Tregs) decreased by 10.83%, 45%, 19.2%, and 34% respectively; CD3$^+$CD8$^+$ and CD3-CD16/56$^+$ cells increased by 49.2% and 14.3% respectively. Comparing immunity three and twelve months after the last dose of radioisotope, results have been shown as follow: CD3$^+$, CD3$^+$CD8$^+$, CD3-CD16/56$^+$, CD3$^+$CD16/ 56$^+$, CD4$^+$CD25^{++}FoxP3$^+$ cells (Tregs) decreased by 5,12%, 15%, 12.9%, 6.3%, and 6.1% respectively; CD3$^+$CD4$^+$ cells increased by 6.3%. In PET/CT and CT, partial responses were revealed after twelve months of this combined therapy (^{90}Y-DOTA-TATE + AHCC) in all patients (see Figure 1).

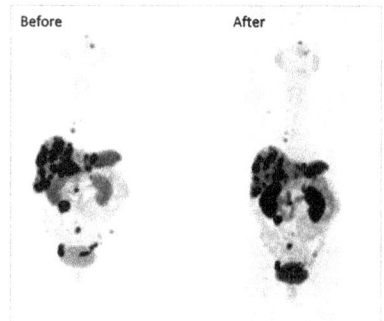

Figure 1. PET-CT with ^{68}Ga-DOTA-TATE before and after therapy of ^{90}Y-DOTA-TATE + AHCC

Based on my past practices of radioisotope therapy, patients have improved their quality of life during AHCC supplementation. In addition, this study with NETs patients showed that AHCC increased the amount of cytotoxic T cells and NK (CD3-CD16/56$^+$) type cells and decreased CD4$^+$CD25^{++}

FoxP3[+] with suppressor activity (see Figure 2 below) after three and twelve months of radioisotope therapy. The increase of NK cell means better results of therapies against of cancer.

Under normal conditions, FoxP3[+] Tregs are essential suppressors of antitumor responses and maintain immunological tolerance to host tissues.[1] High infiltration of FoxP3[+] Tregs is expected to be associated with an unfavorable outcome. Thus, FoxP3[+] Tregs are investigated as potential prognostic factors and they may also represent novel therapeutic targets.[2] This is the first study that revealed decrease of suppressor cells FoxP3[+] after therapy with AHCC. According to Katz et al (See Figure 3 below) the presence of high amount of Tregs correlate with shorter Overall Survival (OS) after treatment of NETs[3]. Our initial result suggests that AHCC may improve OS in NETs patients. Further studies are needed to confirm these results in other patients.

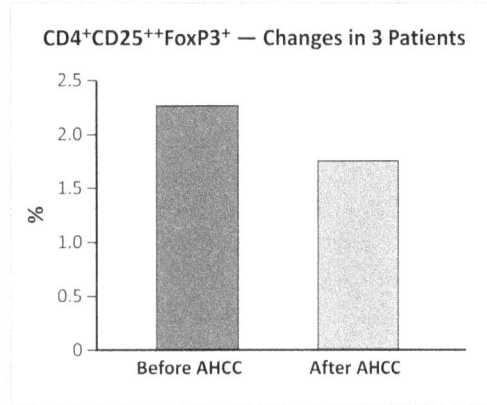

Figure 2. Decrease of CD4[+]CD25[++]FoxP3[+]

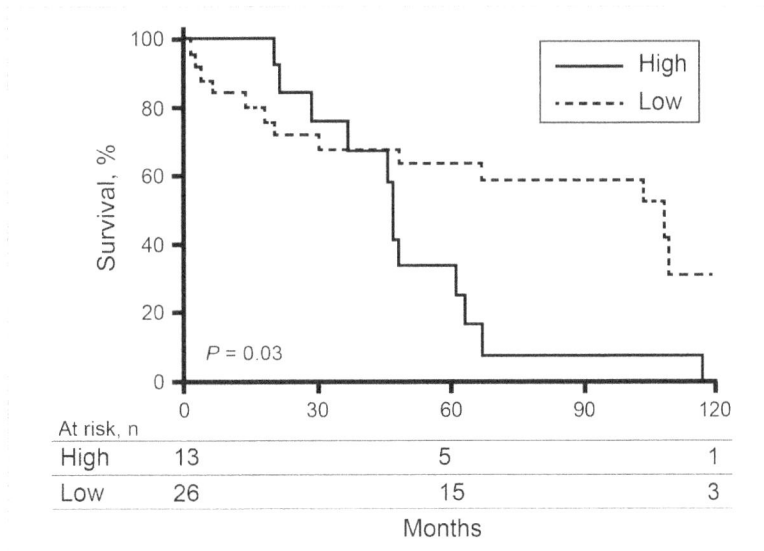

Figure 3. OS Differences between Treg levels (high/low) in NETs patients
Note: This figure is reproduced from Katz et al., 2010.

CASE B REFERENCES

1. Sakaguchi S, Yamaguchi T, Nomura T, and Ono M. "Regulatory T cells and immune tolerance." *Cell* 133 (5): 775–787, 2008

2. Shang B, Liu Y, Jiang S-J, and Liu Y. "Prognostic value of tumor-infiltrating FoxP3+ regulatory T cell in cancers: a systematic review and meta-analysis" *Scientific Reports* 5, 2015

3. Katz SC, Donkor C, Glasgow K, Pillarisetty VG, Gönen M, Espat NJ, Klimstra DS, D'Angelica MI, Allen PJ, Jarnagin W, DeMatteo RP, Brennan MF, and Tang LH. "T Cell Infiltrate and Outcome Following Resection of Intermediate-Grade Primary Neuroendocrine Tumours and Liver Metastases." *HPB?: The Official Journal of the International Hepato Pancreato Biliary Association* 12 (10): 674–683, 2010

Case C: Left Atrial and Ventricular Spindle Cell Sarcoma Treated with AHCC, Selol, and Chemotherapy

Primary cardiac neoplasms are rare with an incidence varying between 0.001 and 0.28%.[1] Among primary cardiac tumors, approximately 75% are benign. The remaining 25% of cardiac neoplasms are malignant; sarcomas are the most common, accounting for half to three quarters of the cases.[2] Cardiac spindle cell sarcomas are classified as undifferentiated sarcomas. They typically involve the left atrium and may extend to the pericardium, resulting in a hemopericardium.

Cardiac sarcomas have poor prognosis with a mean survival of less than one year. In rare cases, prolonged survival has been documented. Surgical debulking is the mainstay of the treatment. It serves as palliative treatment to relieve symptoms, and the role of heart transplantation for malignant cardiac tumors is controversial.[1] Neo-adjuvant chemotherapy to reduce the tumor mass and facilitate surgical excision can be tried, and adjuvant chemotherapy (with regimens combining several agents, usually including doxorubicin) or radiation therapy may play a role in some cases.

An original discovery of Polish researchers, Selol has no equivalents in treatment. The clear demand for new compounds of selenium of lower toxicity than that of sodium selenite (IV) resulted in preparing a synthesis of selenitetriglycerides from chemically modified sunflower oil. Selol is a mixture of selenitetriglycerides obtained by incorporating selenic acid (IV) into molecules of fatty acids from plant oil. After

Selol therapy, the DNA degradation was mostly present in HL-60/Dox cells, which were most extensively affected by Selol. This can be caused by nucleases present in lysosomes, since the complete dispersion of lysosomal content was observed in these cells. The degradation of DNA was probably not the effect of caspase activity, since we have not detected caspase activation.[3]

A 44-year-old female, presented in May 2013 with symptoms of heaviness in the chest on exertion and dyspnea on exertion NYHA grade III. 2D Echocardiography and MRI showed a large mass on the lateral wall and the left atrium (diameter approx. 55 mm). Due to clinical status, she was excluded from operation. From August 2013 to November 2013, she was treated three times with ADIC (Adriamycin: 1,335 mg, dacarbazine: 335 mg) scheme chemotherapy. The control MRI (see Figure 1 below) showed progression of disease, and therapy with chemotherapy was stopped until February 2014.

From the beginning of the third chemotherapy, she began taking AHCC 3 g/day. After two weeks, her quality of life significantly improved. Then she started to intake Selol. The control MRI in January showed regression of the disease (see Figure 2 below). In February 2014, the doctors started a next-step chemotherapy in addition to Selol and AHCC. In April 2014, the next control in MRI revealed a stabilization of the disease (see Figure below 3). After the next chemotherapy, she decided to stay with the therapy AHCC and Selol. The patient died in April 2015.

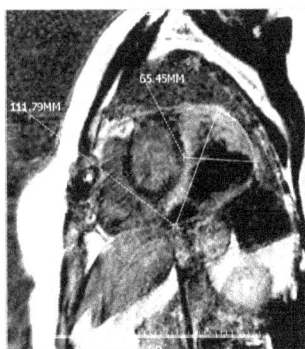

Figure 1. MRI (November 2013) showed progression after ADIC chemotherapy.

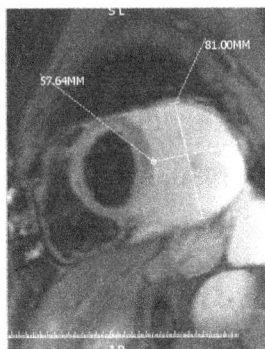

Figure 2. MRI (January 2014) revealed shrinkage of the tumor after AHCC and Selol treatment.

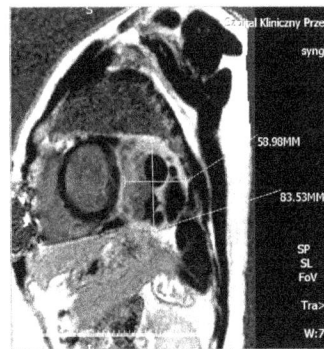

Figure. 3. MRI (April 2014) showed stabilization after 6 months therapy.

CASE C REFERENCES

1. Chahinian AP, Gutstein DE, and Fuster V. "Chapter 95. Tumors of the Heart and Great Vessels." *Holland-Frei Cancer Medicine.* Ed. Donald W Kufe, Raphael E Pollock, Ralph R Weichselbaum, et al. 6th ed. Hamilton: BC Decker, 2003.

2. McManus B and Lee C-H. "Chapter 69. Primary Tumors of the Heart." *Braunwald's Heart Disease.* Ed. Peter Libby, Robert O Bonow, Douglas L Mann, et al. 8th ed. Philadelphia: Saunders, 2008. 1815-1828. Print.

3. Suchocki P. et al: "The activity of selol in multidrug-resistant and sensitive human leukemia cells." *Oncology Reports* 18: 893–899, 2007.

Case D: Anti-inflammatory Action of AHCC in Mild and Moderate Asthma Patients Based on Exhaled Nitric Oxide (eNO)

Asthma is a chronic inflammatory airway disease. According to Schott, incidences of asthma in Europe amounts to approximately 30 million people.[2] In Poland (in a study between 2006 and 2008), Samolin'ski et al. showed that 30 to 40% of the population suffers from periodic or chronic symptoms of allergic diseases. Symptoms of asthma found an average of 13.6% in the study population. This includes 19.3% of children aged 6–7 years, 10% of children aged 13–14 years of age, and 12.4% of adults aged 20–44 years.[3] Epidemiological studies in Europe showed that only 5.1% of patients achieved good control of asthma.[1]

Exhaled nitric oxide (eNO) is produced by the human lung and is present in the exhaled breath. It has been implicated in the pathophysiology of lung diseases, including asthma. The measurement of eNO has been standardized for clinical use in asthma patients. eNO testing is a quick and easy way to measure inflammation (swelling) in the bronchial tubes of the lungs.

We evaluated five patients with clinically confirmed asthma, who were included in the study. The measurement of eNO was taken before and after taking 1 g of AHCC daily (500 mg x 2 times), 40 minutes before every meal. The median time of the observation was 8.4 weeks. Before the study, median value of the eNO in patients was 38.4 ppb (parts per billion). The normal range in healthy subjects is between 20 and 30 ppb. After study, the median of level of the eNO decreased from 38.4 ppb to 19.8 ppb. We showed that AHCC can decrease the amount of eNO in mild and moderate asthma patients.

AHCC is a promising extract, which decreases the amount of eNO in mild and moderate asthma patients, and can be considered as an alternative to traditional steroid treatments for this disease. This effect may be explained by its anti-inflammatory character which is described in the Chapter 7.

Case D References

1. Schott M and Seissler J. "Dendritic cell vaccination: new hope for the treatment of metastasized endocrine malignancies." *Trends Endocrinol. Metab.* 14: 156–62, 2003.

2. European Allergy White Paper, The UCB Institute of Allergy: Allergic diseases as a public health issue in Europe. UCB Institute of Allergy, 1997.

3. Samolin'ski B, Sybilski AJ, Raciborski F, et al. "Prevalence of asthma in children, adolescents and young adults in Poland—Results of the ECAP study." *Alergia Astma Immunologia,* 14(1): 27–34, 2009.

Case Report #3

Edwin A. Bien

CLINICAL SIGNIFICANCE OF AHCC
IN CASES OF ADVANCED STAGE CANCER

The recognized clinical management in the Philippines presently for malignancies is 1) surgery, 2) chemotherapy, and 3) radiation therapy. Admittedly there is an increase in incidence of cancers in the Philippines—whether due to early detection or a change to more Westernized habits among Filipinos. There is a debatable improvement in life span but also a noticeable shift in morbidity from infectious diseases to lifestyle diseases. For the majority of patients and relatives concerned, the decision to choose a treatment protocol lies not only on what is medically accepted but also in their capacity to pay for adequate healthcare.

Even with the most sophisticated instrumentation, surgery of cancer still poses a risk of transporting microscopic malignant cells to other organs via the vascular or lymphatic system. Radiotherapy machines have advanced to being pinpoint sensitive, but they may still damage some surrounding non-affected tissues. Lastly, even with recent advances in cancer-specific chemotherapy drugs, there have been many anticancer medications being recalled after years of use for toxicity to the heart and other functioning organs.

These treatments, though evidenced based, have drawbacks and limitations that must be recognized and discussed. This is where *immunotherapy* counts. Quality-of-life enhancement is just as important to the patient as is the cure. Citing *The European Charter of Patients' Rights* (Rome, November 2002), Article 5 *"Each individual has the right to freely choose from among different treatment procedures and providers on the basis of adequate information."* Personally I believe the basic human right is to receive the best medical service under the suggestion and assistance of medical practitioners and respect one's wish or choice in order to recover, maintain and improve health. For those who have accepted their advanced-stage cancer, finding an improvement in many of the symptoms with the use of AHCC is a big factor—both for the patient and the physician.

Case A: Rectal Carcinoma

Emily N., a 54-year-old businesswoman traveled to Manila all the way from Sultan Kudarat, a remote island in Southern Mindanao, which involved a boat ride and a three-hour flight. A relative from Singapore had referred her, and Emily visited our clinic in May 2014 (see Figure 1 at right).

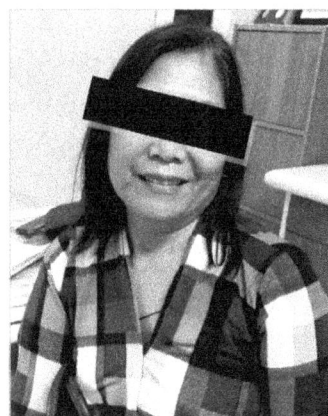

Figure 1. Obstructing rectal carcinoma with post-radiation proctitis and ileitis.

In early 2013, she had noticed increasing weight loss and suffered from general weakness. A chest x-ray revealed that she had pneumonia and minimal pulmonary tuberculosis (PTB). Antibiotics were given to her, but her weight loss continued despite six months of treatment. Thyroid hormone tests revealed normal values. A CT scan of the abdomen done in July 2013 showed that she has hepatic cysts on segment 4 and a mid-lying 8-cm rectal carcinoma blocking the lumen. After colonoscopy was done to confirm the tumor, she underwent twenty-eight fractions of external beam radiation therapy using an Elekta Synergy Platform machine. Even after completing her therapy cycles, she had unrelenting symptoms of abdominal pains and bloating with passage of blood when she moved her bowels. A repeat CT scan of the abdomen done in January 2014 revealed that she had post-radiation proctitis and ileitis. This prompted her to seek advice

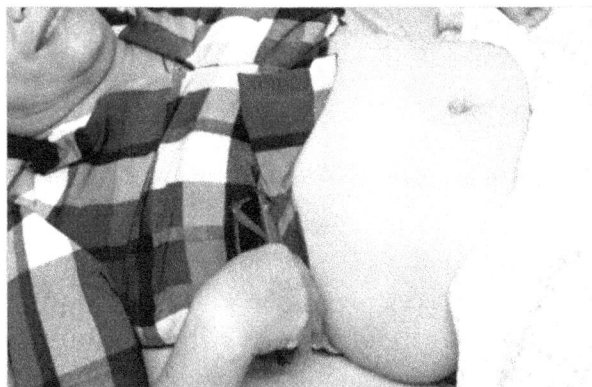

Figure 2. Inflammatory reactions, severe abdominal pains, and melena reduced with use of AHCC.

from a nutritionist, which led to her visiting our clinic in May 2014 (see Figure 2 on the previous page).

After further examinations, we administered intravenous and parenteral medications. She was also started on 3 g/day of AHCC with other immunotherapy programs. Blood chemistry was monitored, including liver function tests (elevated ALT/SGPT of 79 u/L compared to normal of 14 – 54 u/L) and CEA (elevated at 4.1 ng/mL against a normal of <3.4 ng/mL). With continued use of AHCC daily, her liver enzymes and tumor markers went down from June to November 2014. She continued taking AHCC at 3 g/ day until the present time. Her symptoms of pains, bloating, myalgia, loss of appetite, and melena also subsided. In February 2016, she showed a marked improvement in her pallor, negative for ascites, no tenderness in the abdomen, and notable weight gain.

Case B: Lymph Node Malignancy

Ofel M., a 58-year-old female from Quezon City, was referred by a friend who co-owns one of the prestigious hospitals in the metropolis. Both Ofel and her friend believed that the series of antibiotics issued to her by her doctors might not be enough to treat her problem, which had no specific diagnosis to date.

Her condition started in August 2015 with stiffness and masses in the neck, which were increasing in size. She was referred to a laboratory for Sputum AFB test to check for possible tuberculosis. Three repeated tests were done, and the final report in September 2015 revealed negative for acid-fast bacilli. She was then referred for a CT scan of the neck and the mass measuring 6.4 × 6.4 × 10.4 cm on the right lateral side extending from the submandibular to subclavicular region, with no calcification, was diagnosed as malignant primary neoplasm. She was scheduled for surgery.

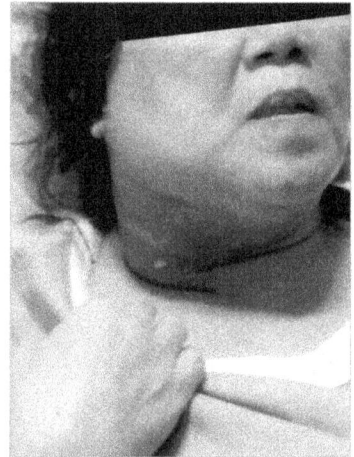

Figure 3. Antibiotic-resistant purulent submandibular and supraclavicular mass.

The painful and continuously enlarging mass was exuding a yellowish-white puerile discharge. She was then referred for immediate incision and drainage prior to further evaluation and management. (See Figure 4 on the facing page.)

Ofel came to our clinic in October 2015 in severe distress. Examination revealed positive rales on her lungs and elevated blood sugar. She was initially given intravenous medications with antibiotics and hyperglycemic agents. AHCC was started at 3 g/day with other medications. She is on continuous follow-ups monthly at our clinic and with her other physicians. With the help of AHCC taken daily in varying doses depending on the patient's condition, we can see a marked improvement in her lateral neck mass with resulting drying of the lesion. She is presently energetic and without pain. The mass has subsided in size with minimal evidence of inflammation. We are currently working on the darkened area of her neck and managing her other metabolic problems.

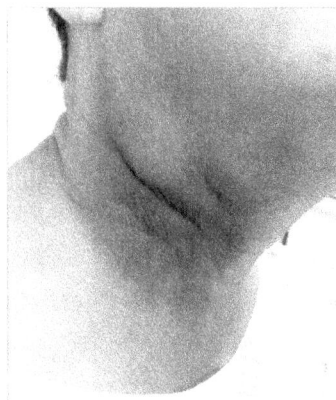

Figure 4. Post surgical neck mass discharge resolved with concomitant use of AHCC.

Case C: Pancreatic Cancer

Rosita B., a 59-year-old office worker, was given devastating news at work, which many of her coworkers believed was a death warrant. In fact, when Rosita absented herself from work for several weeks, one of her coworkers began cleaning up her office space, believing Rosita would not return to work.

After a battery of tests, Rosita had been issued a medical certificate by RPG Medical Center with a final diagnosis of pancreatic (head) cancer stage IV with pleural effusion of the left lung. She was given only a few months to live. Upon much prodding by former patients who have visited our facilities, Rosita reluctantly agreed to come to our clinic in January 2012. Accompanied by several family members, including a daughter who works abroad but came home to give her mother moral support, Rosita endured an eight-hour ride to our facility. Having no desire or strength to undergo further therapeutic modalities, she and her family agreed on nutrition and immunotherapy to support her remaining days. She was easily fatigued and frequently caught her breath as she tried to answer our history-taking questions. Upon examination, it was evident that she was markedly jaundiced with an enlarged abdomen filled with fluid (see Figure 5 at right).

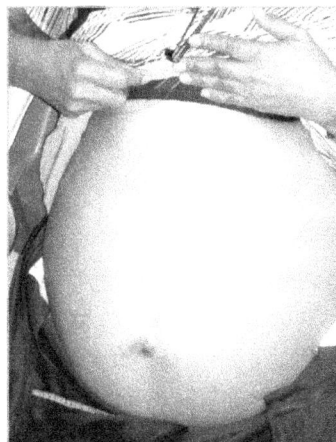

Figure 5. Pleural effusion, hepatomegaly, and pancreatic cancer stage IVA, resulting in dyspnea and cachexia.

Several 2–4 cm masses could be palpated in her abdomen, including an enlarged liver. She was initially given medications to relieve edema and parenteral treatments for her hypoalbuminemia. She was in moderate pain (grade of 5–6) so analgesics were prescribed. To help relieve abdominal fullness and discomfort, dietary restrictions were advised.

Together with other complementary medicines, Rosita was advised to integrate oral intake of AHCC in varying mega dosages. She was to continue this until her monthly trips back to Manila for follow-ups. Her blood chemistry was regularly monitored, particularly the enzyme levels. A 2D echo done in February 2013 showed left ventricular hypertrophy and aortic and mitral stenosis. Her condition gradually improved with the laboratory values subsiding. She resumed work early in 2014 to the surprise of her coworkers. She even regained control of her office desk. Because of her positive response with the treatments and increasing energy with AHCC, we allowed her to travel to Canada last April 2015 to visit her daughter and grandchildren. Her abdomen had markedly shrunken in size, and the

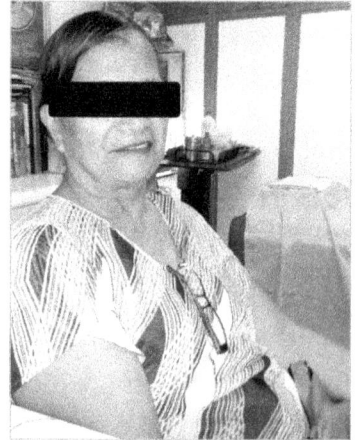

Figure 6. Palliative treatments and immunotherapy with AHCC extends life and relieves symptoms.

jaundice is resolved; she is presently asymptomatic (see Figure 6 above). Although she continues intravenous medications, her AHCC intake is now down to maintenance level of 3 g/day. Her last follow-up in our clinic was in January 2016.

Case D: Metastatic Bone Cancer

Victor M., a 63-year-old male, in severe pain, was brought to one of our branch clinics in Metro Manila in October 2013, by his wife, Ines, after she heard of our services through some members of the Camillian Sisters (of Italy). (See Figure 7, facing page.)

Victor had had an orchiectomy for stage IV testicular cancer compounded by uncontrolled elevated blood sugar level and hypertension. He had already been diabetic and hypertensive many years prior to the discovery of the cancer. He underwent radiation after the surgery and was on hormonal therapy, which made his breasts engorged and painful. His complaints included a burning sensation in both lower legs and an inability to sit for a long time due to a great discomfort caused by a pinched nerve in the lower back. We reviewed and adjusted his medications for blood sugar and blood pressure. We continued his tramadol and paracetamol, as the couple did not want to use opiates. To assist his treatments, we added AHCC at 3 g/day among other medications. We also initiated a form of magnetic and moist heat therapy for his legs and back.

Three-month intake of these medications was continued, and he came back for a checkup with me smiling. He was able to resume one of his favorite hobbies, which was driving. The burning sensation in his legs and severe back pains were greatly reduced. Although he was on strict low-calorie diet, he had a great appetite. He was also able to sleep better at night. Despite our instructions to visit our clinic monthly, he did not return. Subsequently, we heard from his wife that Victor had suffered a heart attack due to uncontrolled elevated blood pressure and passed away. During this call, she expressed her gratitude to us for improving her husband's quality of life, despite his terminal cancer with bone metastases.

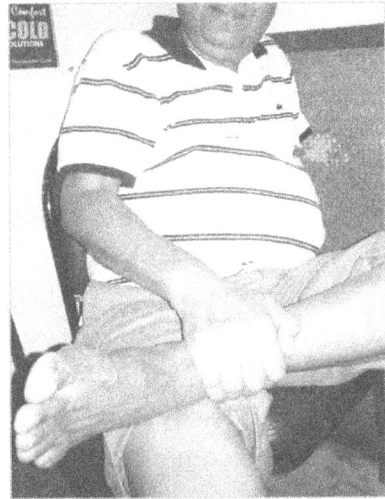

Figure 7. Known diabetic with post orchiectomy and osteoblastic metastatic bone disease provided QOL with AHCC.

Case E: Adenoid Carcinoma

Christopher B., a 39-year-old overseas worker, was experiencing a non-healing cough accompanied by bleeding in the nose and mouth. He had stopped smoking about five years earlier, and was surprised by his symptoms. He returned to his home country to have himself checked and treated.

He was diagnosed with adenoid carcinoma and underwent his first operation in July 2009. A permanent tube was placed in his nostrils extending to his throat to continuously drain exudates. His epistaxis did not abate so he underwent a second operation in February 2012, followed by twenty-eight cycles of radiation starting in May 2012.

Christopher came to our clinic in July 2012 with

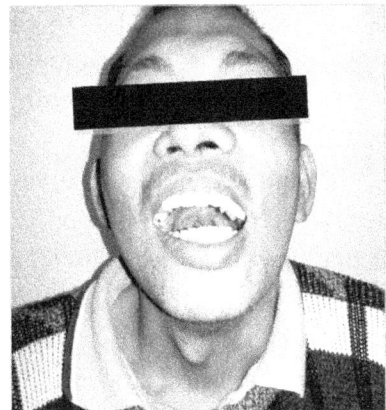

Figure 8. Adenoid cystic CA s/p tumor debulking, lateral rhinotomy, epistaxis and dysphagia resolved with use of AHCC.

241

the tube still attached to his nose (see Figure 8 on the previous page). Blood with mucoid discharge could be observed in the tube. It was also painful to the touch. Upon inspection, his upper palate had been removed, and this is where blood was coming from. He could not eat well due to difficulty swallowing, and he spoke in a nasal tone. He agreed to regularly and consistently take AHCC. We found a sponsor through AHCC Nutrients in the Philippines to provide him the monthly supply of AHCC.

Christopher took AHCC for almost six months. We noticed an improvement in his color from pale to pinkish every time when he visited to collect his supply. He was more animated and talkative, informing our nurses that he was able to eat better. By December 2012, we were able to remove his nasal tube successfully to his great relief. The epistaxis was also resolved. By August 2013, he has already gained 8 pounds and continued to be grateful to those who helped him.

Case F: Nasopharyngeal Cancer

In December 2013, I received a call from a long-lost cousin. His father-in-law had been recently diagnosed with nasopharyngeal carcinoma and had multiple enlarged lymph nodes in his neck (see Figure 9 at right). He had totally lost his voice and communicated only by writing on a slate board. Lamberto C., a 71-year-old, had been a chronic smoker for more than forty years at almost a pack per day. He had the nodes checked and was advised of his terminal case. With his consciousness and blood pressure going down, the family feared for his life.

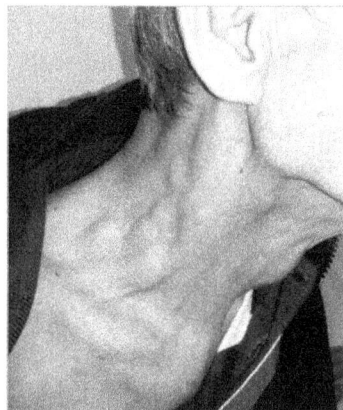

Figure 9. Nasopharyngeal carcinoma with unilateral lymph node metastasis, supraclavicular fossa.

At our clinic, we observed that Lamberto was frail for his height, weighing only 130 pounds. His repeated blood pressure was at 90/60 and falling. An immediate intravenous fluid was inserted due to dehydration signs and medication for the hypotension was given. His relatives reported that his doctors advised that only supportive care should be given for his vocal cord paralysis due to his advancing age, so no aggressive treatment modality was offered.

We placed him on nasogastric feeding with high-protein intake regimen. An initial weekly follow-up was initiated with the administration of intravenous immune stimulants. AHCC capsules were mashed and mixed with food round the clock until oral intake was tolerated. With the nutritional support and immunotherapy, his color and demeanor improved. We still communicated mostly through writing, but his voice, although raspy, returned. We suspected that the inflammation in his vocal cord had decreased, which allowed him to talk in short sentences. We continued seeing him in our clinic for almost six months, during which he was smiling and seemed comfortable. He was able to swallow soft foods, and the regular intake of blended fruit with vegetable juices with AHCC did wonders for him until his last breath. We went to his wake and were warmly thanked by his surviving family for the quality of life he received as a result of the treatment.

Case G: Breast Cancer

Feliza S., a 73-year-old female, could not believe that a simple solid nodule detected by ultrasound done in June 2011 on her right breast would suddenly grow to the size of a small orange within a couple of months (see Figure 10 below). She did not seek further consultation and treatment, hoping the nodule would disappear if she ignored it.

She was brought to our clinic in November 2012 by a Christian pastor to help with her finances. She was asymptomatic except for the discomfort of her breast mass rubbing against her clothing and slight stiffness of the involved shoulder. Physical examination showed a 2.5 x 2.5 cm non-tender, non-movable, hard mass above the areola. The skin was normal with no evidence of lymph nodes. The nipple also exhibited no discharge upon pressing. She refused any form of prescription, insisting that she preferred to shift to a vegan, half-cooked greens and fruit diet, and a lot of prayers. We respected her decision but made her promise to come back if she discovered any untoward

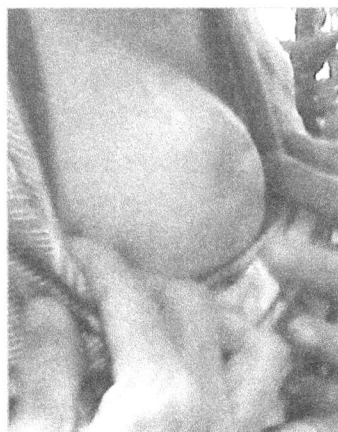

Figure 10. Solid nodule, right breast, with irregular and lobulated border (Birads 4C).

changes. She came back just before the end of December 2012 when she noted that the nodule had grown to the size of a man's fist. This time, there was already a change in the skin texture from previously smooth to orange peel appearance surrounded by redness. The veins were also engorged and were causing tenderness (see Figure 11 on the following page). We suggested a fine needle biopsy for the purpose of determining appropriate treatment, such as possible neo-adjuvant chemotherapy and modified radical mastectomy, all of which she declined, citing personal spiritual beliefs.

Respecting the patient's right of choice regarding her healthcare, we compromised on her taking AHCC at 3 g/day. We also advised her to take an anti-estrogen tablet because we suspected an estrogen receptor positive tumor. To date, she continues taking AHCC. Her last consultation in December 2015 showed a marked decrease in the size of the tumor and an improvement in the surrounding tissues. We saw her last in February 2016; she was still in high spirits with a gift of green leafy vegetables in a basket for our staff and nurses. She even shared her prayer leaflets with the other waiting patients.

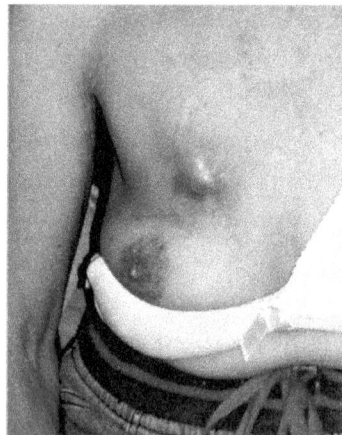

Figure 11. Tumor size reduction (T1N0M0) with use of AHCC.

Case H: Liver Cancer

Segundino D. was a retired 2nd lieutenant with the Armed Forces. He had been fond of drinking alcohol with his military buddies. They had been frequently sent out on dangerous missions in the southern part of the country where there was an ongoing armed conflict with the rebels; they often resorted to drinking to calm their nerves. This went on for many years. Cancer runs in Segundino's family. His younger sister had recently died of colorectal cancer after going to Dubai for a form of stem cell therapy at a non-medical facility. Segundino was devastated by the news.

Upon retirement, Segundino had reported the passage of blood in his stools. He was also losing a lot of weight, weighing 30% less than his original body weight (see Figure 12 at right). He thought he might have the same cancer as his sister, so he agreed to get an abdominal CT scan. In the back of his mind, however, he suspected his case was more severe than his sister's. The results of the CT scan revealed a right hepatic lobe

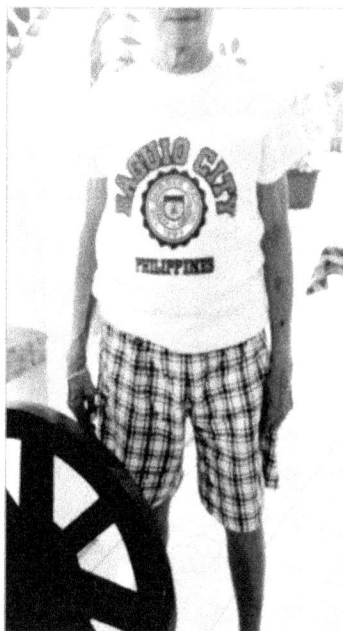

Figure 12. Severe weight loss associated with right hepatic lobe mass, possibly neoplastic. Appetite and weight regained with continuous use of AHCC.

mass, neoplastic process being considered. He decided not to undergo the conventional treatments of surgery, chemotherapy, and radiotherapy, remembering the fate of his sister Bernal.

The whole family came to our clinic in August 2013 with results on hand. Upon examination Segundino's blood pressure was elevated at 180/90 and presented with abdominal ascites. We discussed medical treatments to help his condition. He readily agreed to take, along with other medications, a gradually increasing dose of AHCC from 3 – 6 g/day. Over the course of continuous follow-ups and adjustment of necessary medicines, his symptoms slowly disappeared and his condition markedly improved in less than a year. His last ultrasound in October 2015 still showed the same liver pathology, but he was fully asymptomatic. His last picture taken in January 2016 shows him looking healthy, doing his normal activities of daily living and back to his former self.

Conclusion

In general, quality of life (QOL) is the perceived quality of an individual's daily life taking into consideration the assessment of their well-being or lack thereof. This includes all emotional, social, and physical aspects of the person's life. In healthcare, health-related QOL is an assessment of how their well-being may be affected over time by disease, disability, or the treatments employed for the disorder. Several ways of measuring QOL have been proposed and written. Early simple assessment of physical abilities includes ability of the patient to get up, eat, drink, and take care of personal hygiene without outside help. QOL is now usually assessed using questionnaires both for the patient and family members. The Functional Living Index-Cancer is one designed for easy, repeated patient self-administration. It is likewise important to measure a patient's response to other significant functional factors, such as depression and anxiety, sociability, and family interaction.

I conclude that AHCC has been of great benefit to many of my patients to achieve not only QOL but assist whatever form of treatment that is decided upon. Not only are side effects reduced, but efficacy of therapies is also improved. We are grateful that AHCC is now available for physicians to consider in complementing and integrating with our medical practice.

Case Report #4

Massimo Bonucci

The study of cell neoplastic transformation is based on the identification of the enzyme processes induced by gene modifications that occur throughout human life. Many neoplastic conditions result from originally abnormal genetic patterns (e.g., children neuronal and endocrine tumors, Ewing's sarcoma, etc.), but many others are related to gene changes that take place in older age due to extra-genetic causes: this phenomenon is known as *epigenetics.*

The environment we live in can be the agent of a wide range of gene modifications that in turn may induce the production of so-called carcinogenic substances; they can modify, activate, or inhibit onco-suppressor genes, thus initiating and promoting the neoplastic transformation.

By understanding what happens inside the modified cells, we will be able to learn which molecules are able to reset the system or prevent cell changes, making it possible to design truly preventative measures. In the meantime, we can thoroughly explore the role of the immune system and understand how it is able to fight against tumors.

The human immune system is formed very early in life and consists of two well distinct portions. One is "innate" and operates to protect us from external attacks (due to bacteria, viruses, protozoa, fungi, etc.) by producing immunoglobulins; the other is "adaptive" and is designed to defend us against fiercer threats posed by infected cells and abnormal or neoplastic cells with all their load of cytotoxic lymphocytes and cytokines. Through the stimulation of the innate and adaptive immune system, the body's immune response can be modulated. In the case of cancer, the immune system comes at a standstill and is often affected by either a quantitative (drop in the number of lymphocytes) or qualitative (cytotoxic and NK cells become less active) deficit.

What we need to understand is how our immune system can be brought back to proper functioning. There are many ways to stimulate both immune growth and activation so that the immune system can be better able to tolerate and support antiblastic cancer treatments. The combined use of chemotherapy, radiotherapy, biologic drugs, and natural substances is known as *integrated oncology* and appears to be a promising new approach to deal with cancer-related diseases.[5]

The recent international literature tells us that the use of antiblastic agents, target-specific biologic drugs, and radiotherapy has reached a peak, leading to an improvement in survival but badly affecting the patients' quality of life that too often becomes extremely poor. As we all know, a final remedy to cancer is not yet available. This is why research is now being focused on integrated care in order to improve the quality and extend the duration of survival.

Modern science is paying renewed attention to traditional medicines, and time-old remedies are being explored under a different focus. New laboratory technologies make it possible to identify the active principles of natural remedies and to include them in clinical protocols to be scientifically validated. This is how the interesting properties of the shitake mushroom have been discovered and its active ingredients identified, leading to the isolation of AHCC. AHCC has a wide range of beneficial and specific actions, including antiviral, anticancer, antidiabetic, and immune-stimulating (see Table 1 below), besides its restorative and reinvigorating properties, which convinced us to include it in our integrated cancer-care schemes.[2]

TABLE 1. **A WIDE RANGE OF BENEFICIAL AND SPECIFIC ACTIONS OF AHCC**

Anti-Diabetes

- reduce blood sugar levels
- reduce A1C
- prevents complications

Anti-Hepatitis

- Decrease amount of virus
- Decrease AST and ALT
- Induce enzymes for detoxification and metabolism
- Inhibits decrease in platelet level

Antitumor Effects

- Increased lymphocytes and leucocytes, NK
- Production of cytokines (IL 12, TNF-alpha, IFN)
- Downregulate tumor markers
- Stimulate dendritic cells (1 and 2)

Improvement in Quality of Life

- Prevent side effects of anticancer drugs
- Increase weight
- Calm nervousness

AHCC has been used in oncology in cases of hepatocellular carcinoma with very satisfactory results.[1] We know that this molecule has no negative interaction with the antiblastic agents because its pharmacokinetics, pharmacodynamics, and liver metabolism are well studied (see Table 2 below) and has also been used for its immune-modulatory action.

TABLE 2. **AHCC AND LIVER METABOLISM PATHWAYS STUDIED**

AHCC Is Not an Inhibitor		AHCC Is Not an Inducer	
AHCC Is Not an Inhibitor	• GST Pathway	AHCC Is Not an Inducer	• COMT Pathway
	• UGT Pathway		
	• UGT1A3	AHCC Is an Inhibitor	• QOR Pathway
	• UGT2B17	AHCC Is a Potential Inducer	• UGT 1A3 Pathway
	• UGT1A6		• UGT 1A6 Pathway

It is because of this encouraging data that we decided to engage in an observational study. The preliminary trial involved forty-three cancer patients divided into two groups: group A with thirty-one operated subjects disease-free at the time of recruitment; group B with twelve subjects with metastatic disease. Patients in both groups received AHCC at doses of 3 and 6 g/day respectively. The study was carried out for a preliminary phase of three months and concluded after one year of treatment. Both groups were controlled with hematologic and instrumental tests such as CT scans and ultrasonography every three months. Interesting results were reported both in terms of immune response and clinical objective response. The twelve patients with metastatic disease showed an increase in CD4+ T helper cells

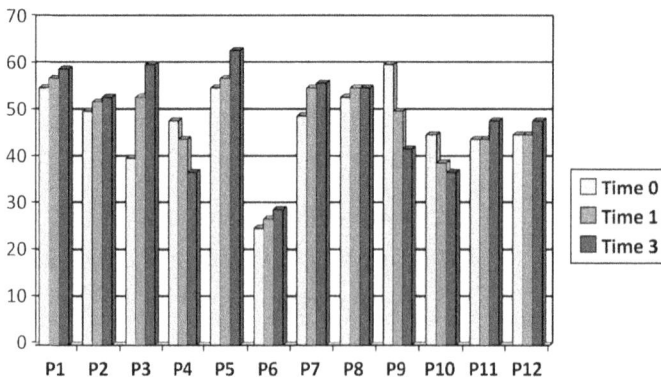

Figure 1.
CD4+ T helper cell (The unit of Y-axis is "cells/μl". The unit for Time 0, 1, 3 is "months.")

(see Figure 1 on the previous page) and a reduction of CD8$^+$ T suppressor cells (see Figure 2 below) with an overall increase of NK lymphocytes (see Figure 3 below), as well as a significant reduction of metastatic lesions.

Following this observational study, which enabled us to gain a deeper under-

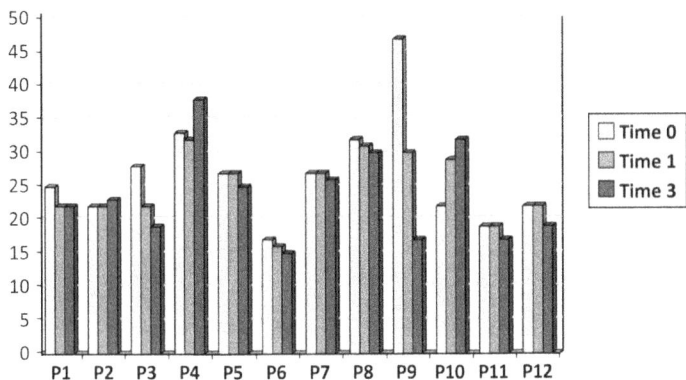

Figure 2.
CD8$^+$ T suppressor cell (The unit of Y-axis is "cells/µl". The unit for Time 0, 1, 3 is "months.")

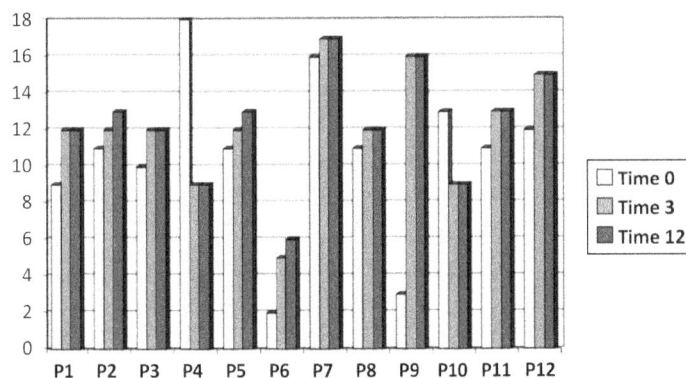

Figure 3.
CD16$^+$CD56$^+$ NK cell (The unit of Y-axis is "cells/µl". The unit for Time 0, 3, 12 is "months.")

standing of AHCC action in the human body, we began to use the product systematically in patients with neoplastic lesions and metastatic diffusion. Two of the cases are reported here: two female patients respectively of 54 and 55 years of age, who came to us in 2014 both with pancreatic cancer and liver metastases.

Case A: Pancreatic Cancer and Liver Metastases

The first case concerns the integrated treatment of a woman with cancer of the pancreas with metastatic involvement ab initio peripancreatic lymph nodes and liver parenchyma with numerous secondary lesions greater than 9.5 cm (see Figure 4 below). The patient underwent during each chemotherapy cycle (FOLFIRINOX: Fluorouracil + Irinotecan + Oxaliplatin with outline 1/8/21) plus capacitive deep hyperthermia treatments. The patient was monitored with blood counts and instrumental techniques. In combination with chemotherapy, the patient was treated with natural substances and AHCC as the mycotherapy, at the dose of 3 g/day, as studied and reported.[3] At the end of the fourth cycle, the patient conducted an audit CT scan that showed a net reduction of pancreatic injury and secondary liver lesion (see Figure 5 below). Side effects were almost absent in this period, with only a mild asthenia the day after the administration of chemotherapy. Alopecia disappeared in the third cycle. Throughout the period of anticancer treatment, the patient did not suffer from any problem. All blood counts remained stable, without the need for referral of the program of administration of the chemotherapeutic. At this point, it was decided to continue with chemotherapy for two cycles, removing a drug (oxaliplatin). The

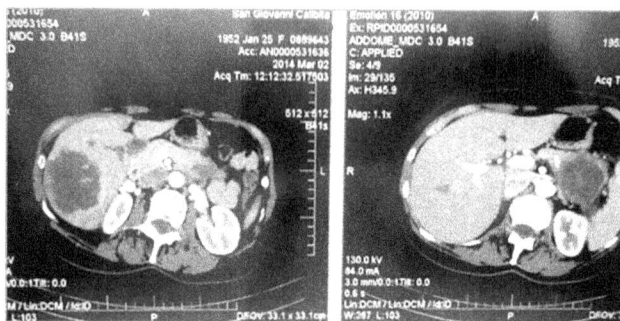

Figure 4. Case A: Cancer of the pancreas with metastatic involvement ab initio peripancreatic lymph nodes and liver parenchyma with numerous secondary lesions.

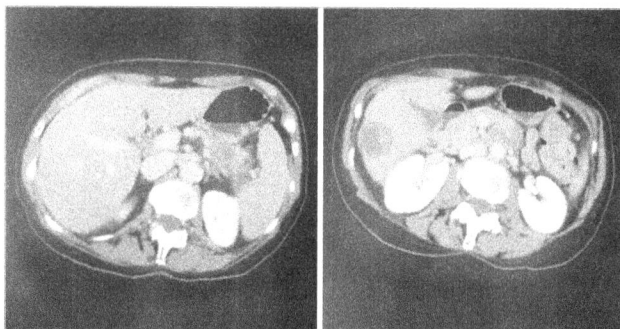

Figure 5. Case A: A net reduction of pancreatic injury and secondary liver lesion.

result was the disappearance of the nuanced liver (see Figure 6 on the facing page). In combination with chemotherapy, the patient was treated with natural substances and AHCC as the mycotherapy, at the dose of 3 g/day.

Case B: Pancreatic Cancer and Liver Metastases

The second case concerns the integrated treatment of a patient with cancer of the pancreatic body with metastatic involvement of the liver parenchyma with small lesion secondary. A 55-year-old female patient was operated on for pancreatic

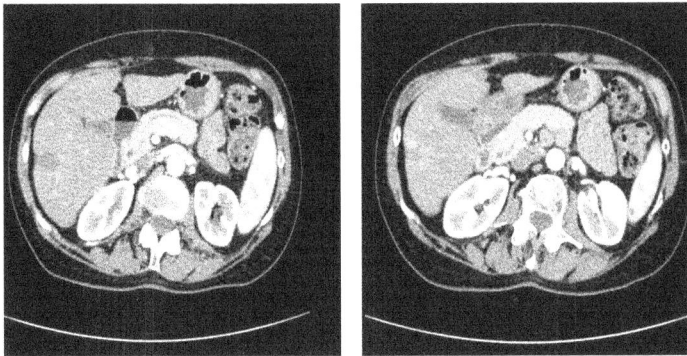

Figure 6.
Case A: The disappearance of the nuanced liver.

pseudo cyst in 2013. Following an abdominal ultrasound and a CT scan, patient was diagnosed with a lesion of the pancreatic body and liver metastases (see Figures 7 and 8 below). A biopsy of the lesion was performed with the pancreatic histology of "moderately differentiated adenocarcinoma, G2, the pancreatic parenchyma." Given the patient's young age and good patient compliance, patient was chosen for treatment (FOLFIRINOX: fluorouracil + irinotecan + oxaliplatin with outline 1/8/21) plus capacitive deep hyperthermia treatments. The patient started taking AHCC at a dose of 3 g/day, simultaneously with chemotherapy. The patient was monitored with blood counts and instrumental techniques. At the end of the third cycle,

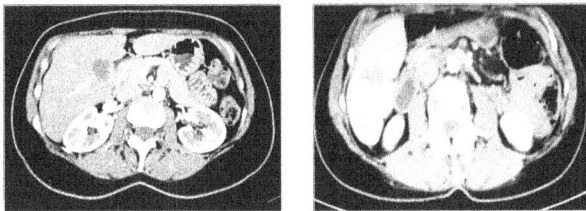

Figures 7 and 8. Case B: A lesion of the pancreatic body and liver metastases

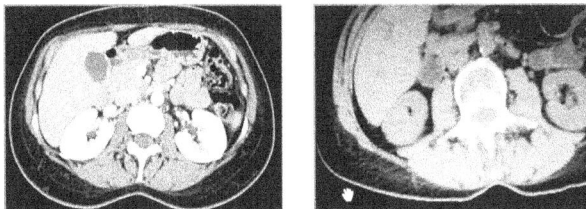

Figures 9 and 10. Case B: The almost disappearance of the pancreatic injury and of all the hepatic lesions.

a CT scan was carried out, which showed a clear reduction (60%) of pancreatic lesion. She continued both treatments. To the control of the sixth cycle, a new CT scan showed the almost disappearance of the pancreatic injury and of all the hepatic lesions (see Figures 9 and 10 below).

Thanks to the adoption of this integrated treatment, the quality of life of both subjects was very good (no nausea, no vomiting, mild asthenia, and negligible episodes of dyspepsia and diarrhea). So far, the patients are doing well and remain disease-free.

In both cases the primary pancreas lesion and liver metastases disappeared in less than one year. Our daily experience shows that we definitely need new and effective agents for the treatment of neoplastic lesions. AHCC is one of them, by virtue of its immunomodulatory and antineoplastic effects, but also of its ability to stimulate the bone marrow function during chemotherapy. Furthermore, AHCC can be used for primary prevention and to avoid the onset of recurrences. We are aware that more scientific evidence on AHCC efficacy is needed, and we are committed to produce new data to confirm the promising results obtained so far. Our short-term goal is to design new protocols to defeat cancer, and we believe that this will soon become possible by combining all the remedies currently known: chemotherapy, radiotherapy, biologic agents, phytotherapy, and nutrition.

Obviously the ideal situation would be helping people not to get sick in the first place. We all know that prevention is the best treatment, and this includes living in a healthy environment with appropriate nutrition and a correct supplementation of substances beneficial for our health: we believe that AHCC is an ideal solution to meet these requirements.

Integrative treatment: Viscum Album Fermentatum "Qu"- Polydatin- Curcumin- Lactoferrin- Astragalus- Ganoderma Lucidum- AHCC mushroom- Graviola
For vomiting, nausea, fatigue: Acupuncture; Ginger; Panax quinq.

REFERENCES

1. Matsui Y, et al. "Improved prognosis of postoperative hepatocellular carcinoma patients when treated with functional foods: a prospective cohort study." *J. Hepatol.* 37, 78–86, 2002.

2. Ahn GH and Han US. "Prospettive, randomized, clinical evaluation of QOL & immune index of AHCC in advanced metastatic cancer patients." AHCC Research Association 8th Symposium, Sapporo, Japan, 2000.

3. Iwamoto M, et al. "A study on dose-dependence of AHCC for cancer patients," The 2nd Annual Meeting of the Japanese Society of Alternative Medicine and Treatment, Oct. 1999.

4. Ishiguro A, et al. "Anti-carcinogenic activity of AHCC and PMP," The 2nd Annual Meeting of the Japanese Society of Alternative Medicine and Treatment, Oct. 1999.

5. Bonucci M. *Integrative Oncology: Scientific Research in support of patients: useful, possible, valid multi-targeted approach to treatment of cancer.* Springer International Publishing, 2015.

Chapter 11

HEPATITIS Treatment of Chronic Hepatitis B with AHCC Combination

Anuchit Chutaputti

Globally, around 240 million persons have chronic hepatitis B (CHB) with a varying prevalence geographically, highest in Africa and Asia. Despite the availability of effective vaccines for three decades and improvement of treatment, the prevalence of chronic hepatitis B viral (HBV) infection worldwide has declined minimally from 4.2% in 1990 to 3.7% in 2005.[1] Moreover, the actual number of persons who are chronically infected is estimated to have increased slightly from 223 million to 240 million during this same period. Treatment for this infection, while advancing to the stage that viral replication can be effectively suppressed and disease successfully controlled, is still far behind compared to hepatitis C virus (HCV) treatment.[2]

Natural History of Chronic Hepatitis B

The course of chronic HBV infection has been grouped into four phases: the immune tolerant phase, the immune active/hepatitis Be antigen (HBeAg) positive chronic hepatitis phase, the HBeAg-negative inactive phase, and the immune active/HBeAg-negative chronic hepatitis phase. However, these terms may not accurately reflect the immunological status of patients in each phase but are useful for prognosis and determining need for therapy.[3,4] (See Figure 1 on the following page). The duration of each phase varies from months to decades. Transition can occur from an earlier to a later phase, but regression back to an earlier phase can also occur.[5] It should be noted that not all patients go through all four phases.[6]

Resolved CHB infection is defined by clearance of hepatitis B surface antigen (HBsAg) with acquisition of antibody to HBsAg. Approximately 0.5% of persons with inactive CHB will clear HBsAg yearly; most will develop antibody to HBsAg (anti-HBs). Low levels of HBV DNA are transiently detected in the serum in the minority of persons achieving seroclearance.[7,8] Clearance of HBsAg, whether spontaneous or after antiviral therapy, reduces risk of hepatic decompensation, hepatocellular carcinoma (HCC) and improves survival. Risk of liver-related complications is variable. Among untreated adults with CHB, cumulative five-year incidence of cirrhosis is 8% to 20%, and among those with cirrhosis, five-year cumulative risk of hepatic decompensation is 20%, and risk of HCC is 2%–5%.[5,9,10] HBV DNA levels, ALT levels, and HBeAg status are among the most important determinants of risk of progression to cirrhosis,[11,12] whereas HBV DNA levels (>2,000 IU/mL), HBeAg status, and cirrhosis are key predictors of HCC risk.[11–14]

	Immune tolerant	Immune active	Immune control	Immune escape	Occult
HBeAg PEIU/mL	Positive 2000-5000	Positive 100-1000	Negative	Negative	Negative
Anti-HBe					
HBsAg Log IU/mL	4.5-5	4.0-4.5	2.9-3.0	3.3-3.9	Negative
Anti-HBs					
HBV DNA IU/mL	>>> 20,000	> 20,000	< 2,000	> 2,000	< 200
Viral diversity Precore/core					
Serum ALT U/L	Normal	Elevated, fluctuating	Normal	Elevated, fluctuating	Normal
Liver histology	Normal, mild	Moderate to severe CH	Normal to cirrhosis	Moderate to severe CH, cirrhosis	Normal to cirrhosis
Intra-hepatic cccDNA/cell	>> 1	0.1-10	0.001-1	0.1-10	<< 0.001

Modified from Dandri M & Locarnini. Gut 2012

Figure 1. Natural history of chronic hepatitis B

Immune Mechanisms of HBV Control and Implications for Therapy

The pathogenesis of chronic HBV infection involves not only viral mechanisms by which HBV establishes a persistent infection but also the host responses to infection. The latter includes the response of hepatocytes to HBV infection as well as the interplay of the virus and infected cells with the other parenchymal and nonparenchymal cells in the liver (i.e., Kupffer cells, endothelial cells, fibroblasts, and nonresident immune cells that are recruited to the site of infection). HBV has evolved mechanisms to counteract and escape these different host responses to establish a chronic infection. Recent studies point out a critical role of the liver microenvironment in the elimination or control of HBV.[15,16] While much has been learned about the HBV-specific adaptive immunity, the early and innate immune response during acute HBV infection remains largely unknown. In addition, few studies have examined intrahepatic immune responses in patients with chronic HBV infection. Available data suggest impaired responses, but the mechanism of this impairment is unclear.[16]

In CHB, the antiviral B- and T-cell responses are quantitatively and/or qualitatively defective. For example, anti-HBs is generally undetectable in the setting of excess circulating HBsAg. Furthermore, antiviral T cells show impaired antiviral effect function in vitro. However, this host immune response, despite being dysfunctional, exerts at least partial viral control in vivo because immune suppression with immunosuppressive therapies results in increased viremia.[17,18] HBV persistence with antiviral immune dysfunction is also associated with the induction of immune-inhibitory pathways, including PD-1, CTLA-4, Bim (BCL-2-interacting mediator of cell death), arginase, and FoxP3+ regulatory T cells.[19–24]

Based on our knowledge of the immune mechanisms of chronic HBV infection, several approaches to restore innate or adaptive immunity or both to control HBV infection in combination with other direct antiviral strategies have been applied. These approaches can be broadly divided into virus-nonspecific and virus-specific modalities. The first involves general immune modulatory agents, and the latter aims to activate the HBV-specific immune response by applying the technologies of therapeutic vaccination. As discussed above, the efficacy of IFN-α therapy can be partly attributed to its immune stimulatory effect. A promising approach emerges from the field of toll-like receptors (TLRs). Various TLR agonists with potent immune stimulatory effects have been developed.[25] Their administration to HBV patients leads to both intrahepatic and extrahepatic induction of type 1 interferons and other cytokines that may contribute directly to antiviral activity or indirectly result in activation of innate and adaptive immune responses.

The second approach involves the blockade of negative immune regulatory pathways (i.e., coinhibitory signals, inhibitory cytokines, regulatory T cells), which may induce a partial restoration of HBV-specific T cells. Third, engineering of redirected T cells may result in a *de novo* reconstitution of functionally active HBV-specific T cells and activation of heterologous T cells. Whether inhibition of a suppressive effect(s) of HBV can lead to restoration of HBV-specific innate and adaptive immune responses remains a challenging question. Several lines of evidence suggest that HBV interferes negatively with these host immune responses. A more detailed understanding of the specific mechanisms is mandatory before new ways of restoring immune responses by targeting virus-specific factors can be explored. HBV-specific strategies may prove more effective and safer than virus-nonspecific approaches. (See Figure 2 below.)

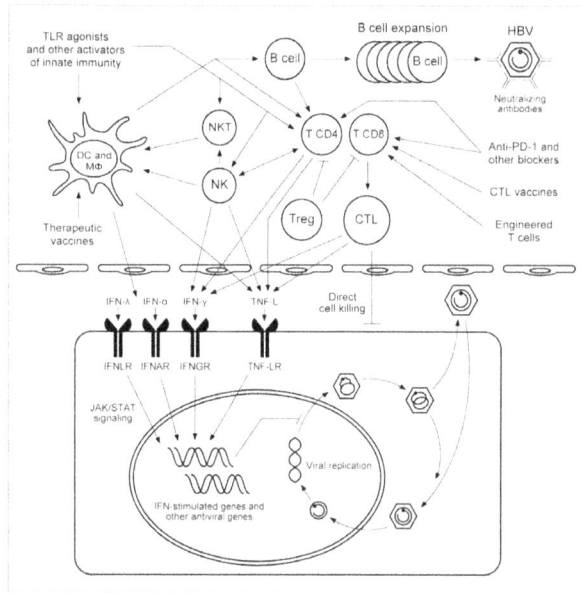

Figure 2. Innate and adaptive HBV-specific immune responses and immune-based therapeutic development. **Note:** This figure is reproduced from Liang et al., 2015.

The goals of antiviral treatment are to decrease the morbidity and mortality related to CHB. The achievement of a sustained suppression of HBV replication has been associated with normalization of serum ALT, loss of HBeAg with or without detection of (anti-HBe), and improvement in liver histology. Historically, the term *cure* was avoided in treatment of CHB, given that persistence of covalently closed circular DNA (cccDNA), the transcriptional template of HBV in the nucleus of hepatocytes, even in persons with serological markers of resolved infection, poses a lifelong risk for reactivation of infection (see Figure 3 on the facing page).[26,27]

The Efficacy of Current Chronic Hepatitis B Treatment

Currently, there are two different treatment strategies for both HBeAg-positive and HBeAg-negative CHB patients treatment of finite duration with pegylated interferon (PEG-IFN) or a nucleos(t)ide analog (NA) and long-term treatment with NA(s).

The main theoretical advantages of PEG-IFN are the absence of resistance and the potential for immune-mediated control of HBV infection with an opportunity to obtain a sustained virological response off-treatment and a chance of HBsAg loss in patients who achieve and maintain undetectable HBV DNA. Frequent side effects and subcutaneous injection are the main disadvantages of PEG-IFN treatment. PEG-IFN is contraindicated in patients with decompensated HBV-related cirrhosis or autoimmune disease, in patients with uncontrolled severe depression or psychosis, and in female patients during pregnancy. Entecavir and tenofovir are potent HBV inhibitors with a high barrier to resistance.[28–33]

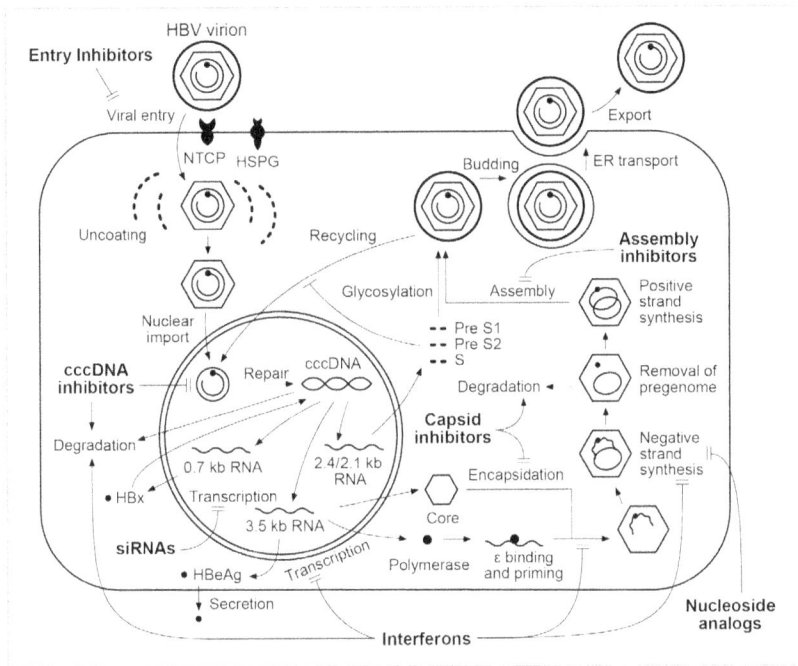

Figure 3. HBV life cycle and targets of therapeutic development. The complete HBV life cycle including entry, trafficking, cccDNA formation, transcription, encapsidation, replication, assembly and secretion is shown. The functions of the HBV gene products are incorporated into the life cycle. Drugs or biologics, in clinical use or development, targeting various steps of the HBV life cycle, are illustrated in bold. See text for details of these drugs. Abbreviations: ER, endoplasmic reticulum; HSPG, heparan sulfate proteoglycan; siRNA, small interfering RNA. **Note: This figure is reproduced from Liang et al., 2015.**

The treatment of finite duration with PEG-IFN or a NA is intended to achieve a sustained off-treatment virological response. A 48-week course of PEG-IFN is mainly recommended for HBeAg-positive patients with the best chance of anti-HBe seroconversion. It can also be used for HBeAg-negative patients.

There are six therapeutic agents approved for the treatment of adults with CHB (see Table 1 on the following page).

Response rates at six months following twelve months of PEG-IFN and at twelve months of NA therapy with HBe seroconversion, 30% with PEG-IFN and approximately 20% with NAs. Anti-HBe seroconversion rates increase with continued NA therapy, but are affected if resistance occurs. Rates of HBsAg loss following twelve months of treatment were 3% to 7% with PEG-IFN, 1% with lamivudine, 0% with adefovir, 2% with entecavir, 0.5% with telbivudine, and 3% with tenofovir.[34]

TABLE 1. APPROVED ANTIVIRAL THERAPIES IN ADULTS AND CHILDREN WITH DOSES, PREGNANCY CATEGORY AND SIDE EFFECTS

CHILDREN*	DOSE IN CATEGORY	USE IN SIDE EFFECTS†	PREGNANCY	POTENTIAL DRUG ADULTS*
Peg-IFN-2a (adult) IFN-α-2b (children)	180 µg weekly	≥1 year Dose: 6 million IU/m² TIW‡	C	Flu-like symptoms, fatigue, mood disturbances, cytopenias, autoimmune disorders in adults Anorexia and weight loss in children
Lamivudine	100 mg daily	≥2 years Dose: 3 mg/kg daily to max 100 mg	C	Pancreatitis Lactic acidosis
Telbivudine	600 mg daily	—	B	Creatine kinase elevations and myopathy Peripheral neuropathy Lactic acidosis
Entecavir	0.5 or 1.0 mg daily§	≥2 years Dose: weight-based to 10–30 kg; above 30 kg 0.5 mg daily**	C	Lactic acidosis
Adefovir	10 mg daily	≥12 years 10 mg daily	C	Acute renal failure Fanconi syndrome Nephrogenic diabetes insipidus Lactic acidosis
Tenofovir	300 mg daily	≥12 years 300 mg daily	B	Nephropathy, Fanconi syndrome Osteomalacia Lactic acidosis

*Doses need to be adjusted in persons with renal dysfunction.

†Per package insert.

‡Peg-IFN-α-2a is not approved for children with CHB, but is approved for treatment of chronic hepatitis C. Providers may consider using this drug for children with chronic HBV. The duration of treatment indicated in adults is 48 weeks.

§Entecavir dose in adults is 1 mg daily if lamivudine or telbivudine experienced or decompensated cirrhosis.

**Entecavir doses in treatment-naive children older than 2 and at least 10 kg are: 0.15 mg (10–11 kg), 0.2 mg (>11–14 kg), 0.25 mg (>14–17 kg), 0.3 mg (>17–20 kg), 0.35 mg (>20–23 kg), 0.4 mg (>23–26 kg), 0.45 mg (>26–30 kg), and 0.5 mg (>30 kg). For treatment-experienced children older than 2 and at least 10 kg, the entecavir doses are: 0.30 mg (10–11 kg), 0.4 mg (>11–14 kg), 0.5 mg (>14–17 kg), 0.6 mg (>17–20 kg), 0.7 mg (>20–23 kg), 0.8 mg (>23–26 kg), 0.9 mg (>26–30 kg), and 1.0 mg (>30 kg).

Abbreviations: CBC, complete blood counts; TSH, thyroid-stimulating hormone.

Rates of sustained off-treatment virological response were of the order of 20% at six months following twelve months of PEG-IFN therapy and <5% following discontinuation of twelve months of NA(s) therapy. In patients adherent to treatment, virological remission rates of >95% can be maintained with entecavir or tenofovir at > 3 – 5 years. Rates of HBsAg loss following twelve months of treatment were 3% with PEG-IFN-2a (at six months after the end of therapy) and 0% with lamivudine, adefovir, entecavir, telbivudine, or tenofovir. HBsAg loss rates increase to 9% at three years and 12% at five years following PEG-IFN-2a therapy In contrast, HBsAg loss is exceptionally observed during the first four to five years of NA(s) therapy in HBeAg negative CHB patients.[34]

The usages of both PEG-IFN and all five oral antiviral agents (OAA) on CHB are still unsatisfied. Even majority of long-term OAA can achieve HBV-DNA suppression, HBeAg seroconversion occur in less than 40% on long-term treatment, and high rate of HBV-DNA recurrent in HBeAg negative patients, especially when HBsAg titer remain > 1,000 IU/ml at the time treatment is withdrawn.

The burden of the long-term treatment with OAA includes the cumulative cost of medicine and drug resistance, which requires an add-on or change in treatment. Renal injury caused by nucleoside and nucleotide analogues is also a major concern in long-term treatment, especially in patients with comorbidity such as older age, type II diabetes mellitus, hypertension, and chronic kidney diseases. The recent observation report found as high as 17% significant renal injury in CHB patients on tenofovir treatment.[35] Many studies using different combinations of PEG-IFN and lamivudine or entecavir could not demonstrate the beneficial effect on HBeAg or HBsAg seroconversion when compared to OAA alone. As PEG-IFN and OAA have different mechanisms of action (immunostimulant and HBV DNA inhibition), the recent study with 740 patients using PEG-IFN with tenofovir achieved 9.1% HBeAg seroconversion and 2.8% HBsAg seroconversion, bringing back the concept of dual action medication in CHB treatment.[36] However, PEG-IFN treatment comes with many side effects and is not suitable for elderly or cirrhotic patients.

Study of AHCC Treatment in CHBeAg Positive

AHCC is known to stimulate systemic immunity as a biological response modifier.[37] The immunostimulant mechanisms of AHCC is supported to mediate to TLR2 and M cell, helper T cells, and B cells, which stimulate IgA production and immune response.[38]

Based on the pathophysiology of HBV eradication, which requires both antiviral and immune-modulating effects, the addition of AHCC in CHB patients who are on long-term OAA serum appears to be promising and interesting. Especially, the usage of AHCC in CHBeAg positive patients on long-term antiviral treatment is an attractive option for shortening the duration of treatment.

From September 2011 to May 2012, we conducted a prospective and observational study on ten CHBeAg positive patients (seven female and three male; mean age of 45.30 years) who were on long-term nucleoside or nucleotide analogue treatment

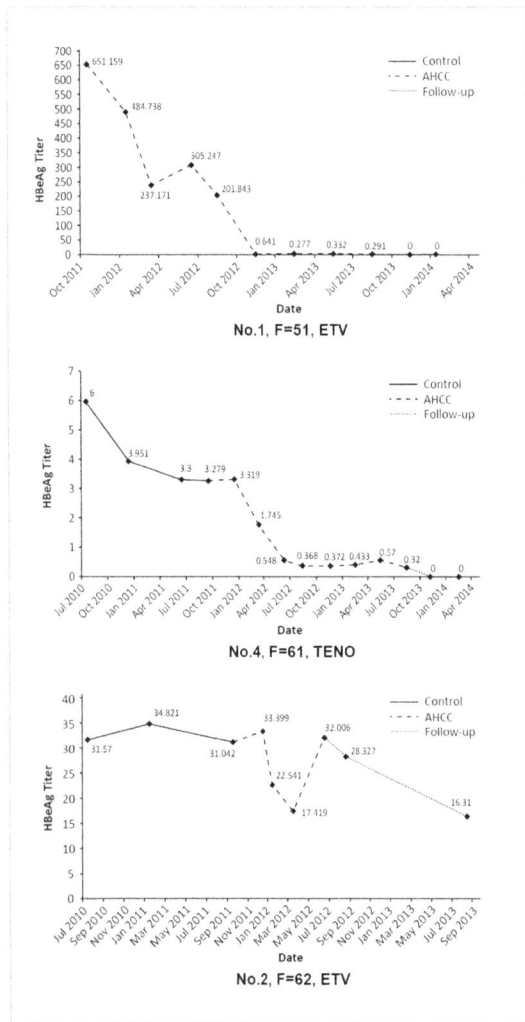

Figure 4. Faster decline, 3 cases

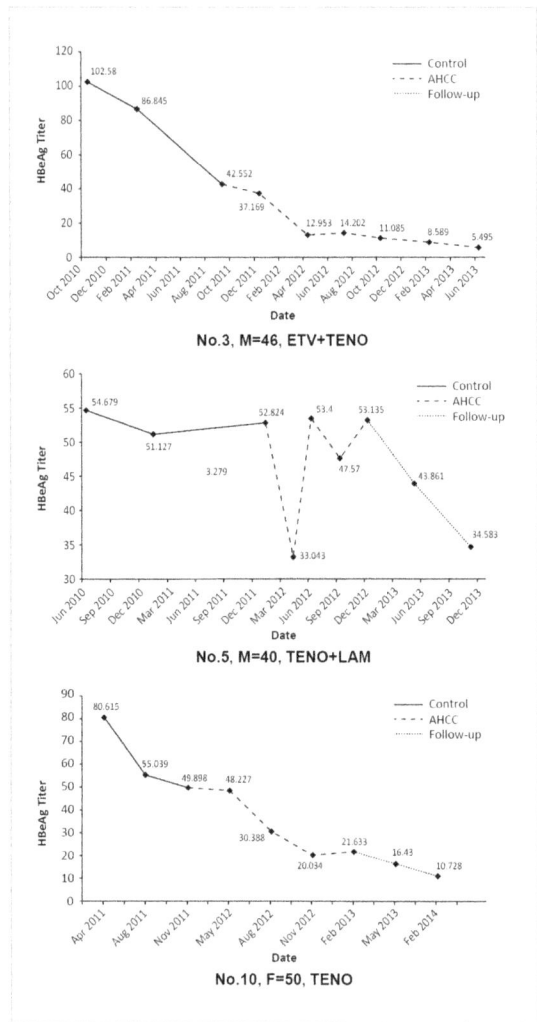

Figure 5. No effect, 3 cases

and persistently had HBV DNA suppression. All the patients were assigned to take 1,000 mg of AHCC three times daily before meals for twelve months. The patients had follow-up laboratory test and their HBe Ag level was tested by chemiluminescent immunoassay (Abbott) every three months for twelve months and three months follow-up after treatment for another six months. All the patients had good compliance, consuming more than 95% of the AHCC dose.

The ten patients in the study were on entecavir or tenofovir or entecavir with tenofovir or lamivudine with tenofovir. The dose of entrcavir was 0.5 mg/day, tenofovir 300 mg/day, and lamivudine 100 mg/day. We found three patterns of HBeAg decline during the twelve months of AHCC combination, faster decline of HBeAg level in three cases (see Figure 4 at left). Of these three cases, two developed HBe Ag loss during period of the add-on AHCC. Three cases had no difference in HBeAg decline (see Figure 5 at left) and four cases with fluctuation of the HBe Ag level (see Figure 6 at right). All the patients tolerated the treatment well without major adverse event.

In this pilot study, we found 30% of cases showed rapid decline in the HBeAg level after the addition of AHCC; In two-thirds of the cases, HBe Ag was eradicated. When compared

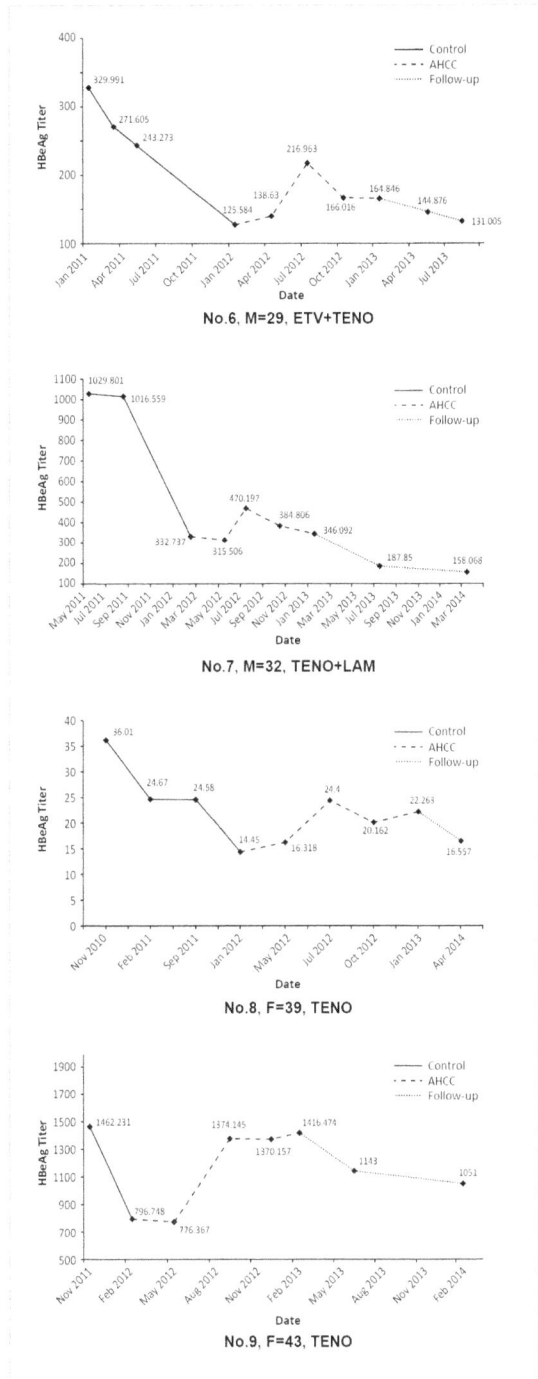

Figure 6. Fluctuation, 4 cases.

261

with another immunomodulatory substance such as interferon, AHCC seems very promising as an oral medication with minimal or no serious side effects—much unlike interferon, which needs to be in injected and has severe side effects, such as fever bone marrow suppression, alopecia, thyroid dysfunction, or psychiatric problems.

In conclusion, the addition of AHCC with CHBeAg positive patients on long-term antiviral treatment is very attractive; it should be considered in combination treatment, especially in patients with very high HBeAg levels or a slow decline of HBeAg levels during the OAA treatment.

Study of AHCC Treatment in CHBeAg Negative

In light of the study described above which demonstrated positive effects, we also studied the effect of AHCC in CHBeAg negative patients by monitoring HBsAg levels during combination treatment. This prospective and derivation study was carried out with subjects who were treated with nucleotide or nucleoside analogues without HBV DNA detectable in serum for more than two years. AHCC treatment with a dose of 3 g/day before meals for twelve months was studied. HBsAg level was measured by chemiluminescence immunoassay (Roche), at baseline, on the third, sixth, ninth, and twelfth months during the treatment and six months after termination of AHCC. We compared the slope of HBsAg decline before the treatment, during the AHCC treatment, and after termination of the AHCC treatment.

There were thirty-nine cases (thirteen female and twenty-six male; mean age of 53.69). The patients were on entecavir 0.5 mg/day or adefovir 10 mg/day or telbivudine 600 mg/day or tenofovir 300 mg/day. After the twelve months of the treatment of both OAA and AHCC, we found three patterns of HBsAg level decline: five cases had rapid decline after AHCC treatment in the first six months (see Figure 7 at right); five cases had delayed decline after six months of the AHCC treatment (25.64%) (see Figure 8 at right); and twenty-nine cases showed no effect of AHCC during the twelve months of treatment compared to the level of HBsAg before the AHCC. There was no rebound of HBsAg level after termination of AHCC. There were also no serious adverse events.

With the available data, it is suggested that AHCC is beneficial to about 25% of the CHBeAg negative patients who have very high or slow HBsAg level decline. Further study with a large number of case and early add on AHCC may give us more information about the benefit of AHCC in CHBeAg negative patient.

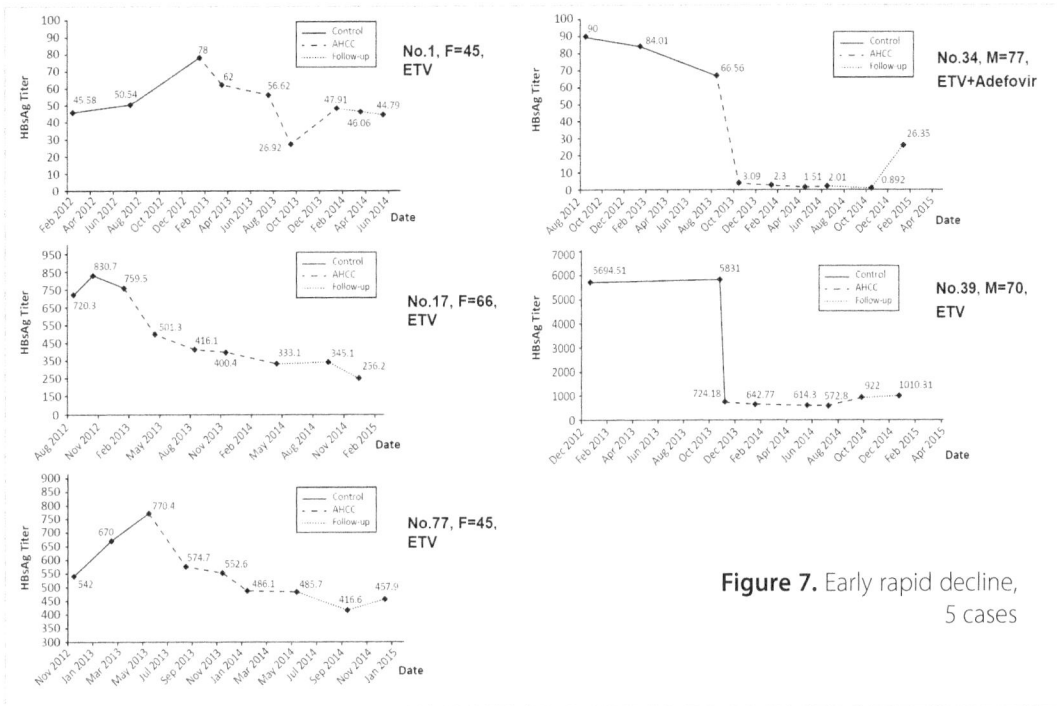

Figure 7. Early rapid decline, 5 cases

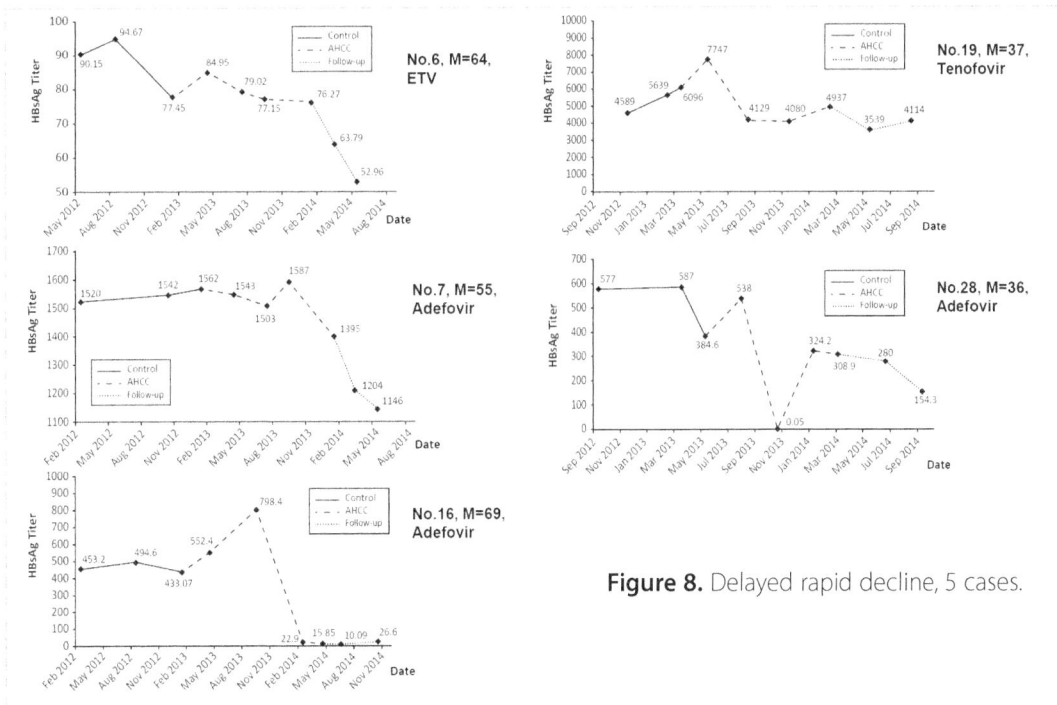

Figure 8. Delayed rapid decline, 5 cases.

Conclusion

The treatment of CHB with new direct oral antiviral agents has a finite time of treatment and efficacy. While our patients are still on available OAA medication, we await new HBV medication such as HBV entry inhibitors, HBV capsid inhibitors, HBV-gene expression inhibitor, HBV-cccDAN formation inhibitor, or new the therapeutic vaccines. AHCC is well tolerated with no serious adverse events or rebound effects and seems to be promising in combination with OAA. From our studies, the benefit from AHCC was not conclusive for all patients. Further trial with a larger number of patients, longer duration, or a higher dose of AHCC is required to conclude who would be a good candidate for combination treatment.

REFERENCES

1. Ott JJ, Stevens GA, Groeger J, and Wiersma ST. "Global epidemiology of hepatitis B virus infection: new estimates of age-specific HBsAg seroprevalence and endemicity." *Vaccine* 30: 2212–19, 2012.

2. Liang TJ, Block TM, McMahon BJ, et al. "Present and future therapies of hepatitis B: from discovery to cure." *Hepatology* 62: 1893–1908, 2015.

3. Kennedy PT, Sandalova E, Jo J, Gill U, Ushiro-Lumb I, Tan AT, et al. "Preserved T-cell function in children and young adults with immune-tolerant chronic hepatitis B." *Gastroenterology* 143: 637–645, 2012.

4. Vanwolleghem T, Hou J, van Oord G, Andeweg AC, Osterhaus AD, Pas SD, et al. "Re-evaluation of hepatitis B virus clinical phases by systems biology identifies unappreciated roles for the innate immune response and B cells." *Hepatology* 62: 87–100, 2015.

5. McMahon BJ. "The natural history of chronic hepatitis B virus infection." *Hepatology* 49: S45–S55, 2009.

6. Prati D, Taioli E, Zanella A, Della Torre E, Butelli S, Del Vecchio E, et al. "Updated definitions of healthy ranges for serum alanine aminotransferase levels." *Ann. Intern. Med.* 137: 1–10, 2002.

7. Seto WK, Wong DK, Fung J, Huang FY, Liu KS, Lai CL, et al. "Linearized hepatitis B surface antigen and hepatitis B core-related antigen in the natural history of chronic hepatitis B." *Clin. Microbiol. Infect.* 20: 1173–80, 2014.

8. Kim GA, Lee HC, Kim MJ, Ha Y, Park EJ, An J, et al. "Incidence of hepatocellular carcinoma after HBsAg seroclearance in chronic hepatitis B patients: a need for surveillance." *J. Hepatol.* 62: 1092–99, 2015.

9. Fattovich G. "Natural history and prognosis of hepatitis B." *Sem. Liver Dis.* 23: 47–58, 2003.

10. Yim HJ and Lok AS. "Natural history of chronic hepatitis B virus infection: what we knew in 1981 and what we know in 2005." *Hepatology* 43(2 Suppl 1): S173–S181, 2006.

11. Chen CJ, Yang HI, Su J, Jen CL, You SL, Lu SN, et al. "Risk of hepatocellular carcinoma across a biological gradient of serum hepatitis B virus DNA level." *JAMA* 295: 65–73, 2006.

12. Iloeje UH, Yang HI, Su J, Jen CL, You SL, and Chen CJ. "Predicting cirrhosis risk based on the level of circulating hepatitis B viral load." *Gastroenterology* 130: 678–686, 2006.

13. Yang H, Lu S, Liaw Y, You SL, Sun CA, Wang LY, et al. "Hepatitis B e antigen and the risk of hepatocellular carcinoma." *N. Engl. J. Med.* 347: 168–174, 2002.

14. Fattovich G, Stroffolini T, Zagni I, and Donato F. "Hepatocellular carcinoma in cirrhosis: incidence and risk factors." *Gastroenterology* 127(5 Suppl 1): S35–S50, 2004.

15. Protzer U, Maini MK, and Knolle PA. "Living in the liver: hepatic infections." *Nat. Rev. Immunol.* 12: 201–213, 2012.

16. Bertoletti A and Ferrari C. "Innate and adaptive immune responses in chronic hepatitis B virus infections: towards restoration of immune control of viral infection." *Gut* 61: 1754–64, 2012.

17. Seto WK, Chan TS, Hwang YY, Wong DK, Fung J, Liu KS, et al. "Hepatitis B reactivation in patients with previous hepatitis B virus exposure undergoing rituximab-containing chemotherapy for lymphoma: a prospective study." *J. Clin. Oncol.* 32: 3736–43, 2014.

18. Lau JY, Bird GL, Alexander GJ, and Williams R. "Effects of immunosuppressive therapy on hepatic expression of hepatitis B viral genome and gene products." *Clin. Invest. Med.* 16: 226–236, 1993.

19. Das A, Hoare M, Davies N, Lopes AR, Dunn C, Kennedy PT, et al. "Functional skewing of the global CD8 T cell population in chronic hepatitis B virus infection." *J. Exp. Med.* 205: 2111–24, 2008.

20. Lopes AR, Kellam P, Das A, Dunn C, Kwan A, Turner J, et al. "Bimmediated deletion of antigen-specific CD8 T cells in patients unable to control HBV infection." *J. Clin. Invest.* 118: 1835–1845, 2008.

21. Chang KM. "Hepatitis B immunology for clinicians." *Clin. Liver Dis.* 14: 409–424, 2010.

22. Bertoletti A, Maini MK, and Ferrari C. "The host-pathogen interaction during HBV infection: immunological controversies." *Antivir. Ther.* 15(Suppl. 3): 15–24, 2010.

23. Xu D, Fu J, Jin L, Zhang H, Zhou C, Zou Z, et al. "Circulating and liver resident CD41CD251 regulatory T cells actively influence the antiviral immune response and disease progression in patients with hepatitis B." *J. Immunol.* 177: 739–747, 2006.

24. Boni C, Fisicaro P, Valdatta C, Amadei B, Di Vincenzo P, Giuberti T, et al. "Characterization of hepatitis B virus (HBV)-specific T-cell dysfunction in chronic HBV infection." *J. Virol.* 81: 4215–25, 2007.

25. Baxevanis CN, Voutsas IF, and Tsitsilonis OE. "Toll-like receptor agonists: current status and future perspective on their utility as adjuvants in improving anticancer vaccination strategies." *Immunotherapy* 5: 497–511, 2013.

26. Moraleda G, Saputelli J, Aldrich CE, Averett D, Condreay L, and Mason WS. "Lack of effect of antiviral therapy in nondividing hepatocyte cultures on the closed circular DNA of woodchuck hepatitis virus." *J. Virol.* 71: 9392–99, 1997.

27. Wong DK, Seto WK, Fung J, Ip P, Huang FY, Lai CL, et al. "Reduction of hepatitis B surface antigen and covalently closed circular DNA by nucleos(t)ide analogues of different potency." *Clin. Gastroenterol. Hepatol.* 11: 1004–10.e1., 2013

28. Chang TT, Gish RG, de Man R, Gadano A, Sollano J, Chao YC, et al. "A comparison of entecavir and lamivudine for HBeAg-positive chronic hepatitis B." *N. Engl. J. Med.* 354: 1001–10, 2006.

29. Marcellin P, Heathcote EJ, Buti M, Gane E, de Man RA, Krastev Z, et al. "Tenofovir disoproxil fumarate versus adefovir dipivoxil for chronic hepatitis B." *N. Engl. J. Med.* 359: 2442–55, 2008.

30. Chang TT, Lai CL, Kew YS, Lee SS, Coelho HS, Carrilho FJ, et al. "Entecavir treatment for up to 5 years in patients with hepatitis B e antigen-positive chronic hepatitis B." *Hepatology* 51: 422–430, 2010.

31. Heathcote EJ, Marcellin P, Buti M, Gane E, de Man RA, Krastev Z, et al. "Three year efficacy and safety of tenofovir disoproxil fumarate treatment for chronic hepatitis B." *Gastroenterology* 140: 132–143, 2011.

32. Lai CL, Shouval D, Lok AS, Chang TT, Cheinquer H, Goodman Z, et al. "Entecavir versus lamivudine for patients with HBeAg-negative chronic hepatitis B." *N. Engl. J. Med.* 354: 1011–20, 2006.

33. Marcellin P, Heathcote EJ, Corsa A, Liu Y, Miller MD, and Kitrinos KM. "No detectable resistance to tenofovir disoproxil fumarate (TDF) following up to 240 weeks of treatment in patients with HBeAg+ and HBeAg– chronic hepatitis B virus infection." *Hepatology* 54: 480A, 2011.

34. European Association for the Study of the Liver. "EASL clinical practice guidelines: management of chronic hepatitis B virus infection." *J. Hepatol.* 57: 167–185, 2012.

35. Sobhonslidsuk A, Wanichanuwat J, Phakdeekitcharoen B, et al. "Nucleotide analogue-related fanconi syndrome and severe proximal renal tubular dysfunction during the treatment of chronic hepatitis B." *DDW* Abstract No.731, 2015.

36. Marrcellin P, Ahn SH, Ma X, et al. "Combination of tenofovir disproxil fumatate and peginterferon α-2a increase loss of hepatitis B surface antigen in patients with chronic hepatitis B." *Gastroenterology* 150: 134–144, 2016.

37. Terakawa N, et al. "Immunological effect of active hexose correlated compound (AHCC) in healthy volunteers: a double-blind, placebo-controlled trial." *Nutrition and Cancer* 60(5): 643–51, 2008.

38. Zhinan Y, Walshe T, et al. "Effects of active hexose correlated compound on frequency of CD4+ and CD8+ T cells producing interferon-γ and/or tumor necrosis factor-α in healthy adults." Human Immunology, 71:1187–1190, 2010

Chapter 12

INFLAMMATORY BOWEL DISEASES
Crohn's Disease and Ulcerative Colitis

Francisco J. Karkow

nflammatory bowel diseases (IBD), such as acute ulcerative colitis (UC) and Crohn's disease (CD), usually present a myriad of manifestations when active that cause affected patients many consequences. The origin of IBD is unknown, but there is relation to genetic and autoimmune diseases. In IBD, loss of weight is frequent, and nutritional support is taken into account when it is necessary to correct malnutrition, to replace macro- and micronutrients, and to reverse metabolic consequences.[1] CD can cause multifactorial manifestations such as malnutrition, joint pain, erythema nodosum, pyoderma gangrenosum, and more rarely, ocular and liver disorders. At this moment, there is no specific treatment for this kind of illness.

Both UC and CD are the most common IBD; they feature immune disturbances with chronic relapsing inflammation of one or more small segments on the small bowel and/or the large bowel, although other gastrointestinal viscera may be involved as systemic complications. The disorders often start in adolescence or early adult years, although very early cases along with delayed maturity puberty exist. The disorders remain for the entire life.

Clinical Manifestations

Clinically, UC may be milder even though life-threatening complications such as acute colitis and toxic megacolon may occur. The main complaint is diarrhea with mucus and blood. Other manifestations include abdominal pain and steatorrhea with anorexia, malaise, and weight loss, eventually combined with extraintestinal manifestations such as rheumatological, dermatological, and ophthalmological symptoms. Tissue damage is typically limited to the mucosa, and either just distal segments (rectum and left colon) or whole of the large bowel is compromised. Colectomy with complete resection of the injured mucosa may be curative.

CD is harder to eradicate, and it mostly begins in the small bowel (*regional ileitis* was the first denomination in the 1930s). The colon and rectum are not necessarily resected, but there would be deep inflammation over the visceral segments expanding by the serosa. For CD, stricturing, penetrating, and general inflammation patterns are recognized as three basic clinical models. Symptoms such as inflammations, fever, abdominal obstruction, abdominal distention, fistulae, perineal disease, vomiting, diarrhea, and weight loss would be observed, and in children and adolescents, growth retardation may occur. In the treatment, nutritional management may be required enterally or parenterally.

Pathophysiology

The pathophysiology of IBD is complex and involves the immune system, genetics, gut microbiota, and environmental factors. More than 150 of IBD susceptibility gene loci have been identified. However, two-thirds of the patients have no genetic defect.

The role of inherited factors was suspected because of the highly uneven distribution of the abnormality. Incidence of CD is 12.7 per 100,000 person-years in Europe, and 20.2 in North America. For UC, the incidence is 24.3 in Europe and 19.2 in North America. On the other hand, incidence is much lower in regions populated mainly by non-Caucasians. However, IBD is still considered a worldwide scourge, and no ethnic group is spared. Socially, IBD can be an economic burden, which leads to elevation of medical costs, reduction of productivity, and increase in unemployment.

Environmental factors should not be underestimated. Rates have been rising in the last fifty years, especially in developed countries. Therefore, IBD could be associated with the modern lifestyle, which often includes high-fat and high-sugar diets, as well as high stress levels induced by a highly socialized life and shorted relaxation time, certain medications, and economic status. Interestingly, appendectomy in childhood and smoking habit may reduce the incidence and disease severity. The gut plays a relevant role in this context. It is very important to protect the microbiota because an impaired interaction between the host and the intestinal microbiota is the primary pathophysiologic aberration.

Protective Drugs and Other Resources

The most effective treatments for both CD and UC are corticosteroids and biologic therapies, even though other pharmacological agents such as 5-aminosalicylates, aza-thioprine, cyclosporine, methotrexate, and antibiotics may be an option.

The pro-inflammatory cytokine TNF-α is believed to be a crucial mediator of the inflammatory response. It is produced by lymphocytes, monocytes, and macro-phages along with other immune and non-immune cells. Anti-TNF-α therapy has been used for approximately twenty years. The reduction of pro-inflammatory cyto-kines and mediators such as interferon gamma, TNF-α, IL-1β, CD40, CD40-L, chemo-kines, chemokine receptors, and adhesion molecules is achieved in the responsive patients with inhibition of local inflammation, including less recruitment of leuko-cytes and other inflammatory cells, less activation of T cells, and endothelial cells, as reduced angiogenesis.

It is important to emphasize that the addition of the dietary immune modulator AHCC to treatments of these illnesses has been very promising; AHCC has function not only at the bowel but also all over the host body. AHCC was used for patients with IBD, and the treatments with AHCC showed great results such as illness remis-sion without relapsing for long period. For example, one CD patient has not expe-rienced relapse in more than four years and his quality of life (QOL) has been kept in good condition. Patients with UC had much more milder relapse of illness, and it was easier to deal with them. These results suggest that AHCC can be a treatment for IBD patients.

REFERENCE

1. Nguyen GC, Munsell M, and Harris ML. "Nationwide prevalence and prognostic signif-icance of clinically diagnosable protein-calorie malnutrition in hospitalized inflammatory bowel disease patients." *Inflamm. Bowel Dis.* 14(8): 1105–11, 2008.

Chapter 13

PHARMACORESISTANT EPILEPSY
AHCC for the Treatment of Refractory Epilepsy in Children

Natalia Mikhailichenko, Viacheslav Kulagin

Epilepsy is a neurological condition that causes seizures. The causes of epilepsy can be put into three groups: symptomatic (a known insult or injury), idiopathic (genetic abnormality), or cryptogenic (no identifiable condition or insult).[1] While the majority of epilepsy patients are taking antiepileptic drugs (AEDs), only 68% of patients are satisfied with these medications, as they have side effects and do not always control the seizures.[1] Refractory epilepsy, in which seizures are not controlled by AEDs, occurs in 3% to 5% of the population worldwide with the highest incidence among children.[2] Therefore, other therapeutic interventions are needed to improve the response of children with refractory seizures.

The incidence of refractory and cryptogenic cases of epilepsy suggests the possibility of other etiologies of epilepsy. The role of the innate and adaptive immune systems in epilepsy has been the topic of recent research.[3,4] The immune etiology for certain types of epilepsy, including Lennox-Gastaut syndrome (LGS), also known as childhood epileptic encephalopathy, is under study. LGS has been attributed to specific immunological deficits. The elevation of immunoglobulin G (IgG) and IgM has been observed in LGS patients, and intravenous immunoglobulin (IVIG) infusions were effective in some cases.

We present a case of a five-year-old girl diagnosed with LGS, a severe form of childhood epilepsy that is often cryptogenic. Genetic tests indicate no genetic etiology. The first seizures began at the age of two and were sequential with ten to twelve sequences per day. Change in behavioral changes and psychomotor retardation began to appear following the seizures. Various AED mono- and polytherapy were administered. Valporic acid reduced the seizures to three times a day, but she experienced thrombocytopenia, and the medication was discontinued. Topamax, Finlepsin, Convulsofin, Lamictal, Keppra, Suxilep, and Sabril were also tried. However, they had minimum effect. A course of Synacthen Depot, a long-acting synthetic β^{1-24}-corticotropin, reduced the seizures to once in two days, but after termination, rose again to three to four times a day. Lastly, a combination of 500 mg/day of Depakine and 500 mg/day of Suxilep were used, but seizures remained at three to four times (6 – 8 clusters). Then, 1 g of AHCC was added to the last regimen, and the seizures were reduced to once per day, with clusters reduced (3 – 4 clusters). The effect of this therapy is the most remarkable of all earlier attempts.

Video electroencephalogram (EEG) findings are an essential component in the evaluation of epilepsy as they can help identify the location, severity, and type of epilepsy syndrome. EEGs also provide quantitative measures of treatment effects. EEG results of the patient before and after AHCC administration are shown in Figure 1 below.

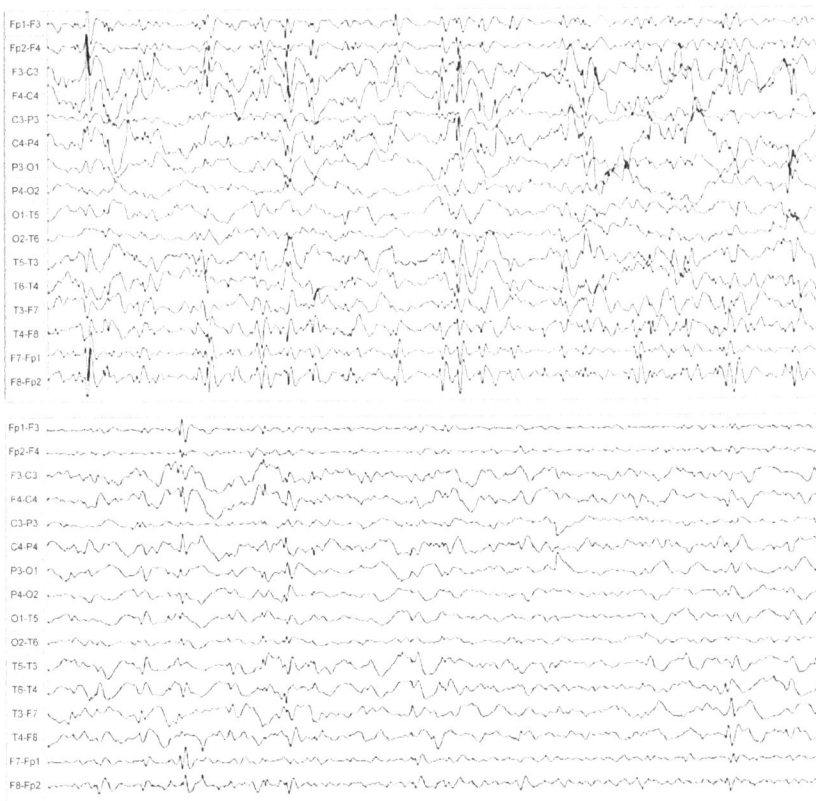

Figure 1. EEGs before (top) and after AHCC administration.

REFERENCES

1. Shorvon SD. "The etiologic classification of epilepsy," *Epilepsia* 52(6): 1052–1057, 2011.

2. Go G and Snead OC. "Pharmacologically intractable epilepsy in children: diagnosis and preoperative evaluation." *Neurosurg. Focus* 25(3): E2, 2008.

3. Xu D, Miller SD, and Koh S. "Immune mechanisms in epileptogenesis." *Front Cell Neurosci.* 7: 195, 2013.

4. Matin N, Tabatabaie O, Falsaperla R, et al. "Epilepsy and innate immune system: A possible immunogenic predisposition and related therapeutic implications." *Human Vaccines & Immunotherapeutics* 11: 8:2021–29, 2015.

Chapter 14

SJÖGREN'S SYNDROME

Francisco J. Karkow

In Sjögren's syndrome, an autoimmune disease, the body's blood white cells destroy the exocrine glands, more specifically, the salivary and lacrimal glands, which produce saliva and tears, respectively.[1] It causes xerostomia (dry mouth) and keratoconjunctivitis sicca (dry eyes).[1] It happens with lymphocyte infiltration of the glands, which can severely damage or destroy the glands. The sicca syndrome also causes vaginal dryness and chronic bronchitis. It is possible that gastroparesis and many other disorders affecting other organs of the body may occur.

This syndrome appears predominantly in females, who usually look for help, with a history of having submitted themselves to many treatments before finally achieving the diagnosis but who have not received adequate results for an extended time. Frequently, these patient are very suspicious, have no faith, no hope, and present many complaints such as bad mood, depression, no tears, no tongue humidity, swallowing difficulty, no vaginal humidity (in men less sperm production), dry skin, constipation, poor sleep, no appetite, weight loss, halitosis,[2,3] and so on.

The diagnosis is made by the history, physical examination, undercount CD3/CD4/CD8, lymphocyte account (diminished), salivary gland scintigraphy (the score shows the level of extraction of the isotope from the bloodstream by the gland), chest X-ray, spirometry, and follow-up.

I had the opportunity to treat nine women and one man, all between the ages of 40 and 55 with the exception of one 84-year-old woman. Only one patient (woman) presented bronchitis. All presented excellent results. The use of AHCC was the focus of the treatment. All patients received 1 g of AHCC three times daily continuously with attention given to all their individual clinical needs. Continued observation of each evaluation item was made taking into account: 1) clinical evaluation including tears, tongue humidity, vaginal humidity (women), swallowing improvement, sperm production (men), appetite, weight gain, mood improvement; 2) lymphocyte account; 3) undercount CD3/CD4/CD8; and 4) salivary gland scintigraphy.

In no more than a month, the sense of taste was gradually improved in association with the improvement in tongue humidity, and gradual tear improvement was also observed. Regardless of the women's age (in the 40- to 55-year-old range), they showed vaginal humidity again. All presented improvement in their mood, appetite, sustaining tongue humidification, and bowel movement, too.

The male patient noticed that his sperm increased in volume in less than two months. What is essential is that all the patients studied regained faith in their normal life with an improved appearance, tidiness, regular bathing, brushing teeth, having normal relationship with their companions, and activities in society.

The oldest subject (the 84-year-old woman) started her case in November 2012 with only 36 kg weight, 1 m 60 cm height, and a BMI of 14.06. At the beginning of April 2013, she weighed 50 kg with a BMI of 19.5. On June 23, 2014, she weighed 55 kg with a BMI of 21.5 with no dry eyes, no swallowing difficulty, and no fatigue; she also regained good sleep, good mood, good appetite, and pleasure of life. There was one curious aspect: the halitosis—one common signal presenting in the patients with Sjögren's syndrome—was usually not seen anymore a few days after the treatment with the AHCC started. Below is the documented evaluation of this oldest subject, which represents the evaluations used in her case as well as in the cases of all the other patients studied in this group.

November 12, 2012

1. Physical examination

   Weight 36 kg / Height 1 m 60 cm

2. Exams:

   - Biochemicals

     ○ TSH 8,11 mIU/L (0,4 – 4,0)

     ○ Cortisol ↑

   - Hemogram

     ○ Macrocytosis

     ○ Lymphocytopenia

○ CD3 ↓

○ CD4 ↓

○ CD8 ↓

- Salivary Gland Scintigraphy

  ○ Parotid, right: **481.806** count / left: **531.931** count

  ○ Submandibular gland, right: **310.466** count/left: **323.961** count

- Very bad QOL

April 6, 2013

1. Physical examination

   Weight 50 kg / Height 1 m 60 cm

2. Exams:

   - Biochemicals

     ○ TSH 3,83 mIU/L (0,4 – 4,0)

     ○ Cortisol ↑ (less higher)

   - Hemogram

     ○ No more Macrocytosis.

     ○ No more Lymphocytopenia.

     ○ CD3 Normal

     ○ CD4 Normal

     ○ CD8 Normal

   - Salivary Scintigraphy

     ○ Parotid, right: **842.623** count/ left: **723.031** count

     ○ Submandibular gland, right: **522.697** count/left: **487.415** count

   - HIGHER ACTIVITY, ALMOST DOUBLED

   - Very good QOL

The scores of salivary scintigraphy shows the level of isotope uptake from the bloodstream by the gland. A higher score indicates better salivation. Figures 1 and 2 on the next page respectively represent the actual salivary scintigraphy images on November 22, 2012 and February 25, 2013. The increases of salivation from both parotid and submandibular glands were observed as the higher level of isotope extraction. The figures capture the significance of AHCC intervention.

In conclusion, the use of AHCC presents an attractive answer for patients without complete havoc of these gland cells, showing: a) presence of tears, b) tongue humidity, c) vaginal humidity, d) improvement in sperm volume (men), e) weight gain, f) improvement in blood count, g) improvement in CD3, CD4, CD8, h) significant improvement in the salivary gland scintigraphy, and i) better mood. AHCC administration must be considered when a patient is diagnosed as Sjögren's syndrome.

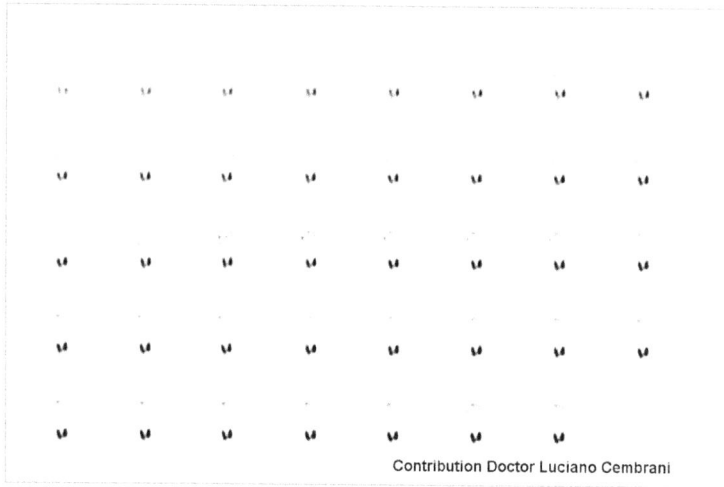

Figure 1. November 22, 2012

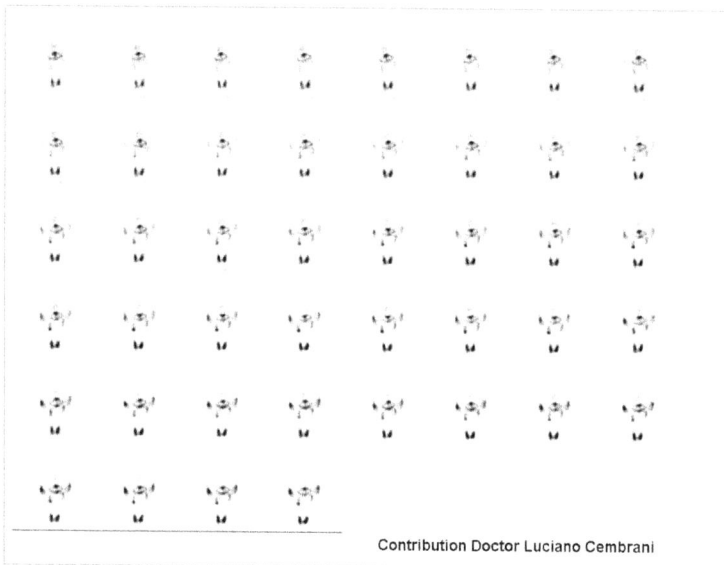

Figure 2. February 25, 2013

REFERENCES

1. Voulgarelis M and Tzioufas AG. "Pathogenetic mechanisms in the initiation and perpetuation of Sjögren's syndrome." *Nat. Rev. Rheumatol.* 6 (9): 529–537, 2010.

2. Ramos-Casals M, Brito-Zerón P, Sisó-Almirall A, Bosch X, and Tzioufas AG. "Topical and systemic medications for the treatment of primary Sjögren's syndrome." *Nat. Rev. Rheumatol.* 8 (7): 399–411, 2012

3. Ramos-Casals M, Tzioufas AG, Stone JH, Sisó A, and Bosch X. "Treatment of primary Sjögren syndrome: a systematic review." *JAMA* 304 (4): 452–460, 2010.

Chapter 15

CHRONIC RESPIRATORY DISEASE
Effects of Alternative Therapy with Fungal Medication at End Stage of Chronic Respiratory Disease

Takayuki Yoshizawa, Akitaka Yoshizawa

Alternative therapies for cancers or other diseases have been the focus of recent interest. In particular, some fungal medications categorized as health food are reported to enhance immunity, prolong life, and reduce the side effects of anticancer drugs. In patients with chronic respiratory disease, including chronic obstructive pulmonary disease (COPD), immune function is reduced and nutritional status is worsened. Thus, the symptoms are repeatedly exacerbated at the end stage and the activities of daily living (ADL) and quality of life (QOL) are reduced. This is often seen in patients with cancers as well.

In this chapter, we describe the effect of fungal medication, a health food, in patients with end stage chronic respiratory disease whose ADL and QOL were significantly impaired due to malnutrition. Here, we report the results with brief considerations.

Subjects and Methods

The subjects were thirteen outpatients with chronic respiratory disease who visited the pulmonology department in our hospital. The cases consisted of the following: six with COPD, three with bronchiectasis, two with pulmonary tuberculosis sequelae, one with pulmonary fibrosis, and one with atypical mycobacteriosis. Their symptoms were repeatedly exacerbated and nutritional status was worsened, and the ADL and QOL were significantly reduced. Of the thirteen patients, nine received home oxygen therapy (HOT). For the ratio of ideal body weight (%IBW), five were 90% or more, two were 80% or more but less than 90%, and six were less than 80%. Moderate or severe malnutrition was suggested in eight cases. Eleven patients received AHCC, and two were administered *Fomes yucatensis* two or three times a day for three through twenty-two months. The changes in body weight, nutritional status, and subjective symptoms were monitored.

Results

Almost all patients noted increases in appetite and body weight, and %IBW significantly increased (see Figure 1A right). As body weight increased, serum albumin, an indicator of nutritional status, also significantly elevated (see Figure 1B right). Serum concentration of cholinesterase usually decreases based on systemic exhaustion, but it was significantly improved along with the improvement of nutritional status after administration of fungal medication (see Figure 1C right). Especially, the patient with less than 80% of %IBW showed a trend of increasing albumin and cholinesterase with a large ratio. For subjective symptoms, eleven of thirteen patients increased appetite, seven showed a decrease in the amount of sputum, and bloody sputum was almost gone in three of the four who had frequently developed bloody sputum. As the amount of sputum decreased, dose frequency of antibiotics was also reduced. Exertional breathlessness was also relieved in three patients.

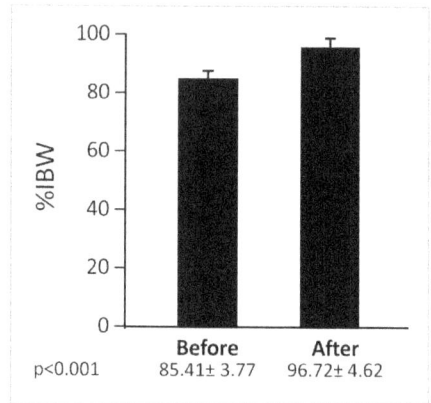

p<0.001 Before 85.41± 3.77 After 96.72± 4.62

Figure 1A. %IBW

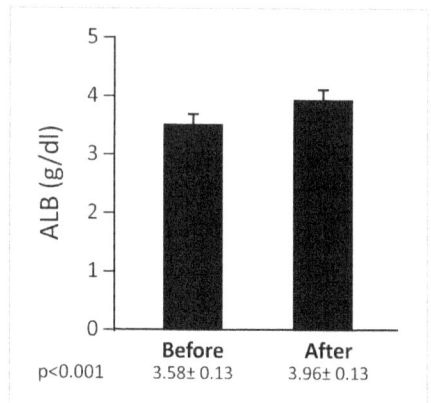

p<0.001 Before 3.58± 0.13 After 3.96± 0.13

Figure 1B. Serum albumin

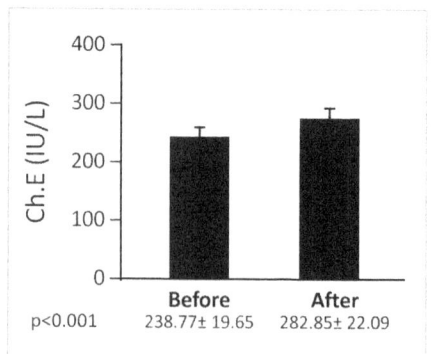

p<0.001 Before 238.77± 19.65 After 282.85± 22.09

Figure 1C. Serum cholinesterase

Patient: T.K. 68 years old, male

Diagnosis: COPD

History: No past medical history

Present illness: The patient was diagnosed as COPD at age 60. He was admitted and discharged two or three times a year due to acute exacerbation since age 64. At age 67, he was referred to our hospital due to acute exacerbation.

HOT was initiated. He was discharged, but rehospitalized due to exacerbation after around three weeks.

Clinical course: When he was rehospitalized, severe malnutrition was seen. Body weight was 39 kg and %IBW was 72%. Walking to a toilet was difficult for him due to general debility (see Figure 2 below). After obtaining informed consents from him and his family, AHCC was started three times a day at meal times to improve nutrition. Two months later, body weight increased to 43 kg, bloody sputum disappeared, and the amount of sputum reduced. He showed an improvement in ADL and was discharged

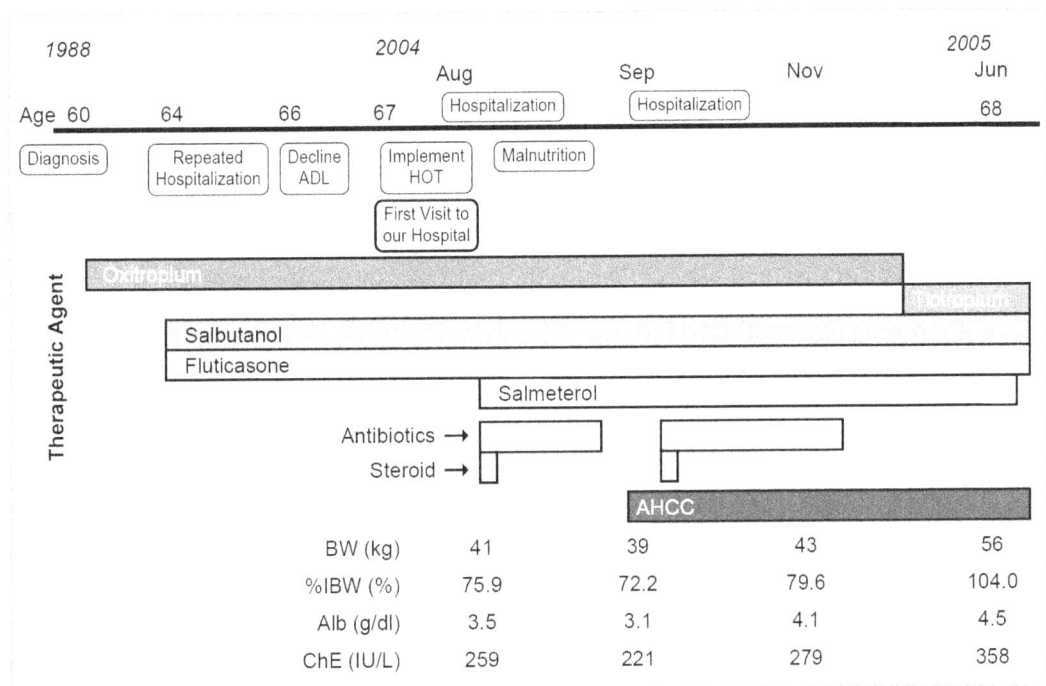

Figure 2. Clinical course of the patient (T.K.)

from the hospital. Nine months later, body weight and %IBW were recovered to 56 kg and 104%. At the time of this report, he did not show any signs of exacerbation, while nutrition and ADL were improved. The patient continued to attend regular follow-ups and participated in respiratory rehabilitation twice a month.

X-ray radiograph had showed a low position and flattening of the diaphragm, but it was resolved as the body weight increased. The improvement in nutri-

Figure 3A. Chest X-ray images of case T.K. August 23, 2004

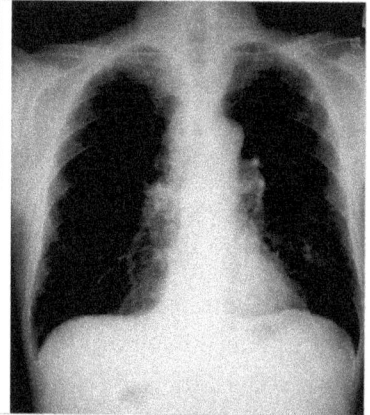

Figure 3B. Chest X-ray images of case T.K. July 15, 2005

tion may lead to strengthening the respiratory muscle and improve shortness of breath (air trapping might cause shortness of breath). ADL was then improved (see Figures 3A and B). Arterial blood gases at rest did not change.

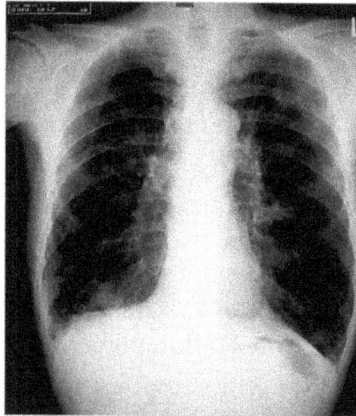

Discussions

The results suggest that fungal medication, a health food, may enhance immunity, accelerate appetite, reduce the patient's subjective symptoms, and finally improve the ADL and QOL. In patients with COPD, malnutrition is a prognostic factor independent from airflow obstruction or exercise tolerability, and relates to underlying systemic inflammation. In our patient, systemic inflammation was improved because the immune system was regulated by fungal medication, and that might have resulted in an improvement of nutrition and ADL.

There is no well-established consensus on nutritional control at the end stage of chronic respiratory disease. However, based on our study, alternative therapy with fungal medication is expected to be useful at the end stage of chronic respiratory disease as well as that of cancers.

APPENDIX

CASE LIST

The following case list is intended to provide an overview of the past clinical use of AHCC. It contains the cases described in this book, as well as some additional cases introduced in the previous publications. Readers can refer to the list to find the expected effects of AHCC in clinical settings.

Please note:

- There are two separate tables:
    1. Various types of cancer (pages 284–289)
    2. Other diseases (pages 290–291)

- The tables are arranged on double spread pages.

- The cases are listed in an alphabetical order.

- There are two types of references in the last column:
    1. The reference numbers 1–7 indicate the references listed at the bottom of pages 290 and 291.
    2. The references regarding "this book" indicate page numbers where the cases are described.

Cancer Malignancy	Gender	Age	Metastasis	Recurrence	Stage	Surgery	Chemotherapy
Adenoid cystic carcinoma	M	39	—	—	—	○	—
Angiosarcoma	F	61	—	○	—	×	rIL-2, local injection of LAK cell, etoposide and steroid after recurrence
Angiosarcoma	F	58	—	—	—	surgical resection	rIL-2, local injection of LAK cell, docetaxel and steroid
Angiosarcoma	M	47	lymph node	○	—	surgical resection	rIL-2, docetaxel after recurrence
Angiosarcoma	M	72	—	—	—	surgical resection	rIL-2, local injection of LAK cell
Bile duct cancer	M	73	—	—	—	surgical resection	○
Bladder cancer	M	60	—	—	—	—	—
Brain stem tumor	F	64	—	—	—	unresectable	—
Breast cancer	F	63	lung	breast	IV with distant metastasis	—	—
Breast cancer	F	54	lung, liver	breast	IV with distant metastasis	—	—
Breast cancer	F	62	rib, chest wall	—	—	mastectomy	○ (UFT)
Breast cancer	F	73	—	—	—	—	—
Breast cancer	M/F	20–64	—	—	—	—	adjuvant chemotherapy
Cervical cancer, HPV infection	F	—	—	—	—	—	—
Colon cancer	M	63	liver	—	IV with distant metastasis	—	○
Colon cancer	F	59	lung, liver	—	IV with distant metastasis	—	○
Colon cancer	F	91	—	—	—	○	—
Colon cancer, Rectal cancer	F	76	liver	liver	IV with distant metastasis	○	—
Disseminated neuroendocrine tumors	—	—	—	—	—	—	—
Endometrial cancer	F	67	pelvis	—	—	○ endometrial cancer × pelvis metastasis unresectable	—
Esophageal cancer	M	76	—	—	—	×(refused)	—
Esophageal squamous cell carcinoma	M	55	—	—	—	unresectable	—
Gastric submucosal tumor	F	64	liver (3 sites)	—	—	total gastrectomy	○ (Imatinib mesilate)

284

Radiation	AHCC Dose	Other Functional Foods	Efficacy	References*
○	—	—	Weight gain	This book, Case E: Adenoid Carcinoma, p241
—	—	—	No distant metastasis	3) p226
○ (electron beam therapy [80Gy])	—	—	No distant metastasis	3) p226-227
○ (electron beam therapy [80Gy] + X-ray [50Gy])	—	—	No side effects; No distant metastasis; No recurrence	3) p227
—	—		No distant metastasis	3) p228
—	3g/day	—	Ease the pain from the side effects of chemotherapy; Improvement of QOL	This book, Case C: Bile Duct Cancer, p219
—	6g/day	—	Disappearance of tumor	2) p140–141
—	—	immunotherapy	Disappearance of the majority of tumor	2) p103
—	—	GCP	Long term survival after recurrence (15y 8m); QOL evaluation; PS=0	1) p191 Table 4-3
—	—	GCP	Long term survival after recurrence (9y 6m); QOL evaluation; PS=0	1) p191 Table 4-3
○ (Linac)	3g/day	—	Suppression of pleural effusion; Survival after metastasis (>2y); Improvement of QOL (cancer pain relief)	2) p125–127
—	3g/day	—	Reduction of tumor	This book, Case G: Breast Cancer, p243
—	3g/day	—	lower usage of G-CSF; Fewer adverse events in TG and T-Chol	This book, Effect of AHCC in Women Receiving Adjuvant Chemotherapy for Breast Cancer: The Present and Near Future, p82
—	up to 9 g/day	—	Clearance of persistent viral infections; Suppression of IFN-β; Upregulation of IFN-γ	This book, HPV and Cervical Cancer, p123
—		GCP	Long term survival after recurrence (>13y 3m); QOL evaluation; PS=0	1) p191 Table 4-3
—		GCP	QOL evaluation; PS=1	1) p191 Table 4-3
—		GCP	Excellent QOL	1) p191-192
—		GCP	Long-term survival after recurrence (11y 4m); QOL evaluation; PS=2	1) p191 Table 4-3
90Y-DOTA-TATE	6g/day	—	Partial remission	This book, Chapter Case B: Disseminated Neuroendocrine Tumors (NETs), p229
× (refused)	6g/day	Other health food	Improvement in inflammation of urinary tract; Weight gain, tumor growth in the pelvis stopped	2) p116-117
○	—	Other health food	Disappearance of tumor	2) p141
—	—	—	Disappearance of tumor, no side effects by radiation therapy	2) p113-114
—		hochu-ekki-to, marine minerals	Disappearance of liver tumor (CT scan); Disappearance of ascites	1) p206-207

Cancer Malignancy	Gender	Age	Metastasis	Recurrence	Stage	Surgery	Chemotherapy
Hepatocellular carcinoma	F	78	—	—	—	transcatheter arterial embolization (TAE); transcatheter arterial injection (TAI)	—
Hepatocellular carcinoma, Stomach cancer	M	64	liver, lung	○	II	—	× (refused)
Huge malignant mammary phyllodes sarcoma	F	53	—		IV with distant metastasis	—	—
Liver cancer	M	54	—	—	—	transcatheter arterial embolization (TAE)	○ (arterial infusion therapy)
Liver cancer	M	—	—	—	—	—	—
Lung adenocarcinoma	F	52	5th rib	○ lung	IV with distant metastasis	—	△ (chemotherapy interrupted)
Lung cancer	F	94	—	—	IV with distant metastasis	—	—
Lung cancer	M	70	—	—	—	unresectable	—
Lung cancer	M	65	right cervical lymph node	—	—	unresectable	× (refused)
Lymph node malignancy	F	58	—	—	—	—	—
Malignant lymphoma	M	61	brain	—	—	—	○ (no effect)
Malignant lymphoma	M	32	—	—	III	—	× (chemotherapy refusal)
Malignant lymphoma	M	74	—	—	—	unresectable	○ (etoposide)
Metastatic bone cancer	M	63	bone	—	IV	—	—
Metastatic brain tumor	F	33	lung	—	—	—	○
Multiple cancer (Sigmoid colon, rectum, cecum)	M	37	—	—	IV with distant metastasis	—	—
Multiple myeloma	F	62	—	—	—	—	—
Myelodysplastic syndrome	M	76	—	—	—	—	—
Nasopharyngeal cancer	M	71	—	—	—	○	—
Ovarian cancer	F	45	inguinal lymph node	—	—	total hysterectomy	○
Ovarian cancer, alveolar epithelial cancer	F	57	multiple metastasis in lung	—	—	○ ovarian cancer	—
Pancreatic cancer	F	60	liver	—	—	—	○
Pancreatic cancer	M/F	18–75	—	—	—	unresectable	Gemcitabine
Pancreatic cancer	F	54	liver	—	—	—	FolFirinOx
Pancreatic cancer	F	55	liver	—	—	—	FolFirinOx

Radiation	AHCC Dose	Other Functional Foods	Efficacy	References*
—	3g/day	—	Improved GSA Rmax by asialoscintigram; Improved nutritional metabolic function of liver; Improved prothrombin time and ICG	4)-7)
—	3g/day	—	Reduction or disappearance of liver and lung metastasis (CT, X-ray); Normalization of tumor marker (AFP and PIVKAII)	3) p215-219
—	—	GCP	Long term survival (>12y 6m); QOL evaluation; PS=0	1) p191 Table 4-3
—		juzen-taiho-to	Stable tumor marker (AFP)	2) p111-112
—	3–6g/day	—	Symptoms slowly disappeared and improved physical condition	This book, Case H: Liver Cancer, p244
—		ninjin-yoei-to, hochu-ekki-to	No observed cancer progression (Chest X-ray); Survival benefit (>5y)	1) p210-211
—			QOL evaluation; PS=1	1) p190
—			Reduction of tumor (CT)	2) p104-106
—			Stopped cancer progression (CT)	2) p106-108
—	3g/day	—	Reduction of tumor	This book, Case B: Lymph Node Malignancy, p238
○ (no effect)		Fucoidan, lactic acid bacteria	Remission of language disorder; Disappearance of tumor (MRI)	1) p179
—		juzen-taiho-to	Disappearance of tumor	2) p119-120
—		juzen-taiho-to	Disappearance of tumor	2) p120-121
—	3g/day	—	Improvement of QOL	This book, Case D: Metastatic Bone Cancer, p240
—	—	—	Disappearance of brain metastatic legion	2) p104
—		GCP	Long-term survival after recurrence (>29y 6m); QOL evaluation; PS=0	1) p191 Table 4-3
—	—	immunotherapy	Improve physical condition; Disappearance of tumor (CT, MRI, X-ray, bone marrow aspiration)	2) p118-119
—	3g/day	—	Excellent platelet count	1) p198-199
○	—	—	Weight gain	This book, Case F: Nasopharyngeal Cancer, p242
—	3g/day	—	Stopped progression of carcinomatous peritonitis; Improvement of lymphedema; Recovery from immobility; improvement of insomnia, anorexia, and anxiety	2) p124-125
—	3g/day	Keishi-bukuryo-gan, Keishi-ka-ogi-to	Disappearance of lung tumor	2) p145
—	—	—	Reduction of primary tumor and disappearance liver metastasis (CT); Survival benefit (>1y); Good QOL	1) p211-212
—	3–6g/day	—	improvement of taste disorder, serum ALB, CRP and mGPS score; The higher disease control rate; The higher tendency for overall survival	This book, Pancreatic Cancer Chemotherapy and AHCC, p90
hyperthermia	3g/day	—	Suppress side effects of chemotherapy; Improvement of QOL	This book, Case B: Pancreatic Cancer and Liver Metastases, p249
—	3g/day	—	Reduction of tumor (60%); Almost disappearance of the pancreatic injury and of all the hepatic lesions; Improvement of QOL	This book, Case B: Pancreatic Cancer and Liver Metastases, p250

Cancer Malignancy	Gender	Age	Metastasis	Recurrence	Stage	Surgery	Chemotherapy
Pancreatic cancer	F	59	—	—	IV	—	—
Pancreatic cancer	F	65	—	—	—	unresectable	○ (5-FU, Cisplatin)
Pancreatic head carcinoma	F	65	—	—	—	○	○ (5-FU, Cisplatin)
Primary brain tumor (medulloblastoma)	M	21	—	—	—	unresectable	○
Primary lung tumor	M	80	—	—	V	unresectable	× (refused)
Progressive papillary pancreatic cancer	M	62	—	—	—	unresectable	×
Progressive recurrent breast cancer (right mammary gland)	F	72	lumbar spine	—	III	mastectomy	○
Rectal cancer	F	60	liver, lung	—	—		—
Rectal cancer, Stomach cancer	M	62	—	○	early	× (refused)	×
Rectal carcinoma	F	54	—	—	—	—	—
Spindle cell sarcoma	F	44	—	—	—	×	ADIC
Stomach cancer	M	50s	—	—	—	○	—
Stomach cancer	—	—	liver, lymph node	—	IV with distant metastasis	unresectable	○ (TS1)
Stomach cancer	M	89	stomach	○	—	unresectable	○ (UFT)
Stomach cancer	F	87	—	×	IIc	×	×
Stomach cancer	M	68	lymph node	—	IV	unresectable	○ (TS-1 and PTX)
Stomach cancer	F	57	—	—	IV	total gastrectomy	○ (TS-a and PTX)
Stomach cancer	F	73	multiple liver	—	IIa and IIc	×	○ (low-dose TS-1 and PTX)
Ureteropelvic cancer, bladder cancer	M	59	—	—	—	nephrectomy (left)	intravesical instillation of BCG solution into bladder
Various cancer	12 patients	—	—	—	III - V	—	—

Radiation	AHCC Dose	Other Functional Foods	Efficacy	References*
—	mega dosage→3g/day	—	Reduction of tumor; Improvement of QOL	This book, Case C: Pancreatic Cancer, p239
○	—	—	Decrease in tumor marker (CA19-9: 92.4 →12.6))	2) p115
○	3g/day	—	No side effects; No gastrointestinal symptom; Reduction of tumor and normalize tumor marker; No recurrence	3) p192-195
—	—	—	Complete remission	2) p102–103
× (refused)	6g/day	Herbal extract	Increasing Th1 cytokines; Reduction of tumor; Decreasing tumor marker	3) p210-212
—	—	—	Improvement of anorexia and physical condition; Disappearance of tumor	2) p139–140
○ (2y before AHCC intake)	6g/day	—	Improvement of physical condition; stop bloody stool; Weight gain; Keep NK cell activity	3) p221-222
—		Fucoidan, Vitamin C	Reduction of tumor size (CT scan); Disappearance of lung metastasis	1) p178-179
—	3g/day	—	Long-term survival (14y); no recurrence; No metastasis	This book, Case A: Stomach Cancer, p213
○	3g/day	—	Improvement pains, bloating, myalgia, loss of appetite, melena; Disappearance of ascites; Weight gain	This book, Case A: Rectal Carcinoma, p237
—	3g/day	—	Improvement of QOL; Reduction of tumor	This book, Case C: Spindle Cell Sarcoma, p232
—	6g/day →3g/day →1g/day		Improvement of QOL	1) p197-198
—		fucoidan	Reduction of stomach tumor (Gastroscope and MRI); PET positive (Liver and lymph node)	1) p207-208
—	3g/day	—	Reduction of stomach cancer; No observed side effects of chemotherapy	2) p136–137
×	3g/day	—	Disappearance of tumor	2) p144-145
—	3g/day (enteral supplementation)	—	Improvement of QOL; Sep. 2014 diagnosis; Feb. 2015 passed away	This book, Case B: Stomach Cancer, p216
—	3g/day	—	Post-operative QOL increased; Meaningfully lived out the rest of her life	This book, Case D: Stomach Cancer, p222
—	3g/day	—	Improvement of QOL; Mar. 2015 diagnosis; Aug. 2015 passed away	This book, Case E: Stomach Cancer, p224
—		Saikoka-ryukotsu-borei-to, tsudo-san, chorei-to	Disappearance of tumor; No recurrence	1) p208-209
—	—	—	Improvement of nausea and pain	2) p127–128

Disease	Gender	Age	Metastasis	Recurrence	Stage	Surgery	Chemotherapy
Asthma	—	—	—	—	—	—	—
Chronic fatigue immune deficiency syndrome (CFIDS)	—	—	—	—	—	—	—
Chronic hepatitis B	—	—	—	—	—	—	—
Chronic hepatitis B	M	32	—	—	—	—	—
COPD (chronic obstructive pulmonary disease)	F/M	—	—	—	—	—	—
Diabetes	13 patients	—	—	—	—	—	—
Hepatitis C	—	—	—	—	—	—	—
Hepatitis C, liver cancer; unresectable tumor near portal vein	M	65	—	—	—	unresectable	—
Idiopathic thrombocytopenic purpura	F	11	—	—	—	—	—
Inflammatory bowel diseases	—	—	—	—	—	—	—
Pulmonary non-tuberculosis mycobacteriosis	—	—	—	—	—	—	—
Refractory epilepsy	F	5	—	—	—	—	○
Sjögren's Disease	F	84	—	—	—	—	—

References

1. 杜 聡一郎 『AHCC のすべてがわかる本・基礎研究からがん臨床最前線まで —All about AHCC from basic study to clinical practice in cancer care』 上山 泰男 監修（現代書林, 2010）(In Japanese)

2. がん医療特別取材班 『21 世紀がん医療のキーワード・ AHCC を科学する —The science of AHCC: keyword in cancer care』（メタモル出版 , 2002) (In Japanese)

3. 山崎 正利, 上山 泰男 編『AHCC の基礎と臨床 —The basic and clinical researches on AHCC』細川眞澄男 監修 (ライフサイエンス , 2003) (In Japanese)

Note: References 1–3 are from books written in Japanese. Please contact the publisher (http://icnim.jpn.org/e/contact/) for any inquiry about the cases and/or references.

Radiation	AHCC Dose	Other Functional Foods	Efficacy	References*
—	1g/day	—	Decreasing eNO	This book, Case D: Asthma, p234
—	—	—	Improvement of chronic fatigue	2) p153–154
—	3g/day	—	HBsAg level decline	This book, Hepatitis: Treatment of Chronic Hepatitis B with AHCC Combination, p253
—	3g/day	—	Disappearance hepatitis B virus; Normalize tumor marker	2) p132–133
—		Fomes yucatensis (2 patients)	%IBW increased, increased appetite, decrease in sputum, exertional breathlessness relieved	This book, Chronic Respiratory Disease: Effects of Alternative Therapy with Fungal Medication at End Stage of Chronic Respiratory Disease, p277
—	3g/day	—	Decreasing blood sugar and HbA1c	2) p134
—	3g/day		Reduction of hepatitis C virus (85%)	2) p152
—		juzen-taiho-to	no interference with daily life After stopped taking AHCC, AFP increased & ascetic fluid accumulated	1) p212-213
—	1.5g/day	—	Increased platelet counts	This book, Case A: Idiopathic Thrombocytopenic Purpura, p228
—	—	—	No relapsing for more than 4 y; Maintained good QOL	This book, Inflammatory Bowel Diseases: Crohn's Disease and Ulcerative Colitis, p267
—	3g/day	—	Condition improved or stabilized; No serious adverse effects	This book, Pulmonary Non-Tuberculous Mycobacteriosis, p120
—	1g/day	—	Seizures and clusters were reduced	This book, Pharmacoresistant Epilepsy: AHCC for the Treatment of Refractory Epilepsy in Children, p270
—	—	—	Weight gain, increased BMI, no dry eyes, no swallowing difficulty, no fatigue, regained good sleep, good mood, good appetite, and pleasure of life	This book, Sjögren's Syndrome, p273

4. Koreeda C, et al., 37th Annual Meeting of Liver Cancer Study Group of Japan (2001).

5. Koreeda C, et al., "Late evening snack, branched chain amino acids, and cirrhosis." *Branched Chain Amino Acids in Clinical Nutrition*. Eds. Rajendram R, et al. 2: 169–179, 2015.

6. Koreeda C, et al., "Effects of late evening snack including branched-chain amino acid on the function of hepatic parenchymal cells in patients with liver cirrhosis." *Hepatology Research* 41: 417–422, 2011.

7. Kawaguchi T, et al., "Branched-chain amino acids prevent hepatocarcinogenesis and prolong survival of patients with cirrhosis," *Clinical Gastroenterology and Hepatology,* 12: 1012–1018, 2014.

INDEX

Mitogen-activated protein
  kinases (MAPKs). *See*
  MAPKs.
Molecular chaperones,
  208–209
Monocyte chemotactic
  protein-1 (MCP-1), 202
Monosaccharides, 25–28
Moods, 188
mRNAs, 109, 111, 116, 118,
  137, 208
Mucous membranes
  intestinal, 15, 73
  oral, 76–77
Multinational Association
  of Supportive Care in
  Cancer (MASCC), 88
Mushrooms, 23, 61
  dried, 24
  shiitake. *See Lentinula
  edodes.*
  See also AHCC.
MyD88, 138, 202, 203
Myeloid differentiation
  primary response 88
  (MyD88). *See* MyD88.

N

National Center for
  Complementary and
  Integrative Health
  (NCCIH), 8, 12
National Center of CAM
  (NCCAM), 11
National Institutes of
  Health (NIH). Office of
  Alternative Medicine
  (OAM), 10–11
NCCAM. *See* National Center
  of CAM (NCCAM).
NCCIH. *See* National Center
  for Complementary
  and Integrative Health
  (NCCIH).

NE. *See* Norepinephrine (NE).
Nervous system
  autonomic (ANS), 184,
  186–187
  sympathetic, 184, 186, 190,
  193
Neuroendrocrine tumors
  (NETs), 229–232
Neuropeptide Y (NPY), 56
Neutropenia, 58, 90, 105
Neutrophils, 105
NF-κB, 136, 137, 138, 198,
  202–203
NF-κB inhibitor α (IκB-α).
  See IκB-α.
NF-κB pathway, 58, 59, 60
Nicotinamide, 174
90Y-DOTA-TATE, 229–232
Nitric oxide (NO), 31, 58, 109,
  134–135, 136–137
NNI. *See* Interactions:
  nutrient-nutrient (NNI).
N-nitrosofenfluramine, 16
Non-nutrients, dietary, 164,
  168–169
Non-tuberculous
  mycobacteriosis (NTM),
  120–122
Noradrenaline, 184
Norepinephrine (NE), 56, 57
NOS2. *See* iNOS.
NPY. *See* Neuropeptide Y
  (NPY).
Nuclear factor κB (NF-κB).
  See NF-κB.
Nutraceutics, 17
Nutrients, 164, 165–166
Nutrinogenomics, 17
Nutrition, 43, 44, 49–51,
  130–133
  cancer treatments and,
  69–81
  See also Diet; Food,
  functional.

Nutrition Labeling and
  Education Act (NLEA) of
  1990 (United States), 5

Obesity, 167–168, 204
Oguri-Shirakawa-Azumi sleep
  inventory MA version
  (OSA-MA), 191–192
Okamoto, Toshihiko, 21
Oligonucleotides, 111
Oligosaccharides, 15, 136,
  197–198, 204
Omega-3 fatty acids, 15,
  71–72
Omnic technique, 17
Ondansetron, 153
Onions, 101
Oral antiviral agents (OAAs),
  259, 260, 264
Oral tolerance, 12–13
Oxidative burst, 48
Oxidative stress, 137, 163,
  184

Paclitaxel, 149
Palliative care, 220, 223–224
Pathogenesis, 132
PEG-IFN, 256–259
Pegylated interferon (PEG-
  IFN). *See* PEG-IFN.
pEL. *See* Pyroglutamyl-
  leucine (pEL).
Peptides, 29, 32
Peripheral nerve disorder, 74
Peyer's patches, 47
Phagocytosis, 45, 46, 51
Phase I metabolic interactions,
  149, 153–154, 158
Phase II metabolism
  pathways, 150, 153–154
Phytochemicals, 168–169
Phytoestrogens, 150
Pineapples, 101
Pitta, 131

www.ingramcontent.com/pod-product-compliance
Lightning Source LLC
Chambersburg PA
CBHW081804200326
41597CB00023B/4137